GRANDPARENTS AS PARENTS

GRANDPARENTS AS PARENTS

A Survival Guide for Raising a Second Family

Sylvie de Toledo
Deborah Edler Brown

Foreword by Ethel Dunn

THE GUILFORD PRESS
New York / London

Published by The Guilford Press
A Division of Guilford Publications, Inc.
72 Spring Street, New York, NY 10012

The following copyright holders have generously given permission
to reprint from previously published works:

Charlotte Observer for quotations from "When Grandparents Start
Over" by Miriam Durkin. Copyright 1991 by *Charlotte Observer*.
Used by permission.

Ethel Dunn for a quotation from "Those Wonderful Abuelas" in
Intergenerational Hookup. Copyright 1993 by Ethel Dunn. Used
by permission.

Grandparents United for Children's Rights, Inc., for suggestions
from *A Walk Through Policyland*. Copyright 1991 by Grandparents
United for Children's Rights, Inc. Used by permission.

Senior Highlights for quotations from "Grandmothers Fill In for
Drug-Abusing Parents" by Miriam Dobbin. Copyright 1990 by *Senior
Highlights*. Used by permission.

U.S. News & World Report for a quotation from "Silent Saviors"
by Linda L. Creighton. Copyright 1991 by *U.S. News & World
Report*. Used by permission.

Printed in the United States of America

This book is printed on acid-free paper.

Last digit is print number: 9 8 7 6 5 4 3 2 1

Library of Congress Cataloging-in-Publication Data

de Toledo, Sylvie.
    Grandparents as parents : a survival guide for raising a second
family / Sylvie de Toledo and Deborah Edler Brown.
        p.   cm.
    Includes bibliographical references and index.
    ISBN 1-57230-011-6. — ISBN 1-57230-020-5 (pbk.)
    1. Grandparent and child.   2. Child rearing.   3.
Intergenerational relations.   I. Brown, Deborah Edler.   II.
Title.
HQ759.9.D423   1995
649'.1—dc20   95-19656
                                                      CIP

To the memory of Nikki de Toledo;
her son, Kevin;
and Andre and Ginette, the grandparents who raised him

To grandparents everywhere
who are struggling to protect their grandchildren

We bereaved are not alone. We belong to the largest company in all the world—the company of those who have known suffering. When it seems that our sorrow is too great to be borne, let us think of the great family of the heavy-hearted into which our grief has given us entrance, and, inevitably, we will feel about us their arms, their sympathy, their understanding.

—Helen Keller

Foreword

The following excerpt is from a letter that I recently received from a grandmother named Charlotte, who catapulted out of the ranks of grandparenthood into that of surrogate parent early one September morning:

> It's 12:00 midnight. A few minutes ago as I walked down the hall toward the kitchen to get myself a glass of water I glanced at my 4½-year-old grandson sleeping peacefully in his bedroom and thought how different our lives were now from only a short time ago.
>
> Calvin's mother brought him to me at 3:00 A.M. the morning of 9/7/92. He arrived with no food; neither did she bring extra clothes. There he stood, a bewildered, scared little boy dressed in a pair of blue jeans with about ten holes in them, no underwear, a shirt that was much too big for his little body, and a pair of dirty white bedroom slippers. She told me that he was my grandchild. We didn't know each other. He was 17 months old when she left without any word. She asked if I would keep him until the following weekend when she would come back for him.
>
> That weekend and many more have come and gone without any word from her. Calvin and I are doing fine because we have each other. We get by on my small Social Security check. We don't know where his mother is. I've gotten an order for temporary custody that allows me to take him to the doctor if he gets sick, and I will put him in school next month. But where is his mother? Will she ever return, and if she does, what will happen to Calvin then?
>
> Please help me. I need some answers and direction.

Grandparents throughout the ages have served as support for their children and grandchildren, and generational interdependence has long been a significant part of American society. The major difference between past generations and the current one, however, is that in the past—except in the event of the death of a parent—grandparents tended to be ancillary in furnishing support to their children's families. Although they certainly provided goods and services to enhance the young family, they, for the most part, assumed a background role in the actual parenting of the children.

Historical tradition has changed, however, and many of today's grandparents now find themselves long- or short-term parents again. Often, they must adjust to being part of a nontraditional family in which parental roles may be reversed: parents may become virtual siblings, aunts, or other kin; parents may not be in the picture at all; or grandparents may have to become parents. Confusion reigns, not only on the part of the children but also in the minds of their caregivers/surrogate parents.

It is to this group of dedicated and caring people that the immensely useful and impressive book you are about to read is directed: the millions of "Charlotte(s)" who daily give of themselves so that their grandchildren may live with love and compassion and without fear of abandonment.

Only a few years ago, little was said about grandparents raising their grandchildren. Today, largely because of social advocacy, we see more media coverage of these circumstances, and we know now that our numbers are large and growing, and that this growth is expected to continue.

What is often not reflected in the media, however, is how grandparent caregivers and their young charges are getting along. What are they feeling, and how are they coping? What are their major concerns and desires? What forms of help do they need when they reach out for support, and what agencies or persons are best equipped to bolster them in times of need? Finally, two people have come along to put some answers to these questions.

When grandparent advocate Sylvie de Toledo first discussed the idea of a book for grandparents who are raising their grandchildren, I was very exctied. I knew that she was just the person who could speak to this audience with empathy and kindness, but also with amazing firmness. I understood that if anyone could offer grandparents a sense of direction it would be Sylvie. From time to time over the three years that it took to complete the book, either she or writer Deborah Edler Brown would call and read half-finished sections to me for input. I have now read the completed book, and can truthfully say that my initial hopes have been surpassed.

What you are about to begin is a reference book that reads like a novel. It is poetic, gentle, and thoughtful, and yet it is brimming with vital information—no page can be skipped.

Furthermore, *Grandparents as Parents: A Survival Guide for Raising a Second Family* could only have been conceived of by someone who has been through the trauma of a family broken by tragedy, by one who has chosen to be there for others who need help and direction. Its availability offers us hope, and validates our personal fears, angers, frustrations, and pain. It points us toward sanity and reason in the face of dilemma and need. We are taken, step by painful step, through the process of learning again how to function as a parent, especially in these complicated times. We are retaught old skills and trained in the process of learning new ones. No topic is too insignificant or cumbersome to be examined, either succinctly or in a thorough manner. Our own personal needs and those of the children that we love and cherish are examined openly and in a straightforward manner.

This remarkable book can be used as a resource not only by those courageous many who have assumed the responsibilities of parenting, loving, and nurturing a generation of potentially lost children, but also by those who serve them—our social service personnel, family therapists, legal professionals, and any others who work cross-generationally with families to help them stay whole.

Ethel Dunn
Executive Director,
Grandparents United for Children's Rights

Acknowledgments

No book of this scope can come to light without the support of a number of people—friends and family, sources, and many outside experts who patiently offered insight and clarification. From the moment this project was conceived to the time the final manuscript was set, we have been graced with heartfelt enthusiasm and help from some very wonderful individuals.

Our first thanks must go to our families for their boundless support and encouragement, particularly our parents, Andre and Ginette de Toledo, Jack Brown and Ana Edler Brown, Sylvie's brother and sister-in-law, Philip and Alyce, Deborah's brother Arthur, and Sylvie's nephew Kevin, who has been very open in sharing his story. Words do not adequately express how deeply they have all affected the success of this project. From the beginning of *Grandparents as Parents*, the program and the book, Sylvie's family members have been case studies, cheerleaders, reseach assistants, volunteers, benefactors, and all-around silent partners. From the beginning of the book project, Deborah's family has been a sounding board, an editorial board, and an ongoing pep rally. Indeed, special credit must go to Deborah's brother Arthur, who carefully read and helped trim an overgrown manuscript with exquisite insight and precision. Our families have offered praise, advice, warm meals, strong shoulders, and even grants when times were lean. We could not have done this book without them.

We owe much to our wonderful editor Kitty Moore. From start to finish, she has been a guide through unfamiliar terrain, a deft ambassador between authors and publisher, and an expert coach whose enthusiasm and clear understanding focused our vision. A similar vote of thanks goes to Wendy Ross, whose preliminary editing helped strengthen and shape the architecture of a complex subject.

JoBeth McDaniel was our matchmaker for this project. An accomplished journalist herself, JoBeth wrote the original proposal for this book but was prevented from actually writing it due to prior commitments. Instead, she eagerly introduced us to each other, and a happy meeting it was. If books have godmothers, JoBeth would be ours.

We have been graced with guardian angels as well. We are indebted to attorneys Larry Hanna, Pamela Mohr, Michael Salazar, Yolanda Vera, Peter Wright, and Ted Youmans, who have shared their time, knowledge, and resources to help us anchor this book in practical, accurate information about family law, government aid, and special education. All have made time in their overcommitted schedules to read drafts of chapters and clarify subtle shifts of meaning. They have also been on call to answer the numerous tiny, detailed questions that came up in the last pressured moments of rewriting. We are equally grateful to Samuel Hananel, Phil Hopkins, Stephen Poe, and Richard Sherer for jumping in as ad hoc editors, proofreaders, and consultants at several critical junctures, offering their expertise and enthusiasm; to Sheila Milnes for her insight on issues of childrearing; and to Pamela Darr Wright for her help in unraveling the IEP process.

We also wish to thank Jacqueline Battle, Alice Bussiere, Leza Davis, Charles Ollinger, Anne Rutherford, Lori Waldinger, Dana Wilson, the ADD+ Forum at CompuServe, and the Department of Health and Human Services and the helpful people who work there. They have all extended themselves to ensure that valuable information reaches the hands of families in need.

Thanks to Karen and Heidi Toffler, as well as Ken Stuckey from the Perkins School for the Blind, for doggedly tracking down the source of the marvelous quote from Helen Keller that starts the book; to Stuart Chapin, for offering up Carl Sandburg as a way to end it; and to Alvin Toffler for his lessons on how to put it all together.

Many others have helped out in quiet but important ways. Deborah would like to thank the close friends and extended family who have offered support, counsel, hugs, and incredible patience with the mental and physical absences of a writer in labor. In addition to those already mentioned, special thanks go to Joe Anthony, Diane Davidson, Josh Gambin, Greg Hughart, Claudia Kazachinsky, Keli Morgan, Kaliko Orian, Donna Pall, Marianne Simon, Andrew Stein, Andrea Trisciuzzi, and Kaki Woods, as well as to Richard Wells, who helped nurture a love of words, to the Browns and the Edlers for funding the first computer, and to Sarah Crane, who so graciously tolerated the wayward schedule of her Aunt Deb.

Of course, none of this would have come together without the wonderful people at The Guilford Press. We thank them for their dedicated work, their enthusiasm, and their patience with frantic phone calls from new authors. We particularly appreciate the careful work of the book's production editor at Guilford, Anna Brackett, and the copyediting of Toby Troffkin. We are grateful to our art director, Ty Cumbie, for giving our book such a beautiful face, and to Lyn Grossman, Rowena Howells, Lori Rothstein, Keisha Simmons, and Kitty Stewart for their parts in turning a manuscript into a book. We also want to thank assistant marketing director Anne Newman for her belief that this is an important book and publicist Phyllis Heller for making sure that people see it.

It's hard to find the right words to describe Ethel Dunn. Friend, colleage, advocate, grandmother, Ethel's exuberance was like food and fresh air when we were weary. She gave us perspective, information, and let us read fledgling chapters to her long-distance. She also lent us her own talents as a writer by writing the foreword to this book. Her excitement has been invaluable.

We are particularly grateful to the past and present board members of Grandparents As Parents (GAP): Carole Bloom, Barbara Castro, Rosalie Cauley, Florence Gilmore, Judith Hirsch, Betty Linstead, Joan McMillin, and Barbara Wasson. There is no way to measure what they have given of themselves in time, money, energy, and heart, to promote the cause of grandparents. They have been our staunchest cheering section, and we couldn't have gotten this far without them.

We deeply appreciate the efforts of all the journalists and talk show hosts who are shedding light on grandparent issues and of all the advocates who are working to improve the plight of grandparents and of children in general.

Finally, no thanks would be complete without remembering the countless grandparents who have so generously shared their stories with us. It was their faces, and the faces of their grandchildren, that kept us going in the bleak hours when the road seemed too long and writing one more word seemed like an inhuman task. They were our humanity, and our light.

Contents

Introduction

In 1983 my sister committed suicide. She locked the doors of her house and overdosed on pills that had been prescribed for depression. She didn't leave a note. She did leave an eight-year-old son. She was 27 years old.

I was away in graduate school, finishing a master's degree in social work. My sister and I had a standing phone date. Every Saturday morning at six o'clock I would call her. My nephew would be asleep, and we could talk without interruption. As a single mother, my sister didn't have much time without interruption. Since Kevin would wake up at some point during the call, I would talk to him, too. Nikki and I were close in age—one year and one week apart—and we were best friends.

That Saturday I called and called, but there was no answer. I finally called my parents to see if they knew where Nikki was. Kevin had spent the previous night at my brother's house and was scheduled to stay with my parents that night to give his mother a free weekend. But she hadn't said anything about going out. We decided they should use the spare key and go in. It didn't work. One lock wouldn't open. It was the one Nikki locked from inside. "She's in there, Mom," I said. "I know she's in there." My parents had the police knock down the door. Nikki was there, but it was too late. I caught the next plane to Los Angeles (by this time, it was early the next morning).

Overnight, we went from a family of five adults to one of four, a hand with a missing finger. We were devastated, and we were in shock. Grief had joined our family.

And then there was Kevin.

Kevin had always been the family child. Nikki dropped out of school at 18 to have him. His father was never part of the picture.

And although Nikki and Kevin had their own apartment, my parents, my brother, and I were always helping out in different ways. Kevin was lovable and he was difficult. Now, at the age of eight, he was parentless.

There was no question of what to do. My parents took Kevin in, and in that moment they became part of a family much larger than ours, although we didn't know it then. They joined the growing ranks of grandparents who are raising their grandchildren.

The media calls them "silent saviors,"[1] "recycled parents,"[2] and, when they are also caring for aging parents, "the sandwich generation."[3] At a time in their lives when they expected to be traveling, enjoying hobbies, and doing everything they had put on hold while raising their first set of children, they find themselves back in a routine of bottles, diapers, and PTA meetings, sometimes 30 years after they last had kids in the house. Instead of doting grandparents who can spoil and coddle and send the kids back to Mom and Dad, they are surrogate parents with all the responsibilities of raising another set of children.

Some are as young as 35, others are in their 70s. Some are even great-grandparents and step-grandparents. They cross economic lines, social lines, and religious lines. They become caregivers because of abandonment, neglect, and abuse, as well as death by illness, accident, suicide, and murder. In some instances their adult children are in jail or mentally ill. By far, the most common reason grandparents raise grandchildren is parental drug and alcohol abuse.

The kids these grandparents get are troubled, burdened with everything from emotional, behavioral, psychological, medical, and academic problems to physical disabilities from a parent's prenatal drug and alcohol abuse.

More than three million children live in the homes of their grandparents. Even so, too many grandparents think they are in this alone. Not a day goes by that I don't get phone calls and letters from grandparents around the country who are looking for a group, a piece of information, or someone to listen to them who will understand their concerns. The letters come typed, written, and scribbled in crayon, on everything from napkins to torn scraps of paper. Some write "Dear Ms. de Toledo" or "Dear GAP [Grandparents As Parents]" and tell their stories; others just write "Help!" One grandparent in Georgia seemed to say it for all of them when he wrote, "I took my grandson when his mother died six years ago.

Ten months ago, his dad died. We need people. My friends call once in a while but don't come around. We are like in a world alone. We need people."

This book had to be done because there was absolutely nothing out there to answer those letters. I talked to thousands of grandparents across the country and realized there was nothing to help these families. People asked me about resources, and because I had nowhere to refer them, I would offer to help start a group in their community.

Before I started my first Grandparents As Parents support group in 1987, I searched a number of libraries for information on grandparents raising grandchildren. I was looking for a foundation. If there was material out there, I didn't want to reinvent the wheel. Unfortunately, I didn't find anything in the professional literature, let alone the consumer press.

Since then, GAP has grown into an organization of nine support groups across southern California and has helped start hundreds of others throughout the country. Local grandparent groups across the United States have joined forces to create a strong national voice on grandparent issues. Various organizations have created pamphlets, brochures, and newsletters. Researchers have just begun to study the grandparenting phenomenon, and a few authors have published books on the changing role of grandparents.[4] Still, there is nothing out there that addresses the broad spectrum of grandparent issues in one place.

So, this is *GAP: The Book*. It is part map, part dictionary, and something of a group hug—a handbook for all grandparents who are raising grandchildren, to help them through the stressful times. Inside you will find descriptions of many of the common problems grandparents face when they take in their grandchildren, as well as practical suggestions for how to cope. You will also find basic information on topics such as government aid, court proceedings, and special education. I hope this book will help get you through the alphabet soup of AFDC, IEP, WIC, and CPS. In these pages you will find guidelines for forming groups and becoming politically active, two sure ways of empowering yourself in a situation that can often make you feel powerless. Here, as in a GAP meeting, I offer support, resource information, and a professional perspective. But it is the other grandparents who will let you know you are not alone, that you can get through this, that whatever you are going through is normal. In the following pages, you will hear their voices and their stories.*

Second-time parenting can be pretty grim sometimes. You face troubled children, uncooperative parents, and a bureaucracy that may not understand your new role or support your new needs. This book does not shy away from those stark realities. It does not suggest that if you follow a prescribed set of steps, your problems will vanish. Life isn't that simple. It does, however, offer hope. By raising grandchildren, you offer them a new future. By learning your options you give yourself choices. By recognizing problems you learn when to adapt and when to fight back. And by joining forces you create hope for the grandparents who follow you.

A NOTE TO PROFESSIONALS WHO WORK WITH GRANDPARENTS

I hope this book will also provide insight for people who work with grandparents: mental health professionals, teachers, doctors, attorneys—anyone who comes in contact with grandparents raising grandchildren and children being raised by their grandparents.

I receive frequent requests from educators and mental health professionals on how to develop groups for grandparents. My work is based on years of observations of and therapeutic work with grandparent families, as well as on personal experience with my own family. This treatment incorporates many aspects: crisis intervention, individual needs assessment, meeting survival needs of individual families, modeling coping skills, teaching problem-solving techniques, and supportive therapy. Some of the work I do is nontraditional for mental health professionals, but I believe it is critical for grandparent families.

Chapter 14 specifically addresses support groups for grandparents: how to find them, how to start them, and what programs and principles have been successful for GAP. The chapter is designed to assist both grandparents and mental health professionals in the rewarding process of developing groups; I hope it helps you.

---

*So as to avoid using sexist language—and so as not to encumber it with an excessive use of "he or she" and "him or her"—we have decided to alternate between masculine and feminine pronouns. We have attempted to do this consistently, and have tried to avoid ascribing the male and female pronouns in a stereotypical way.

HOW TO READ THIS BOOK

Grandparents as Parents is designed as both a book and a manual. You can read it front to back, following the grandparent stories that span the chapters, or you can turn to whatever chapter addresses your immediate questions, without worrying about order.

The book is divided into three sections. Section I, "When the Second Shift Arrives," covers the personal and social aspects of raising grandchildren: the changes, the feelings, and the problems of adult children, grandchildren, and family in general. It starts with an overview of the recent rise in grandparents as parents and looks at some of the myths about the phenomenon. Section II, "Through the Red Tape," addresses the bureaucratic part of raising grandchildren, the legal issues, and the availability of government assistance and special education. And Section III, "Strength in Numbers," focuses on the larger community of grandparents as parents and provides information on finding and starting support groups as well as on the political aspects of the grandparent movement.

Grandparents as Parents represents the work of two authors—myself and journalist Deborah Edler Brown—yet it is written from one point of view. The reason is simple: We wanted this to be a comfortable, personal book, and ten years of working with grandparents has given me an intimate understanding of the subject. As you read through the following chapters, the voice and perspective you encounter will be mine. I hope they help you.

When my sister ended her life, a whole world ended for me. And another one opened. Somehow, when I see the growth of GAP, I feel that something positive is coming from the death of my sister. There is a special place in my heart for grandparents who are parenting again. You all deserve a gold medal for what you're doing. You have sacrificed to be here, and my heart goes out to you.

SYLVIE DE TOLEDO

Grandparents as Parents accurately conveys the themes that are the most central to grandparents who are raising grandchildren, but the names and identifying characteristics of most of the grandparents and grandchildren mentioned in the book have been changed in order to protect their privacy.

When the Second Shift Arrives

CHAPTER 1

Unplanned Parenthood: Why Me?

Becoming a parent again is not a first choice. It's
a last alternative.
—*Barbara Kirkland, founder
of Grandparents Raising Grandchildren*[1]

Sometimes the call comes at night, sometimes on a bright morning. It may be your child, the police, or child protective services. "Mama, I've messed up. . . ." "We're sorry. There has been an accident. . . ." "Mrs. Smith, we have your grandchild. Can you take him?" Sometimes you make the call yourself—reporting your own child to the authorities in a desperate attempt to protect your grandchild from abuse or neglect. Often the change is gradual. At first your grandchild is with you for a day, then four days, a month, and then two months as the parents slowly lose control of their lives. You start out baby-sitting. You think the arrangement is temporary. You put off buying a crib or moving to a bigger apartment. Then you get a collect call from jail—or no call at all.

But whether the arrival is slow or sudden, at some point it dawns on you: You are no longer watching your grandchildren, you are raising them. Take the *grand* out of *grandparent*; you are parenting again, and your life will never be the same.

Emily Petersen knew her pregnant daughter-in-law, Sheila, was a drug addict. She knew the young woman was using drugs throughout her entire pregnancy, and she was prepared to see the effects in her newborn granddaughter—the stiff body, the frantic eyes, the shakes. What Emily was not prepared for was becoming a mother again at 59. But when she and her husband, Carter, arrived at the hospital to see the baby, they found a social worker and two body-guards outside the hospital room. Sheila had been arrested on drug charges, and the baby was being removed. The social worker asked Emily if she would be willing to take the child. "I came in to visit a baby," Emily told her. "I didn't come to take a baby home." But her son was in tears, begging them not to send Amanda into foster care, and neither Emily nor Carter could stand the idea of not knowing where their granddaughter was. A week later they filed for custody.

Ivy Johnson had not seen her daughter Rachel in four years; she had never even met her youngest granddaughter. They lived in Arizona and had no money to travel. Then Rachel left her hus-band and came home with her kids. The minute she came to the door, Ivy knew something more was wrong. Within three days Rachel was diagnosed with liver cancer. Seven months later she died, leaving Ivy to raise five young grandchildren in a one-bed-room apartment.

There is nothing new about a grandparent raising a child in a crisis. For centuries grandparents have taken over when their grandchildren were orphaned by disease or war or when financial troubles split a family. They have also stepped in to support single mothers and widowed or divorced parents of both sexes. Moreover, there is a proud tradition of intergenerational families in working-class neighborhoods as well as in African-American and Hispanic communities of all income levels.[2]

What *is* new are the numbers: of grandparents, of grandchildren, of crises. According to the U.S. Census Bureau, approximately 3.2 million children[3] under 18 were living in grandparents' homes in 1990—a 40 percent increase[4] in 10 years. Nearly one million homes had no parents present at all.[5] And the real numbers are probably higher: Many grandparents don't acknowledge or recognize that they are taking full-time care of their grandchildren; perhaps they only watch them four days a week or are ashamed to admit that their own children can't parent. Many don't believe the situation is permanent. Some estimates put the number of grandparents raising grandchildren at over five percent of American families.[6] That would be approxi-mately 1 in 20 households, or one family per average city block. "What's wrong with my generation that we can't or won't raise our kids?" asks one young mother in Texas. The answer paints a picture of growing tragedy in American families.

AMERICA'S CHILDREN IN CRISIS

Grandparents raise grandchildren for one reason: because the children need someone to raise them. It was true a hundred years ago, and it is true today. Certainly, there are grandparents who try to "steal" their grandchildren, but the vast majority had other plans for this stage of their lives; raising another child wasn't part of them. To quote a grandmother in Oregon: "The bottom line of this whole thing is I didn't need another child; the child needed a mother."

On the other hand, there are many reasons why these children need their grandparents. One writer pinned the cause on what he called the four Ds: drugs, divorce, desertion, and the death of a parent.[7] Indeed, illness, accident, suicide, and murder leave numerous children without parents to care for them, and drugs and alcohol shatter thousands of young families each year. But child abuse, incarceration, joblessness, teen pregnancy, and now AIDS also contribute to the growing number of children without stable homes. Most families suffer from a combination of problems, and the rate at which all these problems are growing is frightening. The statistics point to a nation of children in crisis:

- One in two marriages ends in divorce. Nearly one million children experience divorce each year.[8] Some parents go on to remarry with little interest in their own offspring.
- Teen pregnancy rates are high.[9] Half a million children are born to teenagers in the United States each year.[10]
- Reports of child abuse and neglect are up 300% nationally since 1976.[11]
- The prison population has exploded. Eighty percent of inmates—men and women—are parents of dependent children.[12]
- More wome are using drugs, especially crack cocaine.[13] Every year 375,000 babies are born with drugs in their system.[14]
- AIDS is taking its toll on American families. Nearly 125,000 children will have lost their mothers to the disease by the year 2000.[15]

Many of these children end up in foster care, separated from their siblings and cared for by strangers. But the foster care system itself is in crisis, with a rising demand for care and a shrinking number of qualified foster parents. In some cities, public health officials have talked about a return to orphanages.[16]

All this leaves grandparents, and other relatives, as one of the few buffers between these children and an increasingly precarious future. In fact, as of 1994, 54 percent of children placed out of home in Los Angeles County were placed with grandparents and other relative caregivers.[17]

Whether your grandchild lives with you because of drugs, death, abuse, or abandonment, there are certain factors that are *not* responsible for this second parenthood, despite what people think.

THE MYTHS

There are several reactions that appear, like clockwork, each time a discussion turns to grandparents as parents. They are assumptions that allow people to explain away the phenomenon, to pretend that it doesn't touch them, and to put the blame, somehow, on the victim:

"It's a black problem, right?"
"It's a poor problem—or an urban problem—isn't it?"
"Well, those grandparents probably deserve it if they messed up their first set of kids."

These biases exist as much in the judge deciding a custody case as in the person watching the news. They are responsible for much of the intolerance you may encounter as you try to find help for yourself and protection for your grandkids. These assumptions imply that the "grandparenting" phenomenon is something that happens to someone else, when the sad truth is that each and every grandparent is only one or two tragedies away from the decision to raise a grandchild.

If you and the children you care for are ever to receive the help you desperately need and deserve, we must look through these myths and face head-on the incredible depth and scope of grandparents as parents.

Myth 1: It's an Urban, Minority Problem

Say "grandparents as parents" to people, and, for many, certain pictures come to mind: Black faces. Brown faces. City-dwellers. Families in poverty. These pictures are not inaccurate, but they are incomplete. Raising grandchildren is not strictly an urban, poor, or African-American problem. If it were, it would be no less of a social crisis. But it is not. It is a national problem.

Parenting a grandchild is a necessity born of tragedy, and tragedy has no regard for race, class, ethnicity, location, or religion. Grandparents are raising grandchildren in places as different from one another as New York City, Honolulu, and Paducah, Kentucky. Articles on second-time parenting have appeared in publications as diverse as the *Boston Globe*, the *Katy Times* (in Katy, Texas), the *Cleveland Jewish News*, and a local newsletter in Pottowattamie County, Iowa. More than half of these children are white, and nearly half are African-American,[18] and while Hispanic and other races represent the smallest numbers, they still account for 415,000 children.[19] Grandparenting is color-blind. It is also class-blind. The same can be said of the drug epidemic that drives it.

Drugs and alcohol account for more than 80 percent of grandparent families. They show up combined with teen pregnancy, abuse, neglect, and abandonment. They show up in connection with incarceration and murder. Moreover, suburban, middle-class, and white families are not immune from addiction; they only hide it better. Middle-class addicts may have better access to private drug treatment programs and may be less likely to end up in jail. Private doctors are less likely to question pregnant women about drugs and alcohol than are inner-city doctors in public clinics and county hospitals; private hospitals are also less likely to test pregnant women or newborns for drug exposure.[20]

According to a 1989 study by the National Association for Perinatal Addiction Research and Education (NAPARE), white women are just as likely to use cocaine, heroin, or marijuana during a pregnancy as black women, but black women are ten times more likely to be reported to the authorities.[21] "Physicians were selecting out those women who they perceived as drug abusers to test those babies and then reporting them through the system," says NAPARE president Ira Chasnoff.[22] To quote one grandmother, "Drugs affect us all, whether you live in the streets or in a mansion."

So does tragedy. Both are indiscriminate. Who you are and where you live are not to blame for your situation, and neither are you.

Myth 2: It's Your Fault

Diane Warner is a grandparent activist and founder of Second Time Around Parents in Pennsylvania. She is raising the son of a drug-addicted daughter. It is not uncommon in her lobbying work for her to hear this question: "If you have raised a drug addict, how can we trust you not to raise this child as a drug addict?"[23] It is a question grandparents hear all the time. It is a question that hangs in the air, spoken or unspoken. It floats through the legal system, where judges and social workers question the wisdom of placing children with their grandparents, wondering to what extent the grandparents are responsible for the adult child's inability to parent.

Similar questions haunt many grandparents themselves: "What did we do wrong?" "Is this our fault?" "Are we grandparenting because we failed as parents?" One grandmother feels guilty because she worked nights as a nurse; she fears that may be why her daughter is on drugs. Another is afraid that she didn't love her son enough, that maybe she wasn't there when he needed her and that it drove him to drugs.

Let me set the record straight.* You did not raise your children to be drug addicts, welfare mothers, prostitutes, or even irresponsible parents. Did you make mistakes in childrearing? Probably. Most people do. Are there things you could have done differently? Certainly. We all have 20/20 hindsight. But you did not cause your child's addiction or the abuse or neglect of his or her own child. You did the best you could with what you knew at the time. Again and again, I see families where two or three children grow up to be upstanding citizens and competent parents and one loses control of her life. The New Jersey grandparents who raised a talented musician, a successful accountant, and a young woman who became addicted to drugs. The Montana grandparents who raised three boys: an architect, a county sheriff, and a drug addict. How are these grandparents to be blamed for their children's failings?

---

*Please note that although this book represents the work of two authors, it is written from the point of view of one—Sylvie de Toledo.

Even when child abuse or addiction seems to run in a family—and these problems can be cyclical—grown people have a choice about whether to continue the cycle or break it. There are many adults who were abused as children who do not grow up to be abusers and many children of addicts who take a different path.

Again, the statistics are telling. The recent surge in grandparents raising grandchildren—a 40 percent increase—occurred between 1980 and 1990. That almost precisely coincides with the growth of the crack epidemic. But few grandparents knew much about marijuana, let alone cocaine, when they were raising children. And if you had known, what could you have done? When they caught their teenagers with marijuana, many grandparents marched them off to police stations only to have them slapped on the wrist and sent home. Moreover, many people experimented with drugs and alcohol as teenagers and grew up to be productive adults and parents. Besides, the truth is that most of the grandparents I see are not raising the children of teenagers. In fact, according to one expert, the average age for a crack mother is 25 to 28, and many are in their 30s.[24] "It is the use of substance that creates substance abuse problems," says California psychologist Michael Jones. "We have a whole society that has problems with that, and that is certainly not the making of any particular grandparent."[25]

No one makes a person take drugs, abandon a baby, or abuse a child. Whatever choices you made as parents are past you. You did the best you could. Your children are now adults, and they are making their own choices.

THE REASONS FOR GRANDPARENTING

There are many complicated reasons why grandchildren need grandparents to care for them. But, in the end, the reasons you take them in are straightforward and simple: love, duty, and the bonds of family. Over and over I hear the same refrains: "We want to keep the kids together." "We're all he has." Often you are the only one standing between your grandchild and foster care. I have seen many grandparents disrupt their lives, their finances, and their health to keep their grandchildren together and away from care by strangers.

Anne Sutter's grandson Gregory was born in a crack house, and his mother was arrested on drug-related charges. At 60 years of age and on a limited income, Anne was not prepared to care for an infant, but there was that tiny baby, born stiff and distorted, with drugs in his system, and Anne couldn't say no. She recalls, "I looked at him and thought to myself, 'Nobody else will love my baby; they will look at him and think he's a thing.'"

"Some of our friends say we're crazy, that they would never do this," another grandmother told a reporter. "But if we hadn't done this, in 15 years there might have been a knock on our front door and a young man standing there saying, 'I'm your grandson. Where were you when I needed you, when I lay in bed at night crying for someone to help me?'"[26]

A grandfather calls it a labor of love: "I don't think I could live with it if they went to somebody else."

CHAPTER 2

Taking Immediate Action

I live with my grandma because my mom left me on a hotel bench to go get a cup of coffee. You're not supposed to leave babies by theirselves.
—*Erica, age seven*

Late one Saturday night the phone call came: Leah Croft's 18-month-old grandson had been left unattended in an apartment. The little boy had tried to feed himself dry oatmeal and had started choking. Someone had called the police, and child protective services had removed the baby from his mother. They wanted Leah to take him in. Leah was already raising her daughter Jill's six-year-old twins but, because of Jill's transient lifestyle, had only seen her grandson three times before that night. At 10:30 P.M., Josh arrived in the arms of a social worker. Dressed in a sleeper that had the legs cut off because it was too small for him, he had no socks, no shoes, no bottle, no car seat, and only the diaper he was wearing. The next day was a frenzy. In addition to buying baby supplies, Leah had to find a sitter so she could go to work Monday morning. She had to buy diapers with her credit card because she didn't have enough cash. No one from social services told her she was eligible for government aid for the baby, and when she called to ask about it, she got the runaround. "For five months I didn't get one dime," she fumes. "Not one dime!"

Whether a grandchild arrives in one night or over a period of months, few grandparents plan, anticipate, or prepare for a second parenthood. Your home and lifestyle are geared to adult living. You are not expecting these children or these changes. Instead of one small baby, you may, like Ivy Johnson, acquire several children at once, all at different ages with different needs. Instead of the assured rights of parents, you may find that as grandparents you have no legal right to care for the children you are battling on all fronts to protect. Moreover, you may find your resources tapped in the process. As a grandparent raising grandchildren, you are facing complex emotional, financial, and legal situations that you are rarely prepared for. You may have to resolve problems overnight that most parents address over a period of months, if not years. While each family has different needs, there are a few things that every grandparent should look into as soon as possible:

▪ *Consider other options.* Some grandparents don't have the health or resources to raise a second family, but they do it anyway. A few, however, have been able to place their grandchild with another family member, perhaps a son or daughter who already had children and was willing to raise this child as well. If you have family members who can help out, you might consider letting them step in or at least sharing the responsibility with them. Parenting your grandchildren not only disrupts your life but deprives the children of grandparents who can spoil them and send them home for their parents to deal with. The children have already lost an important relationship with their parents; now they are losing a precious relationship with you.

Most grandparents, however, don't have other options, and the majority don't want to burden their other adult children. Their only choice is to gear up for the changes and the feelings that come along with raising grandchildren.

▪ *Keep records.* One of the most important things you can do when your grandchildren arrive is to start taking notes. I know that buying notebooks and pens sounds more like preparation for school than for grandparenting, but when you take in your grandchildren, you become more than a surrogate parent; you become their advocate. You may be the only voice speaking solely for their safety and their interests. The law will protect the parents, the government will protect its own pockets, and you will be the one trying to protect your grandchildren's rights—in court, in school, and in the welfare system. You are the one who knows that Dad has a drug problem and that the children are being neglected and/or abused whenever they are with him. You are the one who knows that Max throws tantrums in school after Mom comes to visit. Unfortunately, few people will want to listen to the grandparent, which is why you must document everything. The more organized you are, the better your chances that those who listen will believe you (see Chapter 5).

You will also want to use your notebooks to set yourself up as a kind of central headquarters. Throughout this book you will find lists of the kinds of records you will need to keep: names and phone numbers of attorneys, social workers, and welfare workers connected to your grandchild; the names of their supervisors; and information for school, for doctors, and for the welfare office. The more organized you are from the start, the less crazy you may feel later on.

Remember, the best advocate is an organized one. If you ever need to lock horns with the system, you want to be ready. Keep records of the professionals you talk to and what they tell you. Create a paper trail of letters and documents. Keep dates and times of conversations. Try to write letters when you can and keep copies. Knowledge is power; it may be the only power you have. But nothing you know will do any good if you can't present it in a clear, convincing fashion.

▪ *Sort out the legal maze.* Your grandchildren are family, pure and simple. However, family is also a legal relationship, with rights and responsibilities that can be dictated by the courts. Your rights toward your grandchildren will mostly depend on why they are with you. As soon as possible, find out what your legal rights are in this situation and how you can best protect them. Chapter 10 offers a broad overview of custody issues to get you started, but you will probably want to consult an attorney or other legal professional about your individual case.

▪ *Look into financial aid.* Raising children is expensive. Raising children on a fixed retirement income is expensive and stressful. And raising children on a fixed welfare income, as some grandparents must do, can make you crazy. Whatever obligations you feel you have toward your grandchildren, and I know there are many, you do not have an obligation to support them financially. Financial support is a parent's responsibility. If parents don't fulfill that responsibility, their children are entitled to government assistance.

Many grandparents are reluctant to look to the government for help or don't believe they qualify. They have never asked for help before, and the process mystifies them. Still, while government benefits won't make you rich, every little bit helps, especially Medicaid. As soon as you can, find out what assistance is available to your grandchildren. (For more on government aid, see Chapter 12.)

▪ *Arrange for medical care.* One of the biggest expenses with children is health care. Immunizations and the treatment of colds, earaches, and childhood sprains can add up to a small fortune. Many grandparents are shocked to discover that their insurance companies will not add grandchildren to their policies. However, the children can often be covered by Medicaid. Again, apply early (see Chapter 12).

▪ *Keep medical records.* Accurate medical records can be critical when you raise a child. Few children arrive at grandma's house with records of any kind, but if you can somehow acquire them, they will make your life easier. For instance, have your grandchildren had all their immunization shots? If you don't know, you'll have to start all over. Many grandchildren have had to be reimmunized because of lost records. If the children come to you from a foster care placement or group home, ask the social worker for their medical records. At the very least, try to compile a family medical history based on what you do know about your family. You never know what information could be important later on.

▪ *Enroll them in school.* If you can keep your grandchild in the same school or day-care facility, consider yourself lucky. It's one less change for the child and less stress for you. If not, try to get school records and reports of any special education programs transferred with the child (see Chapter 13). Special education plans should be transferable to the new school, even if it is in another state. Granted, school is much easier to handle in an intact family that was hit by crisis, like a death, than in a family where the parents were on drugs and the child rarely made it to school. Just do the best you can.

▪ *Consider counseling.* Few children are raised by their grandparents for happy reasons. Many grandchildren arrive with emotional, psychological, or behavioral difficulties and/or with physical problems caused by parental abuse or prenatal drug exposure. Most arrive suffering from grief and rejection. If your grandchildren are old enough to talk about feelings and events, consider getting them into counseling. Even if they are too young for counseling on their own, you can work with a counselor on their behalf, learning techniques to help them cope with the situation. I have worked with a number of grandparents to address a child's temper tantrums or inability to sleep in his own bed. These children have all had their lives somehow shattered. A support group or family counseling can start the process of gluing them back together.

▪ *Find your own emotional support.* Raising a second family is stressful and exhausting. It wears on your time, your energy, your finances, and your spirit. Like your grandchildren, you have suffered loss. But you also shoulder the responsibilities. Don't try to do this alone. Look around at your resources. Who can be your emotional support? Whom can you turn to for help? My parents were fortunate. They never worried about baby-sitters because my brother and I were there, although they did worry about burdening us. Many families really are alone. Perhaps your new circumstances involve your only child, or your other children live far away or don't support your taking in the grandchildren. If that is true, you may have to look elsewhere for support. Try other grandparents, a support group, or even a therapist to blow off steam, but do look for help.

CHAPTER 3 | # Your Lifestyle: Changed and Challenged

It is not the American Dream of a grandparent
to raise a second family.
                              —*Letter from Texas*

Beth Grafton's life was sweet. Her six children were grown, and she was in a wonderful second marriage to Alan, the man of her dreams. Alan had his own business and a comfortable savings. Beth managed a clothing store. If they needed something, they bought it. Alan's father, whom they had nursed for two years, had died the year before, leaving them with the house to themselves and time to rekindle their marriage. After years of renting they were getting ready to buy a home. On weekends Alan would shop and play golf; Beth would do yard work, work on crafts, and visit her grandchildren. In the evenings they would go out to dinner or dancing. Every other month they would join a group of friends in Cape Cod for the weekend.

And they had future plans. They dreamed of taking cruises, since neither one had ever been on one, and of traveling through the United States together. They worried about their adult children but knew they couldn't control their children's lives.

Then the unthinkable happened: Their daughter Ellen was stabbed to death by an abusive husband. To compound the nightmare, the children, who had witnessed the murder, were placed with the father's family, although they had visited their maternal grandparents regularly since they were born and even had their own rooms in their grandparents' house. In addition to the horrible loss of their daughter, Beth and Alan were deprived of seeing their grandchildren.

What followed was three and a half years of court battles that broke the Graftons' bank account and almost broke their spirits. Beth, 51, was described as "an aging, elderly grandmother" and accused of being manic–depressive. "It was as if they were trying to blame Ellen for the murder, and us for raising her that way," says Beth. The Graftons were eventually awarded custody of the children, but the cost of the battle left them shattered. The stress was so high that Alan had three strokes, although a complete physical the year before had judged him to be in great health. He lost his business, and he and Beth spent all their money on attorney fees. Two sons refinanced their own homes to help them out, but Beth and Alan remain thousands of dollars in debt.

Today Beth, Alan, and the children live on Social Security and the money Beth makes from part-time work; she can't find a good full-time job, and they have no medical insurance. In the evenings Beth does laundry, cooks meals, and reads the mail. There are no more dinners out, and the Graftons rarely see their friends, who have different lifestyles.

And their dreams are gone. "I looked forward to when all my kids were gone," says Beth. "I looked forward to being able to find myself as a person, not as a mother or a grandmother but as Beth. It's like I'm lost again, lost raising children. I miss all the things I thought I would be able to do with my husband. All our dreams were ripped out of our book. The whole chapter of our being adults, friends, and lovers together was ripped out, and we're back to raising kids and school and PTA and cookie sales."

LIFESTYLE CHANGES

Raising a child will change your life at any age, but raising a grandchild will turn it upside down. You are no longer young parents with boundless energy; in fact, you might even be at an age when your body betrays you and your health is questionable. You may find yourself in a hornets' nest of social workers and lawyers that nothing has prepared you for. Your own adult child may be your adversary. The system certainly will be. Your routine, your finances, your social life, and your family relationships will all change radically once you have grandchildren under your roof. Your dreams are on hold. Sometimes you might not even recognize the life you are living as your own.

When my mother talks about raising Kevin, her one wish is that she had known other grandparents raising grandchildren, that she had known that what she was going through was normal. Not only are the changes, and the feelings that go with them, normal, but they are almost predictable. Some grandparents have it worse than others, but each one has stories you will probably recognize.

Your Work Life Changes

Alice Brody had been a schoolteacher for 29 years. She hoped to make it to 30 years before she retired. When her daughter's drug addiction left her with the care of several young grandchildren, she had to quit working without reaching her goal. After her daughter died, Ivy Johnson had to go back to work at a grocery store in order to supplement the government assistance she got for her grandchildren. And although Victor Lane had retired at 62, he had to go back to work when he found himself with three new mouths to feed. It's not an easy age to find work, so Victor, a police service officer, works nights and sleeps days, driving 30 miles to and from work each day. One grandfather jokes that he'll be working until he's 90.

Every aspect of work, from a thriving career to a well-earned retirement, can become a casualty of a second parenthood. Child care is expensive, and so is raising children. Some grandparents quit work to save on child care; others return to work to afford the kids. Many trade jobs or rearrange their schedules in an attempt to both work and care for young children. A Pennsylvania grandmother gave up a career in office management to drive a school bus so she could be home when her grandson is home.

You may have to change your work routine. Maybe you worked at night but have to switch to daytime. Will your job be flexible? Will they lay you off? Perhaps you have to reenter the work force. Will you find a job? Can you handle it? The dilemma of working or not working brings up issues of self-esteem and self-worth for many grandparents, as well as the realities of a more modest income and increased stress.

Your Finances Suffer

You worked your whole life and looked forward to your retirement. You may have pensions, social security payments, and savings you had planned to live on. Then your grandchildren arrived. Now you have to use this money for food, clothes, medical bills, and things for the children. "It seems like I can't save anything," says a Michigan grandmother who remembers when she could spend her money freely. "I don't know when I bought my last outfit. Every time I turn around, she is growing."

Court costs can add to the financial stress of raising grandchildren. Some grandparents have sold their homes and watched their nest eggs empty in the fight to get custody of their grandchildren.

If you are a grandparent who has no savings, you face an even greater challenge. It is a severe financial burden to match a lean fixed income with the "unfixed" cost of raising children. Two grandmothers in my GAP groups each have four grandchildren under the age of eight. They live in one-bedroom apartments and can't afford to move in the near future. One can't afford a car; she walks or takes the bus, towing children to school, the doctor, and the market. The other can't even afford a telephone. For grandparents who are also weathering health problems, the lack of a car or telephone can be a catastrophe.

Your Routine Shifts

You had finally adjusted to living without children in the house. You had your own way of doing things, your own schedule. If you put something down, you knew where it was. Your time was yours to work or not work, see friends, read the paper, take leisurely baths, attend to your hobbies. Now your days have been taken over by diapers, bag lunches, and report cards. While your friends are enjoying the company of adults, you are back to the pediatrician, the zoo, and a string of birthday parties. It's tough to keep the house picked up when you have fingerprints and toys scattered everywhere. And your privacy is shot. You have lost your spontaneity to travel or even to eat out. Your day may start at dawn in the rush to tidy the house, cook breakfast, ship the kids off to school, and get to work yourself. For Grandma, it's a distinct feeling of déjà vu. For Grandpa, who may have seen little of his own children while they were growing up, having kids around for 24 hours a day can be quite a shock. For a single grandparent, it's twice as hard.

I received a letter from a teacher in Massachusetts who is raising her three-year-old grandson alone. She finds it difficult to find time for planning her lessons and grading papers, let alone for herself. "I am mother, father, grandparent, and best friend to this little one," she says. "He is not happy to play by himself while I do my school work. I don't think I'd even have time to attend a support group."

No matter how you make your plans, children change your routine. My mother rearranged her work schedule to minimize the disruptions in her grandson's life. Kevin had had to change schools in order to live with my parents after my sister died. Because his life was already falling apart and any consistency was considered important for him, my mother routinely skipped lunch in order to leave work early and pick him up from the same after-school program he had been in before. A New Hampshire grandmother even left her husband back home and spent eight months in Florida so that her granddaughter wouldn't have to switch schools in the middle of the school year. As a grandparent you make many concessions and sacrifices in your routine and lifestyle for the sake of the children.

Your Social Life Declines

"Our circle of friends has dwindled severely because no one else has children," writes a grandmother in Hawaii. "We don't belong with our old friends, nor do we belong with the young parents of our grandchildren's friends," writes another. "I'm a lot older and a lot wiser parent this time," says a third. "But with the Brownies, the gymnastics, the parents' nights, and the sudden earaches, we've lost our entire circle of friends. Our lives are on hold, indefinitely."[1]

It is a complaint that many grandparents recognize: Your social life and your hobbies decrease when the grandchildren arrive. Longtime friends are caught up with activities they couldn't do when they were raising families; they don't want kids tagging along. Perhaps you live in an older neighborhood with few children. Your friends may no longer have childproof homes. "Our friends raised their kids," says one grandmother. "They don't want hyperactive children in their homes."[2] Even when you can get together with friends your own age, the cost of baby-sitting is one more expense on an already stretched budget.

Single grandparents, particularly single grandmothers, may also struggle with issues of romantic companionship. Many children try to interfere with these relationships. Children may be insecure about a male friend getting Grandma's attention because her dating may bring back memories of their mother's giving more attention to men than to them. One 43-year-old woman who is raising her ex-husband's grandchildren wrote, "My life is on hold because I am never going to find a husband or have a life of my own till they are grown, and by then I will be well into my 60s."

Your Dreams Disappear

More than your immediate lifestyle changes when the second shift arrives; your future changes, too. Plans get put on hold, and some dreams disappear altogether. It's another loss in a long line of losses. Jack and Betty Segal had plans for this time of their lives. Jack would be retired and they would be out on the road together some-where—alone. Instead, they are raising one child of a drug-addicted son and helping a divorced daughter raise three more. "You love the kids," says Betty. "You just resent the fact that you can't be doing what you want to be doing."

Emily Petersen didn't have big plans. She's a quiet person who had looked forward to a tidy home, solitary walks, and presiding over holiday dinners like a traditional grandma. Instead, she is surrogate mother to an active grandchild and can hardly find a minute for herself.

"We planned retirement to do what we wanted to do; it was our time in life," one grandmother told a reporter. "Now we can't even watch the evening news because that's cartoon time."[3] Resentment. It isn't a word we traditionally associate with grandchildren. But when your life changes so radically, it unleashes a torrent of complex and contradictory emotions.

AN EMOTIONAL ROLLER COASTER

As soon as Karlos Gregory heard her grandson was coming, she got in gear: She found a day-care center, talked to an attorney about custody, and turned one room into a little boy's bedroom. When he arrived, she washed his clothes, bought new tennis shoes, and brought a night-light down from the attic. But she wasn't prepared for the feelings that come with the new responsibility and the loss of freedom. "At age 54, all of a sudden I've got a 4-year-old. Nobody seems to understand where I'm coming from," she told a local reporter.[4]

Every grandparent I know would understand. On any given day they can go through a full spectrum of feelings: grief and shame for their grown children, love for their grandchildren, fear for a future in which their health and finances may dwindle, resentment at a juvenile court system that treats them with disrespect, anger at losing their dreams at this time of their lives, and guilt for feeling that anger. The rapid shifts of emotion are like a roller coaster. Your life is in constant turmoil. Of course you feel unstable.

How much these feelings shake you will depend on what kind of resources and support you have. A single grandparent has a tougher time dealing with the ups and downs of second parenthood than a married couple, who can rely on each other to shoulder some of the weight. Two people may not reach their wit's end at the same time; a single grandparent may have no one else to turn to. Either way, it is important to look at these feelings, to really feel them, to give yourself time to deal with the issues they represent. The more you bury feelings, the more likely they are to fester inside you, erupting like a volcano when you least expect it. "It seems to take about a year to stop denying that this unexpected role is not a temporary situation," writes a grandmother from Oklahoma. "From my standpoint, we all need to know and understand that the cycle of shock, resentment, loneliness, guilt and, finally, acceptance is perfectly normal."

Isolation

If there is one theme that runs through every letter and phone call I receive from grandparents, it is isolation. When you parent for the second time, it is a lonely feeling. You feel like you're the only one in the world in this situation. You don't fit in with young parents at school functions, but you don't feel right taking small children to seniors' events. "My husband and I have permanent custody of a four-year-old grandson and find ourselves outcasts in most settings, including visits to the pediatrician," writes one grandmother.

You may also feel alienated from your family and friends. Of course you feel isolated. You *are* isolated. Your world turned upside down, and not many people can accept your new role. Loneliness and even depression are normal, expected reactions to all this overwhelming change. Seek out others who understand, either in a one-on-one relationship or through a support group. It sounds simple, but it's true: The best antidote to isolation is other people.

Grief

Every grandparent raising a grandchild experiences many losses, as well as the deep grief that comes with them. In some cases it is the death of your own child, your grandchild's parent. Your grandchild is a constant reminder of that loss. One grandfather says that the sight of his grandchild always reminds him that his son is dead. "It's a painful thing to live with," he says. In other cases the parent can't parent. This brings a different kind of grief. This adult is not the child you raised. You have lost the bright child with unlimited potential; you have lost the faith that your child would someday be a good parent and a productive adult.

In a sense, you also lose the special relationship with your grandchildren that makes grandparenting so wonderful: the visits, the spoiling, the special treats, the grandparent–grandchild conspiracies. You may feel cheated out of your grandparent role and mourn its loss.

Grandparents whose adult children have died can find solid support and understanding through Compassionate Friends, a national organization for parents who have lost a child. We have also had grandparents and grandchildren benefit from counseling or from bereavement groups, that is, short-term counseling groups that deal specifically with the phases of loss and how to deal with grief. Ask your local hospital or hospice for a referral; social workers, attorneys, doctors, and senior centers may also keep referral lists. Understand that anniversaries and holidays will be emotional times for you, and be on guard against plummeting depression. You need time to grieve, and it is understandable that you might want to grieve in private. However, some people progressively isolate themselves under the weight of depression, and then they can't pull themselves back up. If you can't reach out to people, at least don't push them away. You need loving support to withstand this loss.

It is almost easier to discuss grief when an adult child has died. Grandparents who have lost a child to drugs or mental illness yo-yo back and forth from grief to hope and back again. Here, too, support groups are helpful. Even if your child is living, allow yourself to grieve. Make room for it. You too are suffering severe loss—the loss of your dreams for your adult child, of your relationship with that child, of your lifestyle, and of your grandparent role.

Anger and Guilt

Anger and guilt are familiar companions to many second-time parents. Anger at fate. Anger at the courts and the bureaucracy, which make you feel victimized and penalized for taking responsibility for your grandchildren, especially when you have exhausted your savings and your energy. Anger at your adult child for putting you in this situation. "I could beat that woman for days for what she did to that baby!" said Anne Sutter, whose daughter gave birth to a drug-exposed child and then abandoned him.

You may even get angry at your grandchildren, who are the real victims but who are also the ones who have changed your life. Even when you know that it is not the children's fault, you may still feel resentment—and then guilt for feeling it. "You feel this hostility," says Fay Strassburger. "You feel this frustration. You lose your identity. What are you going to do with these kids? And, then, when they look up at you, you say, 'God, just let me get through another day because they really need me.'"[5]

Lucy Davis is raising her son's daughter, Lindsey. Her son and his girlfriend were both teenagers and drug addicts when Lindsey was born. Lucy took the baby when the mother lost custody for child abuse. Like many grandparents, she thought this would be temporary; she thought that losing custody would scare the parents into shape and that her own life would go back to normal. When that didn't happen, she adopted the child. She loves her completely, but sometimes the frustration is overwhelming: "I should just have to come home and make my bed, and the house should look the way I left it. But it doesn't. There are Barbie dolls everywhere. There's a toy room to be picked up. There's all her laundry to be done. Her dentist appointments. Her eye appointments. She takes up a tremendous part of my time. You can't just call me for drinks; I have

Lindsey. I get angry about it inside, although I don't want to show it. But then when she comes in and breaks a lamp, I'm really angry. And I feel so guilty."

It is okay to feel angry. Your life has been disrupted, and it is normal to resent it. What you don't want to do is take out those feelings on your grandchild. One way to defuse your anger is to write it down. Keep a journal or diary, or write a letter to the child's parents—even if you can't (or wouldn't) send it. Just getting your feelings out on paper can help. Find people who can be a sounding board for your feelings. But don't wait for a crisis to call them; call *before* you reach the end of your rope.

Fear

Grandparents who parent live in a kind of low-grade constant fear, haunted by the courts, the parents, their own health issues, and the steady march of time. Not only are they struggling with severe changes to their lives, but they are often battling the normal aging process, if not illnesses like diabetes, arthritis, cataracts, heart problems, and cancer. The questions buzz around them like mosquitos: "What if something happens to me? Who will raise these children?" "What if the parents resurface?" "What if the system lets the parents take the kids before they are able to care for them?" "How will my grandchildren turn out?" "What effect will all this have on them?"

The hard part about these fears is that they are real and possible. Parents do resurface. Courts do give them priority. Grandparents do get sick and die. And the reality is that many of these children could end up in foster care, separated from siblings, despite every effort to keep them together. A grandmother in one of my GAP groups died of breast cancer this year. Now the family is struggling over her two grandchildren; her other children don't want them, and their mother is still on drugs.

There is not much you can do about these fears. You have to look at them head-on. It doesn't help to put them aside to deal with later—although you may do that for a while. Eventually, however, you need to plan for what you can affect and, as painful as it is, accept what you cannot change. You can, and should, make decisions about who takes the children if something happens to you. If you don't have custody, there really isn't anything you can do if the parents resurface. But living in fear won't prevent it from happening. Although you can't erase your fears, try not to let them overwhelm you.

Doubt

Emily Petersen sometimes wonders if she did the right thing by taking her granddaughter Amanda, if she would have been better off adopted by younger parents. "Maybe we drown in the love for the child—the fear for the child—that we don't stop to think that maybe a younger family, someone a little more prosperous, might give them a better life," she says, pointing out that as older grandparents she and Carter are often not able to do for Amanda what they would like to do. "Some days I get terribly tired," she says.

Doubt, for many grandparents, is a normal part of raising grandchildren. You think it's not fair to the kids that you can't play ball or roller-skate or do many of the things you did as young parents. You do get tired and stressed. But I feel that in most cases children are still better off with family, if the family is able to provide for them. Whether you have made the best choice for yourself, however, is something only you can know.

▪ HOW TO COPE

There is no question that your grandchildren have brought incredible change and challenge into your life. How you approach these changes, and the feelings that accompany them, will determine how well an adjustment is made by everyone involved. As you move into a life with your grandchild, here are a few key points to remember:

▪ *Prioritize.* Decide what is most important and handle that first. Do you need to get back to work to pay bills? Then child care is primary. Don't worry about summer child care if it's just January; think about after-school care.

▪ *Don't just take one day at a time; take one thing at a time.* Get the children ready for school, then make your shopping list and schedule your afternoon. Plan for small increments.

▪ *Take time for yourself.* Structure your life in a way that works for you; find a routine that gives you downtime. What gives you a little bit of pleasure? What can you do to refuel? Is it a movie? Reading the paper? Make time for it. When you are constantly giving, giving, giving, you aren't taking care of yourself. And if you fall apart, physically or emotionally, there will be no one to take care of those grandchildren, and they could end up in foster care. So treat yourself regularly, even if it is just a quiet bath.

▪ *Make life easy.* You don't have to cook full meals every night. You don't have to have a perfect home. Try lowering your standards and lightening your load. It's okay to pop frozen food in the microwave. It's okay to go out for fast food. This is about emotional survival.

▪ *Set limits with your grandchildren.* You will have less resentment about sacrificing your life if you don't give up every aspect of it. Setting rules and limits, like private time or a regular bedtime (earlier than yours!), will give you a little time here and there for yourself.

▪ *Ask for help.* Look for *people* support. If you have supportive friends, use them. Also, find other people who have gone through what you are going through. Check with a senior citizens' group, or ask your grandchild's teacher and pediatrician if they know other people in the same situation. It's important to know you're not alone.

▪ *Get into a support group.* Therapy and support groups are a safe second family. You will be able to talk about your feelings without being judged or criticized. Other grandparents may be able to help you prioritize when you just can't think anymore. You may also find resources in a group: a clothing exchange, grandparents who might be home in the afternoon and willing to watch a child for a few hours. Grandparents who have been in the group for a while are often more than willing to give back to someone in a worse predicament. The fewer resources you have on hand, the more you need to seek outside support. Even if you are well connected in a community, with lots of friends, you can benefit from a support group. The majority of your friends are probably not in the same situation.

▪ *Consider your religious community.* Many people get strength from their faith. I know a number of grandparents who say that prayer and the support of their church or synagogue can help immensely. Some congregations have even provided material support to grandparents in emergency situations.

▪ *Let yourself off the hook.* You need to accept the fact that your adult child's circumstances are not your fault. Your child is making choices, and you have done the most and best with whatever you had. I don't think people intentionally set out to hurt their kids, and when you raised yours, you really thought what you were doing was the best. Understand that your feelings are normal, that you're not alone, and that you will eventually get through this.

▪ *Focus on the positive.* Keep in mind why you are doing this and what you have accomplished. In spite of all the stress, there are rewards.

MOMENTS OF PURE JOY

Grandparents sacrifice a lot to raise grandchildren, but there are rewards: the relief of knowing that the grandchildren are safe and happy, the wonder of watching them grow, the pride in their accomplishments. Some grandparents say their grandchildren keep them young. Alta Edwards believes her three grandchildren gave her a new lease on life. She had diabetes, arthritis, a bad heart, and high blood pressure, and she weighed 300 pounds. "One morning I woke up and realized I couldn't properly raise a two-year-old flat on my back. It was do or die," she says. "They got me back on my feet."[6]

And there is the love. It is the main reason you took in your grandchildren, and it is your greatest reward for raising them. "Nobody has ever loved me in my life the way she loves me," says Lucy Davis of her granddaughter. "She was singing a song one day, when she was three. She was in her toy room, and she was singing, 'I have a mummy and her name is Grammy!'"

Joan McMillin knows the feeling. She remembers the night her granddaughter hugged her and said, "Granny, you're the only person in the world who really loves me." "I had tears in my eyes," she told a reporter. "There's something positively magical in the hugs and kisses that makes it all worthwhile."[7]

CHAPTER 4

Family at Large: Your Spouse and Other Children

You're going to be fighting the battle alone at times. Your friends, even your family, will fight you for raising grandchildren. They each have their own version of how you should handle the situation, and you have to face their advice and their criticism.

—Vermont grandmother

Taking in a grandchild is about family, and the entire family will feel the effects of this new addition. More than your lifestyle changes when you become second-time parents; your marriage and your relationship with your other children may suffer strains you never expected.

ROCKING THE MARRIAGE BOAT

Ivy Johnson's husband left her when the grandchildren arrived. Frank and Gloria Simon fight constantly over their drug-addicted daughter. And my own parents seemed close to divorce on numerous occasions. The burden of raising a child at this stage of life, combined with the loss of or struggles with an adult child (regardless of the reason), often causes deep problems between spouses who have spent most of their lives together. Marriages that have always been stable start to develop rifts, and marriages that were already strained may split wide open.

Sometimes the issue is grief. Everyone grieves differently, and you expect different things of each other in your grief. My parents didn't have time to mourn the loss of my sister before they took in her son. My mother expressed it all openly: She cried constantly and all but lived at the cemetery when she wasn't working. My father, on the other hand, buried his grief deep inside himself, and my mother would get furious at his apparent lack of understanding. Grief can rock the most stable marriage, even without the extra burden of new children to raise.

Sometimes the issue is jealousy: One grandparent gives more attention to the child than to his or her spouse, who resents the change and may then spend more time away from home, become engrossed in hobbies, or generally keep the family at a distance. Growing anger may spark fights and arguments over seemingly meaningless things. Often it is Grandma who devotes herself to the grandchildren and Grandpa who rebels. Says one grandfather from Ohio, "We get along, no fights, no shouting matches . . . but [the child] has caused a deterioration of our compatibility . . . I feel pretty much ignored."[1]

But grandmothers are not immune from jealousy, as Nancy Harper can confirm. "He probably loves her more than me," she says, referring to her husband and the granddaughter they are raising. "My husband was such a wonderful father, and everything was 'the children.' I thought once they grew up I'd have him all to myself. Then Scott presented us with Marissa, and here we are all over again."

The sudden changes to your lifestyle will certainly challenge a marriage. Financial stress is always hard on a couple, and unexpected children's expenses raise new questions about how to spend money and how to set priorities. Adjustments to work and home routines leave you with little time for yourself, for each other, for all the things you planned. And then there is the disruption to your privacy and sexual intimacy.

Rose and Gerald Avery had been married for 30 years. Ever since their son Richard moved out, they had been peacefully on their own. At the end of a long day their house was a haven of quiet, order, and privacy. They liked it that way. They could walk around the house wearing anything they wanted to; they could be intimate and sexual without fear of being heard. When they welcomed Richard and his two young sons into their home, that peace and privacy disappeared. At the end of the day the house is now riddled with the sounds and signs of children: laughter, arguments, toys on the floor. Gerald's office is now the television room. Even their bedroom isn't their own—the boys always want to be with them. Their new circumstances have taken a toll on the couple's intimacy. Even when the children aren't home, they live with the expectation that they could come home at any moment. "At times, it's like we've lost the house and certain things about each other," says Rose. The result is that Gerald is often angry. "It's like having four kids at home, not two," she adds.

The most constant source of marital conflict, however, is the children—both the adult children and the grandchildren. In both cases the issues are overcompensation and setting limits. Each is a normal issue in childrearing, but having to negotiate these boundaries at a stage in your life when you no longer expect to be rearing your child and expect only to be enjoying your grandchild can wear on you and your marriage.

Children, Big and Small

Many couples can't agree as to when enough is enough when it comes to their adult children. Whether the issue is money, visitation, or kicking them out, they are incapable of presenting a united front. One grandparent tries to take a firm stand and the other undermines it. One grandparent feels misunderstood, the other unsupported. If the conflict escalates enough, talk can turn to separation and divorce. That is what almost happened to Frank and Gloria Simon.

Frank and Gloria took in their grandchildren when their oldest daughter, Cheryl, divorced her abusive husband and lost custody of her little girls because of drug abuse and neglect. When I met this family, Cheryl was living at home again, sleeping all day and making Gloria's life miserable. She was verbally abusive to her children and to her mother in front of the children. She felt that her mother had stolen her daughters. When she was under the influence of drugs, Cheryl became violent: She pulled Gloria's hair, threw her to the ground, knocked out windows. But Frank kept supporting Cheryl, and it took forever for Gloria to put her out of the house.

Frank refused to believe the severity of the problem. He worked all day and wasn't home to witness what his daughter was doing. Besides, Cheryl was "Daddy's little girl," and he wanted to believe everything would work out. He gave her chance after chance, undermining his wife: Gloria would reach a breaking point and tell Cheryl she couldn't stay with them, and Frank would let her back in. Or

Cheryl would break a window to come into the house, and Frank would let her stay. He refused to back Gloria on setting limits of any kind, whether expressed verbally or in written contracts.

The Simons' marriage almost collapsed under the strain. When things were particularly bad, Gloria would pile the children into the car and call me from a pay phone. "I can't stand it anymore," she would say, sobbing. "I'm running away and leaving Frank." She always returned home, but she was stuck in a tough situation. As long as the Simons weren't working together, nothing could change. Then one day Frank himself became the target of Cheryl's anger. It was only when his daughter threw a toaster and hit him in the head that Frank put his foot down and joined Gloria in her insistence that Cheryl move out of their home.

When it comes to the *grandchildren,* two problems typically shake a relationship: first whether to take the children, and then how to raise them. Sometimes a grandmother will leave a marriage to be able to take in and protect a small grandchild. Sometimes a grandfather will leave when the children arrive. Writes a woman from Arizona: "I'm 59 and raised seven of my own children and three grandchildren. My husband left me over this last child after 33 years of marriage, but I can't seem to let [this grandchild] go." Emily and Carter Petersen had their marriage pulled almost to the breaking point when their daughter asked them to take her child. Emily and Carter were already raising their son's baby, and Carter didn't want any more. They got into a huge fight about it. "I told him if we can't take care of two, we're not taking care of one," recalls Emily. "If I can care for another girl's baby, I can certainly take care of my daughter's. If you don't like it, you go," she told him. "But the baby's coming in." Faced with that choice, Carter stayed.

The day-to-day task of raising grandchildren is more of a slow wear and tear on a marriage. One grandparent tries to parent, with all the struggle, limit setting, and discipline that parenting entails. Meanwhile, the other one overcompensates for the child's lack of parents and tries to hang on to the role of the sweet, loving grandparent. The result is strife for the grandparents and confused signals for the child.

My parents fought constantly over Kevin, who was not an easy child to raise. My mother overcompensated, giving in to many of Kevin's demands. My father criticized how she handled the child, but he traveled for business and wasn't often there to help. They felt anger and grief; they fought and screamed. Even homework was a horrible scene. Every night for months my brother and I would take turns dropping in to check on them and to smooth things over.

It's true that every couple has its fights and bones of contention, but by the time you are grandparents you don't expect to be arguing about small children. You don't expect to be fighting about your grandchildren: you expect to be loving them, doting on them, and sending them home. In grandparenting you have regressed, and there is an added layer of frustration about the change. To quote one grandmother: "Fifty percent of my anxiety and stress is the old boy [Grandpa]. He fights everything I do."

Strength in a Common Cause

Not every marriage suffers from the arrival of grandchildren. There are couples who find that the challenge of raising a second family draws them together instead of pulling them apart.

Dave and Milly Walsh are raising four grandchildren, and their disruptive daughter is still in and out of the house. Dave works nights, Milly is at home with the children, and the daughter doesn't contribute a dime. Milly's health isn't great. The couple would love to travel alone for once, just the two of them, but it's not likely to happen soon. They're both exhausted. It's fertile soil for conflict, but they don't feel it. "Our marriage is not a flashy thing," says Milly. "It keeps going on." Humor and a strong sense of purpose keep them going. Says Dave, "Every six months we think, 'What are we doing? We're supposed to be retired!' But we laugh at each other when we're blue. We want to be doing what we're doing. It's not duty; we're bonded to these kids. If anything, it made us stronger. We're doing something together. People tend to drift apart as they get older; we have a common cause. We're channeling our energy into something constructive."

▪ HOW TO COPE

How well your marriage survives will depend on how stable it is to start with, how much stress you have to handle, and how committed you and your spouse are to surviving as a couple. The road will be easier, however, if you keep certain things in mind:

▪ *Talk to each other!* Often, when couples disagree, they shut down and withdraw; then they aren't open to compromise and discussion. Taking on your grandchildren will add new dimensions of stress to your marriage; try to keep the paths of communication open.

▪ *Create special time for yourself and your spouse.* It is critical that grandparents take time away from the grandchildren; you need this to refuel yourselves and your relationship. You are both losing out on your plans and dreams for this time together. You must make a conscious effort to do things that make you feel good, or they just won't happen. I know it is hard to plan your own activities when you're overwhelmed by three or four needy, active kids; it's hard to think about yourself when you are so exhausted that you collapse in bed at night and hope you don't have to get up. But you have to make the effort. Your health, your sanity, and your marriage could depend on it.

▪ *Present a unified front to your grandchildren.* It is important not to argue or contradict each other in front of the grandchildren because (1) they already have low self-esteem and feel that everything is their fault and (2) they can manipulate your disagreement to their advantage (children are good at pitting one grandparent against the other to get what they want). When there is an issue to deal with, try to discuss it beforehand, or take a time-out to discuss it. If you are split in your decision, your grandchild may try to play you against each other, which helps neither your decision making nor your relationship.

▪ *Present a united front to your adult children, too.* They are expert manipulators and know which of you to go to when they want something. Discuss limits and boundaries in advance and then stick to them. (For more on adult children, see Chapter 5.)

▪ *Try to keep things in perspective.* It won't make the situation easier, but it can preserve your sense of humor. It also helps when you can lean on each other for support.

SIBLING SUPPORT AND SIBLING RIVALRY: YOUR OTHER CHILDREN

Grace and Marcus Tyler have three grown children. Their only daughter lost custody of her five-year-old son, Jason, because of drugs and neglect, and now they are raising him. Their son Michael, 29, lives out of town with his girlfriend and his daughter. He doesn't see his parents or his nephew often, but he supports their decision to raise Jason. He calls often and takes the boy for occasional weekends. The Tylers' other son, Peter, 25, lives only a few blocks away. In the past, if he didn't see his parents every week, he would at least call two or three times to touch base with them. Now he rarely comes around at all. He says he will help with Jason, but he never does. Moreover, he complains to his brother about their parents' devotion to Jason: "Do you think they would take care of our kids that well? Look at all the attention he's getting. He's spoiled rotten!" "Peter has been jealous from the moment that Jason came into the house," says Grace. "You'd think that he would understand that this is an innocent child who deserves a chance. What are we taking away from a 25-year-old man?"

Two sons, two reactions, and there is nothing surprising about either one. Many lives are touched when a grandchild moves in, and many relationships are disrupted. The other children in your family are not immune to the situation. If they live with you or near you, they may find their own lives altered. Even if they live far away, they may be rocked by unexpected emotions due to this new arrangement. They may be jealous of the drain on your time and attention. They may be afraid of the toll on your health and your marriage. And they may be furious with their sibling for "taking advantage of Mom and Dad." They may even be angry at you for, in their eyes, allowing yourself to be taken advantage of. Some, like Michael, may offer to help out; some may punish you by withholding their support; and others may simply ignore the whole situation, keeping a polite but neutral distance. How your other children choose to handle their feelings will depend on their ages, their circumstances, and their prior relationships with you.

Other Children at Home

Joyce Griffin's children were in their teens when, one at a time, the grandchildren started coming—all from one daughter and all drug exposed. Joyce had already raised five children and had nursed two husbands through injuries and disease. Her other children were not pleased with this new turn of events. "My children thought I was deserving of rest," she says. "They didn't see me starting over raising children, especially drug children." So when the fourth call came, Joyce's oldest son said, "No more." Then he saw the baby, who had been born five weeks early. "When they saw the preemie—how small, how vulnerable she was—then my children became mothers and fathers," says Joyce. "My sons became the fathers to these children; my younger daughter, who is in college, became the mother."

Nancy Harper's daughter, Jennifer, was 16 when little Marissa arrived. Her brother Scott, the baby's father, was 18, and her oldest brother was 22. Jennifer had been the only girl in the family, the light of her mother's life. The baby's arrival was hard for her. Not only was there competition from a needy child in the house, but it seemed as if her life had been taken away: She couldn't run her blow-dryer at night because the baby was sleeping, and she found herself watching her brother's baby daughter while Scott disappeared with his friends. Jennifer was angry at everyone involved. When Nancy asked her to take Marissa for a few hours, her response was, "Why should I, Mom? I'm going out with friends. I didn't have a baby, Scott did. Just because your life stinks, mine won't, too."

Children who still live at home will, of course, be most affected by a grandchild moving in. Like you, they will find their routine and their living space disrupted by the new addition to the family. They may be asked to share their rooms, to limit their activities, and, if they're old enough, to watch a niece or nephew when you need a break. Unlike you, they had no choice in the matter. From their perspective, a new child arrived and began to take over. A child living at home may feel lost amid all these changes. If, like Jennifer, the child has been the baby of the family, she may feel displaced by this new arrival. Younger children may act out to get more of your time and attention, and even young adults may experience jealousy.

Sometimes feelings of jealousy in your children predate your grandchild's arrival. Marlena Hunt's younger daughter already felt ignored growing up, mostly because she was the "good" kid and Marlena was so caught up with her sister Sharon and her problems. Now Marlena is giving her attention to Sharon's daughter.

Of course, the moments of competition and resentment may be much more sporadic once the novelty passes and everyone settles into a new routine. But when you raise a grandchild as one of your own children, you will always get some sibling rivalry.

When Siblings Are Single Adults

Sandra Cobb has two sons and two daughters. She is raising seven grandchildren while their mother is in and out of jail and rehab. Both her sons have been helpful, but her daughter JoAnne has been her right hand. She was 16 when the babies started to arrive, and has been like another mother to them, even though the wear and tear on her 65-year-old mother makes her angry. Although JoAnne now has children of her own, she still lives next door and helps out with her nieces and nephews.

My parents were equally lucky. My brother and I were both single adults when my sister died. We had no commitments, no children, and we were already close to our nephew. Like Joyce Griffin's children, Phil and I pitched in, becoming extra parents to Kevin and taking some of the pressure off our parents. No decision was made without us, and Kevin even lived with each of us at one point or another. Even so, we recognized the differences between the way our parents raised Kevin and the way they raised us. We watched our mother overcompensate, and we watched Kevin get away with things that we would never have gotten away with as children. Phil and I would voice our disapproval and offer suggestions, but these were frequently ignored because my parents thought they were doing the right thing.

Single adults who don't live at home may be less personally affected by your decision to raise a grandchild. Whether they approve of the decision or not, they have the freedom to make their own choices about being involved. Some might even become active aunts and uncles, as JoAnne, Phil, and I did, possibly challenging some parenting techniques, but steadily helping with day care and vacations and acting as parental stand-ins when needed. (My brother even coached Kevin's Little League team.)

Other single adult children, like Grace Tyler's son Peter, may be actively *un*involved. They may vocally disapprove of your choice and may take it out on you by distancing themselves. They may ignore their niece or nephew, neglecting to ask about the child or even send a birthday card. Some may genuinely feel displaced and hurt by the time and attention showered on your grandchild. "But they are adults!" you say in wonder. Yes, but they are still your children.

Many single adults are neither active aunts and uncles nor active critics. These are the neutral ones. They may be caught up with their own lives. They may live far away. They just aren't involved.

When Siblings Are Married with Children

The reactions of married adult children are not very different from those of single adults unless there are other grandchildren in the picture. Then you risk a new kind of sibling rivalry: cousin rivalry.

> "You spend so much energy on Marcia that my kids never see you!"
>
> "You do so much more for Martin's kids than you ever do for mine."
>
> "Grandma, how come you buy so many things for Tommy? Don't you love me, too?"

These are the complaints that can break a grandparent's heart. It is hard enough when they come from small grandchildren who don't really understand the situation, but it can be incredibly frustrating when they come from an adult who knows that Marcia, Tommy, and Martin's kids have no one else spending time and money on them. It is particularly painful when, deep down, you know the accusations are true. And it's not fair.

Sue Ellen Rice would love to indulge all her grandchildren, but she is raising two little ones on a meager income. The rest live several states away, and she can't afford to visit them; she can't even afford to send much in the way of presents. It doesn't make her feel like much of a grandma. Ethel Murray's problem is closer to home. Scott, the grandson she is raising, is the same age as his cousin, Aaron, who lives down the street. Aaron sees that Scott gets special things and thinks that Grandma loves him more. Aaron's mother adds to Ethel's guilt with her own complaints. Ethel has explained to Aaron that he has a mommy to buy him things and Scott doesn't. Although she tries to pick up special things for Aaron when she can, the competition between the cousins still disturbs her.

On the other hand, not every married adult child will resent the time and attention spent on a sibling's child. Some will go out of their way to be supportive, including the child in their own family activities and vacations. Sometimes the same sibling who opposed your grandchild's arrival may, like Joyce Griffin's son, become a doting surrogate parent over time. It all depends on the particular relationships in your family.

Remember Nancy Harper's teenage daughter? Jennifer didn't even want to babysit Marissa, but when Jennifer reached adulthood and married, she and her husband offered to lighten Nancy's responsibilities and raise the little girl themselves. Nancy declined. "Marissa has already felt rejection once," she explains. "She's already had one mummy leave her, and this mummy's not going to." Still, Jennifer had made the offer.

■ HOW TO COPE

The preceding vignettes illustrate just a few of the reactions your other children could have to your raising a grandchild. You may find yourself facing completely different ones, depending on your particular circumstances and your relationships with your children. Moreover, each of your children will have his own individual approach to handling the feelings involved. However they react, there are a few things you may want to consider in dealing with your other children and as a means of keeping peace in your family:

▪ *Listen to your other children.* They deserve to have their concerns heard. First of all, their concerns may be valid. Perhaps you *are* overcompensating with your grandchild; you may be hurting her in the process. Perhaps you are neglecting your teenagers; maybe you can arrange some special time together. See if you can find a compromise without sacrificing yourself. Second, the feelings of your other children are valid even if you can't do anything about their concerns. You may not be able to buy *all* your grandchildren new shoes, but you can try to understand how your other children and grandchildren might feel slighted, however illogical their reaction may seem.

▪ *Validate their feelings.* Everyone reacts differently to crisis, and having your family structure upset is a kind of crisis. It doesn't matter whether your other children are feeling scared about your health, jealous of your time, or sorry for the grandchild you are raising. They are entitled to their feelings, and those feelings are normal. All you can do is try to understand and not take it too personally. You do not, however, have to let them take their disapproval out on you.

▪ *Don't expect their help.* In your heart you will want the support and assistance of your other children. You can let them know you would appreciate it, but don't expect anything from them. They have a right to their own opinions about the situation, and they have to make their own decisions about how they want to participate. Besides, wouldn't you rather have them help because they want to help?

The situation is different when your other children live at home. It is reasonable to have certain expectations of children who live under your roof. Perhaps everyone in your house shares chores and responsibilities; child care may now be one of those responsibilities. However, try to be sensitive to the needs of your children. You don't want to deprive them of time to do their homework or see their friends

▪ *Consider instituting family meetings.* It is easy for members of a family to retire to their own respective corners to nurse their injuries and strengthen their opinions; you could end up as a group of disconnected loners instead of an integrated family. Whether your other children live at home or not, the family meeting can be a way of keeping everyone connected. If your other children feel neglected, you can invite them to participate in certain decisions. If they feel taken advantage of, they can air out their concerns. I can't overemphasize how important communication is in a family, particularly in times of stress.

▪ *Don't forget your other grandchildren.* It doesn't take much time or money to make a child feel remembered, even in another state. Sometimes just a postcard is enough. Be patient if the other grandchildren need repeated explanations about why Tommy gets more toys. It will take them a while to adjust to the situation, too.

▪ *Make your own decisions.* It is good to listen to your other adult children and to recognize their concerns, but in the end you have to follow your conscience, particularly when it comes to taking your grandchild. The bottom line is that when the day is over and the lights go out, the decisions you make have to be the ones you can sleep with.

Remember, there are no perfect families, only people who are striving.

CHAPTER 5 | # Your Adult Child

My son has destroyed all of us and is continuing
to do so. We just cannot get rid of him. He is
just a shell of a person we loved so much. The
hurt is in me so deep, and I always ask why.
—Letter from Missouri

"She was a beautiful, bright, and gifted child, the oldest of my three children," writes Pam Marshall. "She was reliable, sensitive, and unusually creative. During her grade school years, she never gave us any trouble. She studied hard. She helped her younger sister and brother with their homework. Teachers all loved her. In junior high she started to change." Pam is describing her daughter Linda, and at first it sounds like a typical 1960s story of teenage rebellion—flower children, hard rock, heavy makeup and miniskirts, a little marijuana, moving out of the house—the kind of thing a lot of adults today experienced, and outgrew.

But Linda didn't outgrow it. By age 19, she was using heroin. When her parents offered to get her help, she told them her friends were her family now and walked out of the house. Heroin was replaced by LSD, uppers, downers, cocaine, and crack—anything she could get her hands on. Linda got married twice and divorced twice. She was arrested several times on drug-related charges. At 32 she gave birth to a baby girl in jail. Pam and her husband, Robert, took the infant home from the hospital and have raised her ever since.

Linda's story is not an unusual one. In fact, it is all too usual. It is the story of the troubled adult child, the parent of the child you are raising, the author of the situation you are in. No discussion of grandparents as parents is complete without looking at the adult who is still in the picture.

It is a sad fact, but grandparents who are raising the children of dead or absent parents have a much simpler time of it. Except for the cases—and there are some—where grandparents raise grandchildren in cooperation with the parents, adult children seem to have one mission in life: wreaking havoc in your life. For many families it is not the grandchild who is the problem, it is the parent.

A PICTURE OF THE ADULT CHILD

Among the letters I have received is one from a young woman in New York. The picture she paints is a common one: Her mother, a woman in her early 50s, is raising her sister's two toddlers. The sister lives with the mother but doesn't help with the children. She spends any money she has on herself—on drugs, clothing, jewelry, and the boyfriend of the week. She disappears for days at a time, returning only to pick up her welfare check. "My sister has taken the car and told my mom she's going to the grocery store and doesn't come back for a week," the young woman writes. "My sister abandoned the kids one night to go out with friends." The grandmother has bruises from the children's mother, and her jewelry is gone. She needs financial assistance and custody of the children. She needs to get her daughter out of her house, but she is afraid for the safety of the babies.

Some grandparents call them "deadbeat" moms and dads. These are the parents who show up long enough to make promises, break promises, and disappear again. At best, these parents occasionally visit and indulge their children while you and your spouse play Mom and Dad. Linda brings her daughter presents and tries to be a model mother, but her interest doesn't last long. "My daughter loves her daughter," says Pam. "She wants to hold her, dress her up, play with her . . . like a traditional grandparent who comes for two hours." At worst, they can be verbally and physically abusive to you and their children. I heard from Michigan grandparents who took their grandchildren when one of the men the mother lived with, an ex-convict, was preparing a tattoo for their grandson. Because the mother was overheard threatening to blow up the grandparents' car and apartment, the family fled to another state, from which they notified the authorities that they had left, and why.

Many adult children are manipulative. They may use their children as pawns to extort money, shelter, and transportation from you. And if you have no legal control over your grandchildren, you will probably give in. Grandparents are the first to admit that they have bought more drugs than any other class of people by giving into their adult children's demands in order to protect their grandchildren.

Your adult child may also steal, both from you and your grandchildren. Just because it hasn't happened yet doesn't mean it won't in the future. Emily and Carter Petersen came home to find their jewelry gone; they had a lock on their bedroom door, but their son and his drug friends had cleaned them out. Nor is it uncommon for parents to take their children's welfare or Social Security checks for themselves or to sell their kids' food stamps for drugs. In fact, I know grandparents who sleep with purses and wallets under their pillows so that their adult children can't find them.

Some of the mothers are prostitutes, and their parents (with grandchild in tow) may encounter them "working" and then have to handle the grandchild's question, "Isn't that my mom?" Some mothers just keep having babies, who are then taken away because of abuse or neglect. It sounds harsh, but the same stories come up again and again and again. "We're not beating up on parents," explains one grandpa. "We're trying to save the next generation."[1]

The fallout is fierce. Both you and your grandchildren can feel like pawns in a game without rules. The children continuously get sideswiped by conflicting emotions, and so do you. They love their parents and fantasize about living with them yet feel deep rejection, abandonment, and anger. You love your child and hope she will get her act together, yet you hate her for what she's doing to you and her kids. You may experience waves of fear for your grandchildren, suffer guilt that you may be at fault, and spin pipe dreams about the day when your adult child can parent again. Meanwhile, you argue with your spouse and still give your wayward adult child every opportunity to clean up her act, worrying all the while that the phone will ring one day and it will be the police.

Some grandparents use up all their money and insurance policies trying to get their children into drug programs. Some pray they'll end up in jail, where they'll at least be safe. Others, less hopeful, take out life insurance policies on their children so that if anything happens, at least they'll have money to bury them.

And then there are the dark wishes and unspeakable thoughts. The thing a parent never expects to feel about a child, namely, that you would all be better off if he or she were dead. "She is thirty-six years old," says a Texas grandmother of her drug-addicted daughter. "I have honestly wished that she would OD and let her son have half a chance at a normal life." It is a horrible thing to think, but when you reach your wit's end—when the grandkids are in mental chaos and your life feels like an armed camp—the dark thoughts do surface. The painful truth is this: As permanent and terrible a loss as death is, it can seem like a lucky break to grandparents who have to watch their adult children destroy themselves and their families moment by painful moment.

▪ HOW TO COPE

Most adult children are constantly in and out of your life, causing continual disruption. Only you can break the cycle, but it takes determination, fortitude, and a few guiding principles:

▪ *Set firm rules and stand by them.* These parents may look like adults, but sometimes you have to treat them like children. You have to set the same kind of rules and limits you set with your grandchild, being firm and consistent. You need consequences that are clearly stated, and you need to stand by them. Don't make threats you can't follow through on, or you'll open yourself to endless manipulation. Perhaps you have told your adult son that his friends are not welcome in your house. You may not be willing to kick him out for inviting them over, but you could take his key away. And if despite your warnings you come home and find four of his friends sitting on the couch, watching television, and drinking beer, you may have to have the locks changed to keep your consequences. But do it. Otherwise, your adult children get the message that even if you talk big, they can still take advantage of you.

▪ *Learn to say no.* Ruth Castle has a sign on her refrigerator. It says, "NO is a complete sentence." You have to learn to say no to your adult child for the sake of your grandchild. You cannot give your grandchild a stable home if you and your household are at the beck and call of an unstable parent. Your adult child will ask, plead, and demand all kinds of things from you: "Can I borrow the car?" "Can you lend me $20?" "Can you send me supplies in jail?" She will take and take until you have no money left to give, and she will leave you emotionally drained.

Not only is it okay to say no to your adult child, but it is necessary. You will not be abandoning your child; you will be protecting yourself and your grandchildren. Nor do you have to justify yourself. You don't have to give explanations or make speeches. *No* can be a complete sentence.

▪ *Learn to let go.* You need to come to grips with the fact that you cannot really help or change your adult child. This is probably the hardest reality for a parent to face. No matter what this person has done, he is still your child. You gave birth to him and love him, even if you hate what he does. But you have to let go. "My 18-year-old son was getting caught up in drugs. He's left home because he can't do drugs here. He's homeless, but it was his choice," said one grandmother.[2]

BREAKING THE PATTERN OF ENABLING

"One more chance." It's like the magic ring on the merry-go-round. Adult children beg for it: "Give me one more chance, Mom. I'll get it right this time." Grandparents reach out for it: "she's trying so hard now. If I help her, just this once, maybe she'll make it." Like children on a merry-go-round, they go round and round in circles, trying to catch the magic ring, the one that will make everything better. Unfortunately, there are times when helping someone can actually hurt him; when the chances you give your adult child only allow him to continue destructive—and self-destructive—behavior. In the mental health community this kind of help is called "enabling." When you *enable* your adult child, you are doing more than allowing him to continue his behavior, you are actually assisting him.

Grandparents who enable their adult children often only pour good money after bad. They pay for one drug treatment after another, hoping that each new program will be the one that leads to a cure. Unfortunately, true rehabilitation is rare, and the sad reality is that many addicts don't make it. I have set counseling appointments with many adult children as part of their reunification agreements; most don't show up. Some will clean up their acts for a year, even two years, but then they hit a stress they can't handle and they're back to their old ways. It is true that since I see grandparents in crisis, I don't hear many success stories. But when a person abstains from drug use for one or two years and then falls back, at what point do you trust a success story?

"A sure way to cripple a person is to allow her to sponge off you," says one grandparent. "People who are warm, comfortable, and well fed usually have little motivation to change their lifestyles." At one point Pam Marshall decided to keep Linda away from the baby. "I had to choose," she says. "Either Megan or my daughter. My daughter was an adult. The baby wasn't." But it was still difficult for her. Robert finally had to throw Linda out of the house.

No grandparent gets off this merry-go-round until he or she is good and ready. A support group can give you other people's stories to use as a mirror. It can help you find inner strength to say no and mean it. It can prevent you from spinning in circles as much as you would on your own. But only you know when you're truly tired of chasing chances. Even then, there is that extra inning, that last prayer, that last chance before you call it quits.

When grandparents want to let an adult child come home "one last time," I recommend using a written contract. If the contract is violated, the adult child knows that he has to leave.

Try a Written Contract

Verbal promises are tricky; adult children can claim you never told them something or that they didn't understand. Verbal contracts get renegotiated at each stumbling block and have more holes than a colander. With a written contract, everyone knows where they stand. The conditions and consequences are in black and white. By signing the contract all parties are indicating that they understand and agree to accept the consequences if they violate the terms of the contract.

Creating a written contract is like making a behavior chart or a chore chart for your young grandchild. Your rules must be spelled out in detail (for example, "I cannot sleep until 3 P.M.; I must help with the dishes"). It is not enough for a rule to state that the adult child must "find a job in a month." Be specific: "You must not sleep in. You must be out looking for a job from 8:00 A.M to 5:00 P.M., and you must provide me with a list of the employers you have contacted." Otherwise, the adult child could be out all day but spending that time at the movies or in the park.

Each contract item should have its own consequence, one related to the severity of the problem. For instance, if your daughter runs up a $200 phone bill, she can't use the phone until the bill is paid back. I know grandparents who lock the phone in their bedroom so their adult child can't use it. However, your consequences must be realistic. Try not to threaten your adult child with things that you know in your heart you can't do. If the consequence of stealing from you is moving out within 24 hours and if you can't bring yourself to enforce that, then your child will have won. She will immediately start to manipulate you and to ignore her commitments to the contract. The purpose of the contract is to provide incentives to change. If you keep threatening to put your son out but you don't follow through or you let him back two days later, why shouldn't he take $100 from your drawer? Be realistic. What consequences would you really be able to follow through on? Enforcing a contract with your adult child depends entirely on your own ability and willingness to follow through.

Make sure everyone has a copy of the contract. If it is in black and white, no one can misconstrue the rules. Adult children can't say "You never said that" or "I thought you meant such and such." They've read it. They've signed it. There is no gray area. But you must follow through with the consequences or your contract is worth nothing. (See pp. 69–71 for a sample contract.)

Tough Love: One Grandma's Story

"I want my baby to love me. I can't live without my baby," croons Maggie Butler, imitating all the grandparents who can't let go of their adult children. "That's the hook," she says seriously. Maggie knows. She gave her son one last chance to pull himself together, then she finally put him out for good. It was a hard choice. "There is loss there," she admits. "We all lose."

Maggie knew, clearly, that her son's life was in shambles. David was an alcoholic and a drug addict. His marriage had failed years ago, and his two daughters lived in Pittsburgh with his ex-wife and a boyfriend who Maggie suspected was sexually abusing the girls. David had been in and out of detox several times, to no avail, and he had just served two years in jail in West Virginia for assault. But when David's ex-wife abandoned the children on the street one day, he decided to shape up and get custody of his kids. He asked his parents to help him, and they said yes.

Maggie had already done years of work on letting go. She had joined Alanon when she finally accepted the fact that David was an addict; she had gone on to participate in other 12-step programs and had used support groups, as well as individual therapy, in her search to understand herself, her son, and the patterns of addiction. "I had already released David and accepted that he's very much on his own," she said. "But, for some reason, I needed to help him one more time. I said to myself that as his mother I would like to see David get his life together and maybe get his children." It turned out to be a costly lesson: expensive, painful, and emotionally draining.

Since the court would not allow the children to live with David yet, the girls were placed in temporary foster care. David came home, but there were strict terms. He had to go to Alcoholics Anonymous meetings, he had to work, and he could not just sit and watch television. "We will help you," Maggie told him, "but you must help yourself. If you mess up, you're out of here." He said, "Mom, I want to change my life."

When David first came home, he was "good as gold." He got a job at five dollars an hour, although he had once earned three times that amount. He saved his money and bought a car. He got his driver's license, insurance, and a bank account. He made his parole appointments, and he went to meetings religiously for four months. Then something seemed to change. "I think it was just too much good," Maggie says sadly.

One night Maggie's husband went to a meeting David was supposed to attend. He wasn't there. Later, when her son came home, Maggie asked him how the meeting went. "Great," he told her. She didn't say anything, but she was watchful. She was still hoping he would make it. A few days later he went out and didn't come home. He was gone most of the next day, too. That was the last straw for his mother. As she tells it: "He pulls up at six o'clock like a kid with a hand in the cookie jar. 'I guess I messed up, Mom,' he says. 'I guess I should go in and pack.' I said, 'No, your stuff is packed.' That was the deal."

Five days later, after a three-day cocaine binge, David was arrested for kidnapping, robbery, and assault. He was sentenced to 22 years in prison. He was 26.

Maggie now has her granddaughters living with her. She hasn't spoken to David since then, although he writes to her from jail. She loves David, but she chooses not to be in his life right now. She describes herself as a "hard cookie," but it has been a painful process—a lot of grieving, a lot of crying, a lot of letting go. "I used to pray a lot for David," she says. "Now I pray for myself. David will make his own choices. What I have learned from all these support groups is that we have to allow our children to do what they need to do. They have to make all the mistakes. They have to be the ones to pick themselves up. They have to be the ones to find help for themselves. They will always stay crippled if we are the ones to pick them up.

"I have to give up the control and give him the right to live," says Maggie. "Years ago, I said to him, 'David, when are you going to hit your bottom?' He said, 'Mom, I may not have a bottom.'"

Kicking Out Your Adult Child

Putting your child out is the toughest thing in the world. Maggie had 12 years of self-help groups and therapy behind her, and it was still incredibly painful. Some grandparents can't do it until they reach the end of their rope, and even then they need a lot of support. Everyone's bottom line is different. For the Smiths it might be that their son came out of a drug treatment program and relapsed. But the Joneses may still be trying to help a daughter who has been in 16 drug treatment programs and has stolen the car, the jewelry, and the VCR. Each grandparent has a different threshold for feeling that he or she has done everything possible. My rock bottom and your rock bottom can be miles apart.

Some grandparents will talk about the same issues for years and still be unable to act on them. A lot depends on how much support you have from friends and family and how much control you have over your grandchildren. If you kick out the parents, will they—and can they legally—take the child with them? The answer to that question will affect how long it takes you to kick a parent out of the house.

Even after you hit bottom, the obstacles are tremendous. You may find yourself facing guilt, embarrassment, and your own protective feelings. This is, after all, your baby. You gave life to and raised this child, and even if this is not what you brought her up to be, she is still your kid. You might not like this person, but on some level you do love her. Then there are the fears: "Where will my child be? On a park bench? In an alley? Will I get a call to identify a body found in an alley someplace?"

You may also confront strong family pressure: relatives who don't approve of or understand your decision; a spouse who isn't supportive and who undermines your efforts; the grandchildren themselves, who won't understand and who may blame you and cry, "Don't kick out my Mommy! She has no place to go!"

I have seen grandparents who, with support, have managed to let go. Some, like Maggie, pack up their children's belongings and leave them on the porch. Others give their son or daughter a deadline for getting out. Either way, once you tell a child to leave, watch carefully. You might consider changing the locks, in case your child gave copies of the key to friends. Never say, "My child will never do that to me," because you never know. The drugs take control, or friends and lovers exert influence. One couple came home and discovered that their furniture and possessions had been sold. These are things you don't think about until they happen.

Some grandparents persuade their children to move out by setting up apartments for them. They may pay just the first month's rent and deposit, or they may go further and pay the rent and utilities and buy the furniture. It's something many grandparents would like to do, if they could afford it. It is one way for grandparents to get a child out of the house and still reassure themselves that he or she is safe. It's a nice idea; unfortunately, I have rarely seen it work. What I have seen, instead, is this: The apartment gets destroyed; the child invites friends over to "party," sells the furniture for drugs, and eventually gets evicted, often leaving the grandparents with financial liability.

Then there are the adult children who won't leave or who leave but won't stay away. You change the locks and come home to find them on the couch eating ice cream and watching television, the window broken behind them. One grandparent had to go through the eviction process with her own daughter because the police would not evict her.

If you have legal custody of your grandchildren and the parents pose a threat to you or your grandchild, you may be able to get a temporary restraining order against them. How much good it does is debatable. Dorcas King used one to keep her drug-addicted daughter at least 100 feet from her house. Other grandparents have had less success. One thing is certain: It is difficult to call the police on your own child. But if you must, a restraining order may increase your credibility. Remember, you cannot get a restraining order against a parent who has legal custody.

However, all the techniques in the world will be useless until you are ready to let go.

THE CHALLENGE OF CHANGE

Doug and Jane Sullivan's daughter, Mindy, is 28 years old and mentally unstable. She has three children from three different fathers, and her parents are raising them. She started running away at 13 and lived on the street for years. Her parents don't know if she used drugs. Right now she is living at home, but she interferes with the house more than she helps. Once, when Jane asked her to watch the children for an hour, she came back to a house in shambles. Mindy had put the seven-year-old in charge of the little ones and was lying on the couch watching television. The children adore her, but she can't take them for more than two hours.

Mindy repeatedly has horrendous outbursts. She is abusive to everyone in the house. She gets angry at the younger children and swears she will put them in foster care. She tells them they'll never see Grandma and Grandpa again. Once she actually called the police and said, "I want to get rid of my kids." The whole family tiptoes around her. Mindy orders Doug and Jane around like she's the queen of the house and they're her servants. "We spend all our effort and our money and energy on these children, and she doesn't want to help," says Jane. "Unless you watch it, she takes control of the household."

Jane and Doug have made some progress. They now take the kids and leave when Mindy blows up. She still has her outbursts, but at least the children aren't subjected to her threats. This is not the ideal choice. It basically tells Mindy that she can do what she wants and that her parents will leave instead of making her leave. It enables her to continue with the same behavior. However, it does protect the children from her abuse. Until Doug and Jane are ready and able to have their child move out, avoidance is the best choice they have.

Doug and Jane don't lack resolve as much as they are caught in a complex struggle with change. Throughout this chapter we have talked about changing behavior, saying no, setting limits, and even putting your adult child out of the house. But change is never simple. We always have good reasons to change our actions; less apparent are the good reasons not to. To quote psychologist and author Harriet Goldhor Lerner, Ph.D., "Change requires courage, but the failure to change does not signify the lack of it."[3] It took a lot of courage for Maggie to kick her son out of her house. But Jane and Doug, and grandparents like them, don't lack courage. They are still weighing the cost between giving in and giving up. There is a clear benefit to setting limits, but there is also a cost. For most grandparents still struggling with these decisions, the issues at stake are love and fear.

When Love Is at Stake

Love is powerful stuff, and Jane and Doug love Mindy. They raised her, they had hopes for her, and they desperately want to see her get better. Like many grandparents, they are not yet ready to let go. No parent wants to give up the hope that one more chance will save a child. Even 15 or 20 chances later, some grandparents are still trying. A family can deal with these issues for 20 years. When you spend a lifetime loving your child, who can say how many chances it takes to let go of her? There is no magic number. It may take two years in a grandparent support group to get one small change in a grandparent's behavior, but that alone can be a significant thing. Remember, each small change builds a path for bigger change. Until you can make larger strides, keep taking whatever steps you can.

When Fear Is at Stake

Fear is also a powerful motivator, and Doug and Jane are afraid of Mindy. They are afraid she could make good on her threats and disappear with the children. She has done it before. Like many grandparents, Doug and Jane have uncertain custody arrangements. Mindy could easily take her children and wander the streets with them. The grandparents would have nothing to say about it. The only way they can protect their grandchildren is to have them in their home, which means having Mindy there, too. They put up with the mother's behavior for the sake of the children.

Fear and uncertainty are common problems for grandparents who don't have legal custody. They feel trapped and may give in to all kinds of behavior, including extortion or blackmail, to protect their grandchildren. Living without legal custody is like living in an armed camp, always looking over your shoulder; it makes setting limits difficult. If you have this problem, consider what small changes you can make to create pockets of safety for your family. Jane and Doug's leaving with the children when Mindy flies off the handle is their attempt to make the best of a bad situation. Until you are ready or able to make bigger changes, you can only make the best of your situation.

DAMAGE CONTROL: PROTECTING GRANDCHILDREN FROM THEIR PARENTS

As painful as it is for you to witness and suffer the results of your adult child's behavior, it is even harder for your grandchildren. This is, after all, their mother or father, the supposed guardian and architect of their young world. They don't have the age or experience to judge their parent's behavior; they can only react to it and be shaped by it. Chapter 6 will look at the emotional and behavioral problems your grandchildren may face as a result of their circumstances. Here, however, are a few of the questions and problems you may encounter when your adult child interacts with your grandchildren.

What Do I Tell the Kids about Their Parents?

What to tell children and how much to tell them are tough questions for grandparents, and I have heard all kinds of stories about how people have handled this issue. Some grandparents tell the kids that Mom is sick and needs help. Others don't tell them anything, or say they don't know. One grandmother I know tells her grandchildren that Mom and Dad are on vacation whenever the parents land in jail.

I do not advocate lying to children. First of all, they may not believe you. Children pick up on things; they know when secrets are being kept from them. Second, if they do believe you, they will grow up with a distorted view of what life is all about (e.g., that it is common to spend a lot of time on vacation). But, more importantly, if you try to protect children by lying to them and they find out the truth, they'll start to wonder what else you're not telling them.

My parents didn't tell Kevin that my sister committed suicide. They told him she died of a breathing sickness. Later they said she died from smoking too much. Kevin accepted their explanations without question, and as he got older, he assumed his mother had died of lung cancer. When he finally did learn the truth, he was angry. "I felt they lied to me," he said recently. At age 19, the shadow of the lie still lingers. "I don't trust them the same as I might have if they had told me the truth from the beginning. Even if I might not have understood when I was eight, I still would have preferred to know the truth."

Tell the truth, but tell it in bite-size pieces. Think about the child who is asking. How old is he? How much can he understand? What is it that he really wants to know? For example, when a three-year-old asks where babies come from, he's not asking about sex. He just wants to know if he was hatched from a plant or a person. "You came from Mommy's tummy" is all the answer he needs at the moment. This is a conversation a parent will have again and again, over time, as the child's need and ability to understand increase. The same standard applies to grandchildren's questions about their parents. Children need and deserve the truth but in portions they can handle. The answers will depend on their age and maturity, how much contact they have with the parent, what the relationship is with the parent, and what kinds of questions are being asked.

Kids ask a lot of questions that don't require whole explanations: "Where is my mom (or dad)?" "Why can't I be with my parents?" "Will I ever live with my parents again?" Many times grandparents have to admit that they don't know where the parent is. If your grandchild sees her mother, you can tell her Mom has some troubles now. You can reassure her that this is not her fault. If the mother hasn't come by in six years and is remarried in another state, you can tell the child that Mommy is living far away and you don't know when she will come to visit.

Again, consider the age of the child. An eight-year-old will understand that Dad is in jail; a three-year-old doesn't know what jail is. You might tell a very young child that Daddy has gone away and we don't know when he'll be back. As the child gets older, she'll understand more. For instance, Pam Marshall's five-year-old granddaughter, Megan, knows that her mother uses drugs and that drugs make you sick. She knows that Linda's boyfriend hits her, and that's why she isn't allowed to see her mother when he's around. Essentially, she knows enough to understand why she can't do certain things, and in terms that a five-year-old can understand. "We only answer the questions she asks," says her grandmother. "We try to be as honest as we can without burdening too much."

Tell children in pieces, but tell them the truth. They eventually find out, anyway. Children sense a lot of things that they may not be able to verbalize. And be as gentle as possible. These children already have a profound sense of loss, abandonment, and rejection; you don't want to add to that.

What Do I Do When Parents Lie and Make Empty Promises?

Jay and Brenda Saunders are raising their grandson Anthony. Their daughter, Eva, has been abusing cocaine for 25 years. At 40 she is uneducated and homeless; her parents fear she may be selling crack. Eva loves her child dearly, says Brenda, but cannot care for him. "It's a crazy, immature love," she explains. "A child love."

Six-year-old Anthony only lived with his mother for one year, but he adores her. Eva comes to the house and plays with him. She promises to take him away. Sometimes she promises to visit and never shows up; when this happens, she blames other people for the lapse. She also tells her son that Grandma and Grandpa are the reason they can't be together.

Jay and Brenda want Anthony to know his mother. But whenever he sees her, there is a price to pay afterward in regressive behavior or anger at his grandparents. "When she's at the house, we are invisible," Brenda explains. "You can't believe the difference. But when he's with her . . . it's a disaster later on. I think he's furious at both of us because we're not his mother." And it's clear that Anthony suffers. "He's torn," says Brenda. "It's visible. It looks like he's been ripped apart after his mom was here."

Parents promise things: "I'll take you to live with me." "We'll have a house with a dog." "I'll take you bike riding on Sunday." When parents break promises, you get the fallout. Your grandchildren can't help it; you're an easy target. First, because you're there and the parent often isn't. Second, because their feelings about their parents are so conflicted that it is safer to get mad at you.

Broken promises are hard on children, who nevertheless continue to believe in their parents. They wait expectantly for the package or check or for Dad to pick them up at school, and they suffer deeply when nothing happens. Broken promises are equally painful for grandparents, who have to watch their grandchildren suffer each new disappointment as deeply as the first. If you are able to talk to the parents, try to explain the effect of this on the child. Perhaps they can run their plans by you first. If you have legal custody, you can even insist that this happen.

You can also talk to the children. Let them express their feelings about what happens with Mom or Dad. Sometimes they don't want to admit that there's a problem. As they get older, they sometimes come to realize that this is the pattern, that they can't believe what their parents say. Either way, they have strong feelings to express and need safe places to share them. Look to support groups, social workers, and family therapists for feedback about this kind of situation. There is rarely one best way to handle it.

Parents may also lie to their children: "Grandma took you away from me." "Don't listen to Grandpa." "Misbehave with your grandparents, and you can come home." They try to channel their anger and frustration through the children, who don't know whom or what to believe. Lies are even harder for a grandparent to handle. You can't control what a parent tells a child when you're not there, and you don't want to get into debates with your grandchildren about their parents. The best thing you can do is understand the fallout, give the children room to have their reactions, and continue to assure them that they are safe and loved in your home.

Again, if you can prevent the parents from making plans with the child, do; have them make plans with you instead. Tell Mom that you'll be in the park from two to three o'clock, or arrange to meet Dad at the movies. If the parents show up, great. If not, you'll be disappointed, but the child won't be devastated.

What If I Suspect Abuse during Parental Visits?

Continued abuse is a serious concern for many grandparents. Your grandchild may live with you but still have continued contact with unstable or abusive parents. What you can do about it depends on how much control you have over visitation. If you have legal custody of your grandchild and if visitation is at your discretion, you can insist on supervised visits. On the other hand, if court orders call for unsupervised visits and your grandchild comes home with unexplained bruises, contact your social worker immediately. If you suspect any kind of abuse during visits, at least keep a log of what you see and hear, including pictures if you can. Any documentation you gather could be important if a social worker or court becomes involved (see the section "Documentation" later in this chapter for more details).

WHEN THE PARENT IS IN JAIL

Handling your adult child is somewhat easier when she is in jail. As painful as it is, you know your child is safe and you know that, for the moment, she cannot physically disrupt your life or that of your grandchild. But the fact that your child is out of sight does not put her out of mind or out of contact with you. You may get frequent collect calls and letters requesting money for cigarettes and shampoo. Even at a distance, your child can play on your heartstrings. Be careful. If your child says she needs something and you do want to help out, send the item, not the money. Here, too, think about whether you are really helping or only enabling.

The picture changes when the adult child is about to be released from jail. Some will ask to come home at that time. If yours does, and you want her to come home, do not send money; send a nonre-fundable ticket instead. I have seen several situations in which grandparents sent money for a bus or a train ticket for an adult child to come home. They prepared the grandchild to see the mother or father, and the parent never came. Instead, he or she hooked up with old friends and cashed the ticket in. The child and the grandparents were devastated.

This is exactly what happened to Marta Sobol, a grandmother from Poland. Her oldest daughter, Anna, had been in and out of jail and rehab while Marta raised Anna's eight-year-old son, Christopher. Anna was now in jail again and started to write her mother lengthy letters of remorse. She had changed, she said. She wanted to be a good mother; she wanted to know her child, to be a real parent to him; and she wanted another chance. Marta didn't want to give in, but Christopher, always hopeful, begged his grandmother to give his mother another chance. I talked with Marta for months in GAP meetings, preparing her for the possibility that Anna might be using her again and making empty promises to Christopher. Finally, the time arrived. Marta sent Anna a bus ticket and told her that she and Christopher would be at the station. As soon as she saw her, Marta knew her daughter wasn't serious. After all her repentant letters, Anna had made arrangements to have friends pick her up. "I'm going out for a little while," she told her son. "I'll see you when I get home tonight." The child fell asleep at 10:00 P.M. and woke up again at 2:00 A.M., sobbing because Mom wasn't back yet. She never came back. She ended up back in jail after seeing her son for 10 minutes at the bus station.

Barbara Douglas had a similar story. Her daughter, Rhonda, had supposedly recovered in jail and wanted a fresh start. Barbara and her husband, offering to give her one more chance to come home, sent a ticket. The day she was released, Rhonda called to say she would be home the next morning, after she went to get her belongings. Barbara said, "Don't go anyplace. Don't pick up anything. We'll buy you new clothes, whatever you need. We'll start you over. Just come home." She didn't want Rhonda to go back to her old place because she knew that Rhonda's friends would get to her and that she wouldn't be strong enough to say, "No, I don't do this anymore." Rhonda didn't listen, and Barbara only heard from her months later, when she was once again in jail. At that point Barbara and her husband filed for guardianship of their grandson.

Some adult children don't even make a pretense of coming home; they go directly to their old neighborhoods and friends. Their parents may not hear from them again until they're back in jail. One day they get another collect call, and the cycle starts again.

Nevertheless, there are those who truly recover in prison. They get involved in Alcoholics Anonymous or some other program and start to put their lives together. But successful rehabilitation depends on how long an individual is incarcerated and how willing he is to change. Unfortunately, I have seen few cases of successful recovery. More often, I see adult children make empty promises and revert to old habits.

Remember, if there is no court order giving you legal custody of your grandchild, either through dependency or guardianship proceedings, a parent may resume custody when he or she is released from prison. If you have concerns about your grandchild and the system is not involved, you might consider seeking guardianship while the parent is incarcerated (see Chapter 10).

WHEN A DAUGHTER KEEPS HAVING BABIES

Julia Stone's daughter has already lost custody of four children; now she is pregnant again. "We all think maybe it will go away," Julia says quietly. It's a terrible thing to be a mother with a pregnant daughter and to be praying for a miscarriage. But that seems to be the only thing to do when your daughter keeps having babies—often drug babies—she can't care for. You can't force her to use birth control, and you certainly can't reason with her. Yet there are grandparents who are raising as many as six or seven children from the same mother. The babies are all medically fragile, and they just seem to keep coming—partly because the mothers know Grandma will care for them and partly because the mothers don't think about it at all.

The young women who have baby after baby aren't thinking about repercussions or about the fact that they already have five drug-addicted children out there. They are thinking about immediate gratification: the next man, the next fix. Often they are prostituting themselves without precautions. They could get an IUD or contraceptive implant, but they aren't able to plan ahead or follow through. Marlena Hunt's daughter scheduled an appointment for a tubal ligation but was back in jail before she could make the visit. Sandra Cobb's daughter planned to have her tubes tied after her sixth pregnancy but she delivered in a Catholic hospital and they wouldn't perform the surgery. Before she could get around to it, she was pregnant again.

Even the ones who may not be on drugs but who may be mentally unstable are not thinking about birth control. Liz Andersson's family has a history of mental illness, and her daughter inherited the problem. She is not responsible enough to take birth control measures, won't do a tubal ligation, and has already had five sons, ranging in age from 12 years to 18 months. Liz, who is 65, is raising them all.

Some women seem to have children just for the welfare check. I know there are many parents with large families who live just below the poverty level; that doesn't mean they are using drugs or neglecting their children. The parents I'm referring to are the ones who keep having kids but don't parent them. Often there are drugs involved. These are the mothers whose parents are already raising two or three of their children. If the grandparents get government aid for the children, the daughter may have her "own" baby to get welfare. Women who prostitute themselves for drug money may also get pregnant. If the choice is between paying for an abortion or getting welfare benefits during and after the pregnancy, they may have (and keep) the baby—until this one, too, gets removed by the courts. In the mind of a drug-addicted mother, a baby may mean easy cash for drugs.

Some mothers are even self-righteous about their children. One young woman I heard about had seven children taken away from her by the system before she was 30. The last one was removed when she threatened to push him in front of a truck—and she is sure the system is at fault!

Unfortunately, there isn't much you can do when a daughter keeps having babies. The options aren't encouraging. You can keep taking them, although your finances and energy may already be stressed to the limit. You can try to encourage her to get her tubes tied or get a contraceptive implant, but it must be her choice. Or you can let the next one go into foster care. Wanda Davis is one grandmother who managed to make that decision. She only has one of her four grandchildren, her sister is raising one, and two more are in the foster care system. Diane Snyder also has one grandchild, her sister has another, one was put up for adoption, and Mom has the fourth. Still, as much as you tell yourself you won't take the next one, when that baby comes, it's hard. Sandra Cobb has said that many times; she is now 67 years old and is raising seven grandchildren from the same daughter, ranging in age from 2 to 14 years.

One thing you can do is realize that you have no control over your daughter and make peace with what you will or will not do when the next baby arrives. Be realistic about your circumstances and your ability to say no. Your decision is not just about what is best for that baby but what is best for the children you already have and what is best for you. Remember, if you don't protect yourself, you can't protect even one grandchild. Consider what decisions you can live with and make peace with them.

When Mom Has Another Child and Keeps It

There are a number of reactions your grandchildren could have if their mother keeps the next baby; these depend on their age and the degree of contact they have with her. Two common reactions, however, are abandonment and relief.

A child who wants to be with his mother can be totally devastated if Mom has another baby. Feelings of low self-esteem and abandonment are compounded, and the child may wonder, "Why is she having another baby if I'm already here? If she can take care of a baby, why isn't she taking care of me?" He may lash out in anger and may regress to bed-wetting, thumb-sucking, and using baby talk in an effort to become a baby again so Mom will take care of him.

On the other hand, a child who is secure with Grandma and Grandpa might be relieved that Mom has another baby. She may think, "Maybe now Mom will leave me alone." The child may, in fact, feel guilt or anxiety about being safe with you while the new baby is with her mother. A child who is well settled with you might be afraid of being taken away. Unfortunately, you can never guarantee children that they will never be removed, unless you have adopted them. Even legal guardianship can be revoked.

DOCUMENTATION

Emily Petersen saved everything connected with her granddaughter—pictures, letters, birthday cards—because she thought she might need them someday. Lucy Davis kept a notebook documenting every visit with her daughter-in-law, whether it was good, bad, or even a no-show. She wrote down everything that happened and her granddaughter's reactions to each event. She knew that her memory alone would not be enough if she wanted to recount these things later on. Each of these grandmothers came to bless her foresight.

When Emily's granddaughter Amanda was three years old, the child's mother (Emily's daughter-in-law) asked Emily and Carter to adopt her. Sheila became less cooperative, however, as the adoption proceeded, and told the social worker handling the case that neither she nor her parents were ever allowed to see Amanda. It wasn't true, and Emily could prove it. She had cards and letters from Sheila thanking her for watching Amanda and for letting her see her child, as well as photos of the other grandparents at the house for Easter. Her careful documentation put Sheila's accusations in perspective.

Lucy, on the other hand, found herself facing an angry judge. Lucy had canceled visitation one afternoon because Lindsey started vomiting when she heard she had to see her mother. "Who do you think you are?" demanded the judge, who assumed she was arbitrarily refusing parental visits. "Here," Lucy said, pulling out her notebooks. "It is all here. She had thirty-two scheduled visits; she showed up for twelve." The judge agreed that visitation had to be consistent or not at all and ordered that future visits be held at the courthouse in order to monitor the mother's attendance.

Even if you're not currently involved with the system, document everything. If at some point in the future you do find yourself involved with the court or even a private attorney, you may have less of an ordeal if you have records of the parents' behavior and the children's reactions to parental visits. You look more organized and accurate if you have information written down in concrete detail and chronological order. If you have to rely on your memory, your statement to the judge may go something like this: "My daughter drops by unexpectedly and intoxicated. The last visit was maybe six or ten weeks ago." Compare that statement with: "On June 14 my daughter appeared at my door unannounced. She was staggering and slurring her speech." It makes a much better impression in court, and you don't have to rely on your own memory.

How to Document

- Keep a journal or log. Use a bound diary or calendar, and keep a daily record of your adult child's behavior and anything pertaining to your grandchildren. Don't use a loose-leaf notebook; a bound book is a much more convincing document because the chronological order cannot be faked.
- Don't write down what you *think* is happening, only what you can verify with dates, times, and photos. It is one thing to say, "My daughter never visits when she promises to." It is another to say, "On May sixth my daughter said she would come for a visit on May seventh; that was six weeks ago, and we haven't heard from her since."—especially when you have the calendar entries to prove it.
- Write down everything concerning the parent: the time, day, and nature of phone calls and visits; the child's behavior and reactions before, during, and after the call or visit; and the behavior of the parent. Does the parent appear to be in control or under the influence of something when he calls or comes

by? Does the parent ask about the child when he calls? How often does the parent call? Does he visit as promised? Does the parent make promises that aren't kept—ice cream, toys, birthday presents, trips? Write it all down.

- Document what the parent *doesn't* do: when she doesn't visit, doesn't show, doesn't call, doesn't send a card for a birthday or holiday.
- Record everything you spend on the child and keep receipts. This not only verifies what it costs you to keep the child, but could be used later to prove that Mom and Dad are not supporting him.
- Document everything that might be helpful to show a court that the parent is not ready to handle the responsibility of raising a child. If a child comes back from a visit with a parent and has unexplained bruises or resumes bed-wetting or thumb-sucking after being with Mom or Dad, write it down. Write everything down.
- Be forewarned: having documentation won't guarantee a positive court response. I know grandparents who had everything written down but were not permitted to enter their journals as evidence, and I know grandparents whose records, though presented to the court, didn't help. Still, it is better to have records and not be able to use them than to need records and not have them. And if you do get the opportunity to present information, you will look more organized and believable if everything is documented.

Sample Written Contract

The Story

Donna and Hal Smith are raising two grandsons. Their daughter Caroline is 31 years old, divorced, and drug addicted. She has been through numerous drug treatment programs, and she has been in jail several times. Each time she is released, she makes and then breaks the same promises. She has stolen her mother's jewelry and even her kids' piggy bank to buy more drugs. Now she is coming out of rehab again, and her parents want to give her one last chance for the sake of the children. This time,

(continued)

(continued from previous page)

however, they are using a written contract, signed by Caroline and witnessed by their family therapist.

The Contract

Rules of the House

Between Donna and Hal Smith and Caroline Black.

The purpose of this contract is so that we can all live peacefully under the same roof and know what our expectations are of each other.

For Caroline Black to continue to live with Donna and Hal Smith, the following rules must apply. These are not in order of importance.

1. Caroline must strive to lead a sober and productive life. She must prove to her parents that she can be a good mother and a safe provider for her children. She is not to socialize with any of her old friends from the street.

2. This phone number is only to be given out on job applications. Donna or Hal will take all calls. Caroline may use the phone only with permission from Donna or Hal, or she will lose her phone privileges.

3. Caroline must be in this residence by 10:30 P.M. or call by 10:00 if she can't make it on time. She is not to be in the house alone, unless given permission by Donna or Hal. Caroline is not allowed to take any property from this residence unless given permission by Donna or Hal. Caroline shall not give out this address to anyone (unless it pertains to a job). The doors of the house and garage are to be kept locked at all times. Electricity and water are to be used only as needed.

4. Caroline is to start an outpatient drug program immediately. She is expected to comply with any drug testing required by her parole officer or by Donna or Hal. Caroline must also start a counseling program to help begin a new relationship with her children. These counseling sessions must be attended weekly. Alcoholics Anonymous or Narcotics Anonymous programs must be attended three times a week.

5. Caroline is expected to find a job within two months. She may not sleep in. She must be out looking for a job from

(continued)

(continued from previous page)

8:00 A.M. to 5:00 P.M. and must provide her parents with a list of employers she has contacted. Once she has a job, she must then contribute to the expenses of running the house. This includes food and monthly bills.

6. Donna and Hal are to provide food and shelter to Caroline. They will give Caroline a bus pass, but they will not give Caroline any money. Donna and Hal are not responsible for Caroline's transportation.

7. Caroline must share in household responsibilities. She must cook dinner three times a week and do dishes on the other nights. She must do her children's laundry, pack their school lunches, and keep her own room clean.

8. Caroline must not upset her children. She must realize that her children come first, and she may not raise her voice or spank them. She is not to make promises to her children or plans without discussing them with Donna or Hal first. She may not take the children away from the house without supervision.

9. At any time, Donna and Hal have the right to ask Caroline to leave if they think she is under the influence of any drug or alcohol.

10. Caroline must leave this residence if any of these rules are broken. Caroline must also leave if she cannot live by the rules of this contract. This is a firm contract between Donna and Hal Smith and Caroline Black. The purpose of this contract is to restore Donna and Hall's trust in Caroline Black and to assure the safety of Caroline's children.

11. At the advice of Donna's counselor, Martha Steven, Donna and Hal must keep this contract in force.

(Date) _____ Caroline Black

_____ Donna Smith

_____ Hal Smith

witnessed by _____ Martha Steven

A reminder: This is only a sample contract. Your own contract should reflect your own needs and purpose. However, try to write it with tight rules and specific expectations. Then, as trust is restored, you can loosen up a little. It is much more difficult to start loose and then have to tighten the rules later on.

CHAPTER 6 | # Your Troubled Grandchild

You raise your kids; you think it's over. No one
tells us it's just the beginning.
—*Colorado grandmother*

One morning when John and Carol Waters's
daughter didn't answer the phone, John
crawled in her window and found her dead
in her bed with her three-year-old son in her arms. The little boy
was desperately trying to wake his mother, who had died of a heart
attack in her sleep. When I first met this family, Brian was so insecure
he could not let Grandma sit in a chair beside him; he had to sit in
her lap and would have crawled inside her if he could have. Grandma
couldn't be out of his sight even to go to the bathroom. She had to
sleep in his room. Brian couldn't sleep through the night and was
constantly telling Grandma not to close her eyes. He was afraid that
if she fell asleep, she, like his mother, would never wake up.

Carolyn Parker's grandson, Eric, had been living on the streets
with his drug-addicted teenage mother. One day the young woman left
the little boy alone in a motel room, and neighbors called child protective
services, who called Carolyn. He was like "a wild animal" when he
arrived, says Carolyn. At two years the child could barely talk; he only
cried and screamed. He didn't know how to sit down and eat properly,
and he was painfully insecure; he hoarded food and screamed every
time anyone tried to take his new coat away. "He thought he wouldn't
get it back," says Carolyn. "He had nothing he could call his."

72

Four-year-old Heather Pierce was a very sad, frightened little girl when she arrived at her grandmother's house. She wet her bed, she hid under the cushions on the couch, and she had trouble sleeping. But she wasn't afraid of the dark. Instead, she was afraid of the light. She needed everything shut and tightly closed—the windows, the blinds, the door—and complete darkness before she could fall asleep at night. She was afraid that her father, who was in prison for murdering her mother, would come and get her, too.

Not only are you raising a child you never planned for, but you may be raising a child with multiple problems. Many of these children are the walking wounded. They are good kids, but they have not had a good start in life. They may be anxious and insecure. Since the people who were supposed to nurture them have, through choice or accident, left them, they may have a tough time trusting anyone or anything. Many have been left alone in motels and in strangers' homes. They may be used to falling asleep in one place and waking up somewhere else. They have no sense of stability.

Some of the children will defy authority. Some have been responsible for themselves since they were five or six years old. They may have cared for infant siblings, diapering and feeding them; they may have cared for drug-addicted parents. They think they can come and go as they please. Far from grateful, these kids may resent your taking on the role of parent and may rebel when you set rules.

Some grandchildren are physically and verbally aggressive—with you, other adults, and other children. They only know how to get negative attention and may fight, swear, lie, and even commit petty crimes to get noticed. They will push your limits to see how far they can go until you finally push them away. Since everyone else has abandoned them, they reason, it's only a matter of time before you do, too. Children who have been molested may act out sexually, and even very young children will pick up inappropriate sexual behavior if they have been exposed to pornography or have seen their mothers with various men.

On the other hand, your grandchildren might be the best-behaved youngsters, sturdy little ones who seem to have it all together. You may even count on them to help you with their younger siblings. But an excesssivly mature and obedient child is also a source of worry. For healthy, normal development children need their childhood, and that means acting like children. Some of these children may also withdraw and get depressed. They turn their feelings inward and become introspective and shy, isolating themselves from adults and peers. They're your "easy" kids. But don't let this behavior fool you; they may be just as needy as children who overtly act out.

The tricky thing in all of this is that three children who have had the same neglectful upbringing or the same traumatic loss could react in three completely different ways.

WHAT YOUR GRANDCHILD IS FEELING

To understand your grandchild's behavior, it helps to understand what he or she is going through. In the turmoil of a shattered family, children are the most affected and the least prepared to understand or talk about it. A small child can't turn around and say, "I am angry because my mother abandoned me, and I'm afraid it might be my fault." Instead, she may act out her feelings. She may become aggressive at school or depressed and withdrawn; she may have difficulty sleeping, wet her bed, or revert to baby talk. The types of emotional problems a child experiences and their severity will depend on the individual child, on how much trauma she survived, and on the child's age and stage of development when she moves in with you. However, most grandchildren will experience a similar set of intense, overlapping feelings.

Grief and Abandonment

Every case of grandparents raising grandchildren is somehow about loss—for the grandparent and the grandchild. And where there is loss, grief inevitably follows. Whether a parent is absent owing to death or drugs, these children suffer a profound sense of loss, abandonment, and rejection.

Don't let appearances fool you. Children grieve differently than adults do. They grieve like children. One little boy was four the year his father left and his mother died. When his grandmother took him in, he was "a little wildcat." "He suffered a tremendous amount of losses," she says. "Grief in a child is anger."[1]

Nightmares, confusion, and even moments of forgetfulness and joy are also part of a child's grieving process. When my sister died, my mother felt that Kevin wasn't grieving the way he should. He wanted to play with his friends, have a good time. He was trying to put his life back together.

Young children don't have the concept that death is really final. They go from periods of sadness and depression to moments when they block things out. They may not remember what has happened. They may focus on things like toys and friends. They may repeatedly ask if or when Mommy is coming back. The biggest difference between the child who has been orphaned and the one who has been abandoned is the answer to that question. For one, it is certain Mommy is not coming back. Understand, however, that it is normal for children to alternate between overt sorrow and happy self-involvement. It may be hard on you to hear your grandchild's laughter if your own child has just died, but your grandchild is processing the death in his own way. Just as you must mourn at your own pace, allow your grandchild to set the pace for his own grieving process.

There are many books that help children deal with death and that are written on a level they can understand. We used several with Kevin when my sister died, and I highly recommend checking some out at the library (see Appendix A for suggestions).

A child who is orphaned loses his parent once, and it is permanent and tragic. A child whose parents are in jail, in rehab, on the street, or just missing harbors a hope of returning to them but in the meantime loses them over and over again as they wander in and out of the child's life. Strange as it may seem, a sudden death may be easier for a child to handle than months or even years of not knowing. It is the difference between a clean break and prolonged uncertainty, and certainty is extremely important to children.

Reassurance, nurturing, and acceptance are what your grandchild needs, as well as consistency and routine. Children need to be reassured that you will not leave them and that they are safe. These children have a low sense of self-esteem and a high sense of self-blame. Do things to shore up your grandchild's self-image; use positive reinforcement and praise. Remind him over and over that you love and accept him. Predictability and sameness are also important. Try to maintain a consistent, predictable routine so that your grandchild can begin to trust you and his new environment. It takes a while, but it eventually sinks in.

Guilt

Children feel incredible guilt when a crisis happens in the family and a parent is suddenly absent. The crisis can be a divorce, an arrest, a suicide—it doesn't matter. Children have a narrow definition of cause and effect. It is easy for them to believe that the parent would not have left if only they had been "good," if only they had been more helpful, if only they had cleaned their room or finished their dinner. In some distorted way, they blame themselves for their parents' not taking care of them.

The guilt intensifies if a child comes to you from an abusive or neglectful situation. She may feel relieved about being with you and away from her parents, but that same relief feels like a betrayal of her parents. And if she has been placed with you over the wishes of her parents, she may feel like a pawn, split down the middle in her loyalties, caught between her love for her parents and her need to be safe with you. Your grandchild may also feel guilty for being a burden in your life, particularly if she is the cause of friction between you and your spouse. Even when there is no friction, a child may feel guilty for changing your life. "Poor Grandma," six-year-old Lindsey told her aunt. "Daddy is always going to parties. Aunt Dawn and Jason are married now, and they go everywhere. And poor Grandma. . . . You know, she's got me, and she never goes anywhere." "It isn't that I say it," says her grandmother, "but the child is not blind."

It is critical that you help your grandchildren understand that they are not to blame for their parents' absence or the current situation. Again, the key is reassurance and positive reinforcement. You cannot use logic to change children's minds; you can only continually reassure them. Give them affection and frequent praise. One grandmother always looks for something positive to focus on with her hyperactive grandson. Even when he is acting out or misbehaving, she will ask him to take something to the trash for her or to turn on the light; this way she can praise him and continue building his self-esteem.

Anger

Seven-year-old Gabriel is a good kid, but one morning he started throwing things and came after his grandfather with a pipe, saying, "I'm going to kill Grandpa." Yet at the end of the day, he was hugging Grandpa good night. Adam, 15, told his grandmother he would break a window, and he did; he threw his skateboard through it. And four-year-old Monica has started choking cats.

Anger builds up inside children—anger at their parents for not being there or for breaking promises, anger at you for not being their parents, anger at the neglect and abuse they experienced before coming to live with you. They may blame you for sending their parents away (their parents may even tell them that you did). If they had the run of the streets before coming to you, they may also resist your attempts to impose rules, limits, and structure. Very young children lack words and will physically express their feelings, but even older children may act out complex emotions. Grandparents often become the target of the unexpressed anger these children feel, perhaps because the parents are absent or because the children think that if they do express their feelings, their parents will abandon them forever. You're an easy target. Try not to take this personally, however; you are also their lifeline.

Try to direct and channel your grandchild's anger when he gets mad. Help him verbalize his feelings. It is better for a child to say, "I'm mad because my Mommy didn't come to see me today and she promised," than for him to hit someone. Let your grandchild know that it is okay to be angry, that you understand that he feels hurt and confused, but that it is not okay to hit or threaten. Teach the child that feelings and actions are different. If he can't verbalize his feelings, let him get the anger out safely on a pillow or punching bag.

An angry child who threatens someone, even if it is with a plastic baseball bat, has reached a crisis point. It doesn't matter whether or not the threat would have been carried out. The fact that the child was that angry and couldn't channel that feeling is a warning sign. Children who have reached this point could hurt someone; they could also hurt themselves. If the problem isn't addressed, it may only worsen as they get older. Anger that is extreme or disrupts your daily life is a sign of crisis. This is the time to seek professional counseling for the child—and for yourself, so that you can learn to help her.

Fear, Anxiety, and Insecurity

Every child has fears of some sort—of the dark, the boogeyman, being lost. The world is a big place full of dangerous unknowns, and children are particularly powerless in it. But while a night-light can take care of a childish fear of the dark and you can talk about the questionable existence of the boogeyman, what can you do about a child who has already lived the nightmare? Your grandchild knows there are real things to fear because she has seen them. The child may not trust adults because her parents proved untrustworthy. She is probably terrified of being abandoned again, this time by you. "Who will take care of me if Grandma gets sick?" is a scary thought for a kid.

When Marilyn McIntosh first got her grandchildren, they were anxious and insecure. They asked questions like these: "Do you love us as much as you loved your own kids?" "Are you and Grandpa always going to live together?" "Are you going to live long enough for me to grow up and take care of myself?"[2] As time passes and children are exposed to the constancy of a loving, safe environment and a normal, predictable daily routine—having their clothes and toys in the same place each day and sleeping in the same bed every night—the questions come less frequently. But they are probably never far from the surface: Anne Sutter was just flopped across her bed one day, tired after a grueling day at work. Perhaps she dozed awhile. It was enough to panic her six-year-old grandson. Anne woke to a child frantically shaking her foot and yelling, "Mommy! I thought you were dead!"

There are also fears about the parents: "Won't they ever come back?" Or the reverse: "What if they *do* come back?" One little boy was so afraid that his mother would come and take him that he built traps for her; he rigged a gate with rubber snakes so that if she tried to open the gate, the snakes would pop up and scare her away.[3]

Reassuring frightened children takes time, patience, and consistency—not just the consistency of reassuring words and hugs but of three meals a day, regular school hours, a stable routine. You may have to reassure your grandchildren again and again as they slowly adjust to their new situation. Extreme fears, however, may indicate a need for counseling.

Embarrassment

Some children may be sensitive about the fact that they live with grandparents, particularly when other children are around. They may also be embarrassed by their parents. It is difficult for children to accept the fact that their situation is different from that of their peers. Their friends may ask painful questions and tease them. The parents of their friends are probably younger and able to participate in more activities. Although there are increasing numbers of older first-time parents, as well as young grandparents, the age factor can spark embarrassing, if innocent, questions. "Where's your mother?" a little girl in the playground asked seven-year-old Melissa one day. The little girl had heard Melissa call her 70-year-old grandmother "Mommy" and didn't believe mothers had so much gray hair. "Where's your mother?" the little girl persisted. Melissa didn't know how or what to answer. She doesn't know where her mother is—her mother abandoned her when she was 10 months old and she has never seen her. Grandma overheard the exchange and came to her rescue. "Why do you ask so many questions?" she asked the little girl; then she changed the subject.

Perhaps you live in a small community and your grandchild's friends know that the child's parent is in jail or on drugs. The teasing may be far less innocent. Children can be cruel, and they will use whatever ammunition they can find to inflict pain. Fifteen-year-old Vanessa constantly gets into fights at school. The other children say horrible things to her: that her mother was a "jailbird," that her mother didn't want her, that her mother had syphilis. Vanessa says that she gets into fist fights because the taunts make her "crazy."

Sometimes the parent's presence itself is the problem. Sixteen-year-old Mark remembers coming home from shopping one day to find his mother stretched out on the front lawn looking "like a bum." He recalls, "I felt so embarrassed; I never wanted to come back. My friends were standing around and said, 'Who's that?' I said 'Just a friend of the family.' I can't believe I said that. And then someone said, 'That's his mother.' Everybody knew about my mother by then, but nobody ever saw her. And she was lying on the grass, and the neighbors were staring."

These are hard situations to face, and there is no perfect way to handle them. Teach your grandchildren that they don't have to answer questions that make them uncomfortable, that they can change the subject or say, "I don't want to talk about that right now." Teach them to use their words, not their fists, when they are angry. But, most importantly, try not to be hurt by their hurt and embarrassment. When they talk about these feelings at home, it is important to listen and acknowledge their pain. Growing up is hard enough without all these extra problems. What they most need is for you to understand that. You can't make it go away and you can't make it better, but you can certainly hear them.

Hope and Fantasy

Unless they are terrified of them your grandchildren will probably never give up the hope, the fantasy, that their parents will some-day come back and take care of them. Although they love you, the parent–child bond is a tight one that never vanishes–even when a child has been mistreated. Ten-year-old Stephanie was abandoned by her mother when she was two years old. She hasn't seen her in five years, but she still fantasizes about her. One day Stephanie called 911 and asked the sheriff to find her mother. Although five-year-old Marcy was physically and sexually abused, she still talks about going back and living with Mom. Many children want to remain with their grandparents, but they fantasize about having their parents join them. When five-year-old Megan's mother asked Megan if she wanted to live with her, the child replied, "No, I want you to come live with all of us in the same house."

These hopes and fantasies can result in erratic behavior on the part of the child. Some children act out in the hope that their grandparents will be unable to handle them and will send them back to their parents. Others will become depressed and withdrawn. Says one grandmother, "The kids believe their mom will come get them. When it doesn't happen, we get anger." The reverse is also true: Children who are returned to their parents and are unhappy may misbehave so they will be sent back to Grandma's.

It is normal for your grandchildren to have these hopes and dreams and to be disappointed when they don't come true. All you can do is let them know you understand their feelings and that you will continue to be there for them when they need you.

COMMON BEHAVIOR PROBLEMS

Every child who lives with grandparents suffers some part of this emotional kaleidoscope. Children need reassurance that their thoughts and feelings are normal and that most other children in their situation would have similar ones. Encourage your grandchildren to express their feelings in whatever way they can, provided they don't hurt themselves or others in the process. If they can talk about being hurt or angry or frightened, they are less likely to channel those feelings into inappropriate or negative behavior.

Not every child, however, is capable of verbalizing feelings. Sometimes the feelings are too big; sometimes there are too many of them. And many children are too young to understand what they are going through, let alone talk about it.

What follows are some common behavior problems and parenting issues that trouble grandparents. Remember, children act out what they cannot verbalize. These behavior problems are mostly symptoms of underlying emotional issues. Sometimes several behaviors may be related to one issue. For instance, a child who is experiencing eating and sleeping disorders as well as severe "clinginess" may be suffering from a shattered sense of trust and will need your help to restore it. On the other hand, these three behaviors could have three different emotional roots. In any case, both your grandchild's behavior and the feelings behind them will need to be addressed for the child to make a healthy adjustment to his or her new living situation.

Excessive Clinging

Fear and insecurity can make a grandchild excessively clingy. Carol Waters couldn't take a shower without her grandson Brian in the bathroom. He wanted to sit in her lap in public, not next to her. He didn't want to be left at school or with a baby-sitter and cried excessively when she left.

When their grandparents are attending a GAP session, the children will often wander past the door and peek in just to make sure that Grandma or Grandpa is still in the same place. Five-year-old Megan often sleeps in Grandma's lap through the whole session to avoid having to leave her grandmother and go with the other kids. And one day when six-year-old Gregory saw the group members leave the room and his grandmother was not among them—she was in the bathroom—he let out a bloodcurdling scream: "Where is my grandma!?"

Most children have clingy moments, but for these children clinging is almost a way of life. They may also talk excessively as a way of keeping adults not only physically present but also mentally and emotionally present. For a harried grandparent, behavior like this can be hard to handle. Try to understand that your grandchild doesn't want to drive you crazy but is only trying to stay safe. These children are terrified of being left or forgotten, even for a moment. It takes time, reassurance, and consistency for grandchildren to trust again and feel secure. Once they start trusting that you will continue to be there for them, and can see it with their own eyes, the clingy behavior will ease up (although it may reappear again in times of change).

For severe situations like Brian's, however, therapy may be needed. I worked with Carol Waters's grandson Brian in individual and family therapy for several years. At first I had Grandma stay in the office with us for the entire time. Then I told her to say in the middle of the therapy session that she had to go to the bathroom. Brian would scream and yell in a fit of anger and panic. I would hold him at the door of the bathroom while Carol talked to him from the other side. Then she would be silent for a minute and come out. Brian thought she was going to disappear through some secret door in there. He finally reached the point where he could see me without having Grandma in the room and could go off to play in the park with other children during GAP events. But it took time, patience, and a great deal of consistency and reassurance.

Sleeping Problems

Five-year-old Patrick was raised by a mentally ill mother and an abusive father and stepmother before coming to live with his grandmother. He is so frightened and insecure that he can't sleep in his own room; he sleeps on a mat on the floor by Grandma. The same thing happened with Kevin after my sister died. I had temporarily moved in with my parents after graduate school and slept on a mat on the floor next to Kevin's bed. My nephew wouldn't sleep unless I was holding his hand. If I moved at all, he would wake up instantly. If I wasn't there, he would take his blanket in the middle of the night and lie down beside my parents' bed. He was very afraid that people were going to die on him again, and we were all he had.

Sleeping problems are common with children whose lives have been disrupted. They take the form of nightmares, fear of the dark, and wanting to sleep with the grandparents. These are unspoken cries of insecurity and indicate a need for reassurance, nurturing, and trust.

Going to bed can be a difficult time for your grandchild. It means a long separation from you and may tap fears that you could disappear in the night or that she may wake up in a strange environment. Again, reassurance, consistency, and a predictable routine are key. Try to establish a bedtime ritual. Set a bedtime hour and stick to it. As you tuck your grandchild in, talk about how the day went and any plans you may have for tomorrow, letting her know you will be there if she gets scared at night and when she wakes up in the morning. You can even leave a picture of yourself or the family by the bed to reassure her. Bedtime rituals can be a wonderful, secure part of childhood, a time that your grandchild may use to discuss the day or confide in you.

If, on the other hand, you have a grandchild who can't sleep or wakes up with nightmares, there are a number of things you can try to get him back to bed: You can rub his back, sing to him or read him bedtime stories to quiet him down (although you don't want to reward waking up if it becomes a nightly habit). A night-light in the room and hallway can help youngsters who have nightmares. Try to address the problem in the child's room. Children need to feel secure in their own beds, and sleeping alone is an important step in learning a healthy autonomy. Besides, you need your privacy, too. Once you consistently allow a child to sleep in your bed, the habit is more difficult to break.

As children begin to work through their fears and rebuild trust, their sleeping problems should start to dissipate. My nephew Kevin eventually learned to sleep alone in his room, and Heather Pierce has begun to sleep with her windows open. But it takes time, patience, and, with some children, counseling to help them process the trauma and loss they have experienced.

Eating Problems

Food can be the focus of several kinds of problems for your grandchildren. They may not have had enough to eat before they came to you. They may eat too fast or too much, as if each meal might be their last for some time. They may even start hoarding food. When two-year-old Eric arrived at his grandparents' house, he ate so quickly he was in danger of choking. "Eric, take little bites; there's plenty of food," his grandmother would assure him. And six-year-old Daryl hides food under his bed, even cans he can't open.

On the other hand, some children may get depressed and stop eating or may refuse to eat, using mealtime as a way to get your attention. Charlotte Buckley has a four-year-old grandson who turns food into a power struggle. Joey won't take a bite unless Grandma is there to bribe and spoon-feed him; sometimes even that doesn't do any good. He does eventually eat, however, when she ignores him.

When you are dealing with a problem concerning food, whether a child is eating too much or too little, you need to rule out any medical problems. Most likely the problem is related to psychological issues, but you don't want to overlook any physical cause. A change in a child's eating pattern is often a symptom of depression. Consider it in the context of your grandchild's overall behavior: Is there also a change in sleeping pattern? Is the child becoming withdrawn and isolated? If so, you may want to have her evaluated for depression and treated accordingly.

Children who hoard, like Eric and Daryl, need to be reassured that there is plenty of food. They do well with a consistent eating routine. If they know they will have breakfast, lunch, an after-school snack, and dinner at the same time each day, they can start to view meals as something they can count on. If they can tell time, they can see when the next meal will be. Children who eat too fast or too much may need to be monitored for a while. They should be served small portions and encouraged to ask for more if they are still hungry. You might also consider keeping healthy snack foods in a place your grandchildren can reach; this practice will reassure them that if they do get hungry, they can do something about it. It gives them a safe sense of control over their food.

A child like Joey has a different problem. For him, food is a way to manipulate Grandma. Why should he make an effort to eat by himself when refusing to eat earns him Charlotte's undivided attention? If you have a grandchild like Joey, understand that this is a different control issue: It is not about controlling food, it is about controlling you and the environment. If your grandchild can get you to sit in the kitchen for three hours trying to get him to eat, he wins. You can, however, step outside of the power struggle.

Again, the key is firmness, consistency, and patience. Have regular meals that last a usual and reasonable length of time. Let your grandchild know that if she hasn't eaten by the end of the meal, she may have to wait until the next one. Since children have a poor sense of time, it's a good idea to use a timer to let her know when the meal is over. When she realizes she won't have someone sitting and coaxing her to eat—and she misses a meal or two—she'll start eating.

If you do use this technique, you must be consistent. It doesn't do any good if you feel sorry for your grandchild and provide a snack later on. All he will learn is that he can eat whenever, and whatever, he wants. What you can do is remind the child that he can't have a snack today because he didn't eat his dinner, that perhaps if he eats dinner tomorrow, he can also have dessert. Don't forget to check with your pediatrician regarding vitamins and proper nutrients, and, again, make sure the problem isn't medical.

However your grandchild relates to food, don't ever withhold meals as punishment; eating should be a safe and reliable experience for a child, not something to be earned.

Babyish Behavior

Three-year-old Savannah reverts to using diapers and a bottle whenever she sees her mother, although she doesn't use either in nursery school or at home. "I think she thinks Mary wants her to be in diapers and bottles," says her grandmother, who traces Savannah's babyish behavior to the birth of her twin sisters. Ever since that time, Savannah has been possessive of her mother, trying to prevent her from holding the infants.

When young children feel threatened, they may revert to babyish behavior: thumb-sucking, baby talk, using a bottle, bed-wetting, clinging, wanting to be carried, or waking up in the middle of the night. A new sibling is certainly a threat. A child may feel insecure because everyone is paying attention to the baby in the family, a position she held until now. She may feel rejected if Mom keeps the new child but doesn't take her. A sibling is not the only threat a child faces; each time she sees a parent leave, it can feel like rejection. If her mother was nurturing during the child's infancy, an insecure six-year-old, hoping to bring Mom back, might revert to babyish behavior.

Understand that these are normal reactions. Most children will regress briefly, and need to, in order to work through changes in their life circumstances. Acting like a baby may be a sign that they need extra nurturing or need to adopt the role of a baby for a while. Eventually, they return to their more mature selves. Some children, however, will cling to this baby identity and not progress to the next stage of development.

If your grandchild is regressing, allow him some room to be a baby and work out the feelings. If the situation doesn't resolve itself, don't let it continue too long. You can address the insecurities without encouraging the babyish behaviors. You can validate the child's feelings with questions like "Do you wish you were still a baby?" or "Do you wish you still had your bottle?" Recognizing and understanding the feelings is different from encouraging the actions. You can reassure your grandchild that you love him and that he is very special but also remind him that he is no longer a baby. You can point out the advantages of being big and the disadvantages of being a baby: Big children can play with toys and watch television; babies take lots of naps and don't get to make decisions. Remind your grandchild to use words, not baby talk. Be reassuring and nurturing but also firm.

One more thing you can do is create a "life book" for your grandchild, that is, a collection of photos from the past arranged in chronological order, like a story, with descriptions underneath each photo. It is important for children to have a sense of roots and progress, and photos clearly document the passage of time. Your grandchild can see herself when she really was little, and she can see how much she has grown. There is a healing power in being able to hold your history in your hand and look at it, even for a small child. If you want to do a life book for your grandchild and you don't have access to early photos, start with the pictures you have. Add to the life book as often as you can, depending on your time and circumstances. You don't have to wait for major events like birthdays and holidays to take snapshots. Everyday activities can make charming photos and tell a story about a child's life.

Wanting to Call You Mom and Dad

A child who has a relationship with his parents already knows them as Mom and Dad and knows you as Grandma and Grandpa. Other children, however, may want to call you Mom and Dad; all the other kids have mothers and fathers, and your grandchildren don't like feeling different. Older children may even want to have their names changed whereas little ones tend to call anyone who nurtures them "Momma."

The truth is that you will probably have a harder time with this issue than your grandchildren. You may not want the children to forget their parents and may fear that this could erase their memory.

You might feel like you are usurping their parents' place. Or you might just be uncomfortable: You were a parent, now you are a grandparent, and you want the difference to be clear. When the subject of names comes up, don't make it a big emotional issue for a child. It is all individual, and there are no right or wrong answers. Whatever you and your grandchild are comfortable with will probably work fine. If you and your spouse are not comfortable being called Mom and Dad, you can tell your grandchildren that you are doing all the things a parent does but that they still have a mom and a dad and you are Grandma and Grandpa.

"Stuart asks me about how I can be both Grandma and Momma," says Arlene Townsend. "I tell him, 'I am what you want me to be.'" Three-year-old Tamara refused to call her mother "Mommy" when she saw her on visits. Her grandmother asked her why. "Her not my mommy," the little girl replied, "She's just my friend. You're my mommy. You take care of me every day." And Denise, who has lived with her grandparents from the day she was born, has it all squared away: Her grandmother is Grandma, her grandfather is Daddy, her Aunt Carla is Momma, and her mother is Momma Gail.

Tests and Manipulation

All children test limits; it is how they discover the boundaries in their world. They mouth off and act out and then learn from our reactions what is acceptable behavior and what is not. They don't fight fair, either. Children know just what to say, and when to say it, to get you to melt. They use scraped knees and hurt feelings, pouts, whines, and tears to get their way. Some parents handle the tests and manipulations of childhood better than others, but it is all part and parcel of raising kids.

Many grandparents forget this fact. Perhaps you haven't lived with small children in years and have allowed your memories of childrearing to mellow over time. You may be surprised and frustrated when your grandchildren are hard to handle; unfortunately, your grandchildren may be harder to handle than most children their age.

Tragic circumstances have given many grandchildren a distorted sense of limits. If parents were unstable and inconsistent—punishing today behavior they permitted yesterday—your grandchildren may see rules as flexible and changeable. Children who had free reign with their parents may have learned that they can do as they please. They may not think your rules apply to them and may resent your attempts to impose structure on their lives. They will test and retest the limits you set for them, beyond the point where other children would give up. Because these grandchildren struggle with profound feelings of rejection, abandonment, and poor self-esteem, they will also test how far they can go before you, too, reject them. They will push you away before you push them away.

Your grandchildren also have a stronger arsenal than most kids in the "I'm so unhappy; just do it my way" phase of childhood. While the reality of being neglected, abandoned, or abused is tragically painful, it may also be used as a means of manipulating adults. Every child cries "I want my mommy" when someone else—even Daddy—sets limits. (And if Mommy sets limits, "I want my daddy" might do just fine.) But it's a whole new ball of wax when it's a grandchild raised by grandparents. When Mommy might be in jail, on the streets, or even dead, a plaintive "I want my mommy" can just about kill Grandma, and she usually melts.

Don't underestimate the intelligence of children, particularly these kids. Many of them have picked up traits and characteristics from parents who are equally manipulative—addicts are the greatest con artists in the world—but most of these children are smart enough to push your buttons. They play for sympathy. They get Grandma and Grandpa fighting and take advantage of that. They tell their tragic stories to teachers, counselors, and peers as justification for poor behavior or as a means to get their way. When Kevin was in school, he once tried to get himself out of trouble by telling the teacher his mom had died. I think he believed he wouldn't have to be responsible for his behavior if he came up with something tragic.

Meanwhile, you start the game with your defenses weakened. Your grief at the situation, the split in your identity between grandparent and parent, your need to nurture these children and show them they are loved—all these factors make you vulnerable to manipulative behavior. There is, after all, a fine line between being a doting grandparent and a second-time parent with a need to discipline. Often you slip from one role to another almost without noticing it, and the kids know how to get you to do just that.

▪ HOW TO COPE

▪ *Set a clear, daily routine.* Children need consistency, particularly children who have suffered from loss and uncertainty. Try to make some aspects of your daily life predictable. Have clear expectations for each day, and warn your grandchildren about any expected changes. Recognize that change may trigger a repeat of unwanted behavior.

▪ *Offer positive choices.* Build regular choices into your grandchild's life. Allow him to have control over which book he reads at night, what stuffed animal he takes to bed, whether he eats his peas or potatoes first at dinner, whether he wears the blue pants or the green ones to school. Let him make decisions about things that don't matter to you or between two equally acceptable choices. Making decisions will give your grandchild a sense of control and may spare him from needing to seek power in negative ways.

▪ *State rules in the positive.* Whenever possible, tell your grandchildren what you want them to do instead of what you don't want them to do. You don't want to sound like you're constantly criticizing. If children follow positive rules, they feel they are accomplishing something, instead of simply succeeding in avoiding punishment.

▪ *Set limits and stick to them.* Children need firm, consistent limits. As much as they resist them, limits give children a sense of security and help them know what the expectations are in the world around them.

▪ *Present a united front.* Divide and conquer is a classic military maneuver, but kids seem to have an instinct for it. Your grandchildren know whom to go to for whatever they want, and they will play one grandparent against the other to get it. Try to make parenting decisions with your spouse, and stick to them. Otherwise, your grandchild may "win," and your marriage may suffer.

▪ *Learn to recognize manipulation.* One of the biggest problems in handling manipulative behavior is recognizing it, particularly in such troubled children. These children are surviving enormous tragedies, and yet some are arch manipulators. How do you know whether your grandchild is really missing her mother right now or just trying to stay up for another hour (or both, as is often the case)? You will need to rely on your instincts, the advice of counselors, and how well you know this child. Consider these factors: the timing of the outburst, the age of the child, and the child's level of sophistication. Put yourself in the child's place. Why is she doing this? If you have just refused to give the child a candy bar or it is bedtime, she may be trying to push your buttons. It's different when a child scrapes a knee and can't stop crying because Mom, who is no longer here, was most nurturing at such a time.

▪ *Separate feelings and actions.* Whether a child's tears or bid for sympathy stem from manipulation, emotional turmoil, or a combination of the two, there is one important thing to keep in mind: Feelings and behavior are not the same. It is important to reassure your grandchild that all his feelings are valid. He has a right to be sad or mad or upset. But, you can explain, feelings are not an excuse for not following directions or doing what is expected of him. You can certainly say, "I understand that you miss your mom. I miss her, too, and we'll discuss that in a few minutes, but it doesn't mean you're not going to bed on time." Likewise, children will say "You don't love me" as a way of diverting a situation. If it's time to make your bed: "You don't love me." If it's time to go to school: "You don't love me." "That's not the issue," you can tell them. "The issue is that you have to make your bed now because we're getting ready to go to school." Of course, always reassure your grandchildren that you love them. Children can't hear "I love you" too much. They just can't use it to get their own way.

▪ *Try to stay calm.* Sometimes children will push every single button you have, and you won't feel like being nurturing or loving. If you can, stay cool and collected. If you let your grandchildren realize they can get to you, you lose. Once they know they can shake you, it will be an uphill battle to regain control. Also, your grandchildren look to you for security and a sense of order. If you lose your temper, you may just confirm their conviction that all adults, like their parents, are out of control. This doesn't mean that you can't admit fear or sadness or anger, but children need to know that they can trust your stability.

OVERCOMPENSATION

Henrietta Casper has a problem. Her 15-year-old grandson is defiant and disrespectful. When she tells him he can't go out at night, he just walks out the door. Her husband would set firmer rules, but Henrietta can't stick to them. She promised her daughter on her deathbed that she would always care for Adam, and she can't find it in herself even to withhold privileges from the boy. Henrietta is falling into a classic grandparenting trap: overcompensation. She is trying to make up for the pain and the loss her grandchild has suffered by attempting to make him happy every moment, in other words, by always giving him what he wants.

It's an easy trap to fall into. Up until now you have been a grandparent and only a grandparent. You could dote, pamper, spoil, and comfort to your heart's content. It is hard to realize that you are now a surrogate parent and must also discipline and educate your grandchildren. It can take time for this new reality to sink in. Some grandparents can spend years caught between roles; they stay indulgent grandparents, rarely letting a day go by without buying something, however small, for their grandchildren. Then they don't understand why they can't get respect as parents. If you let your grandchildren have french fries and ice cream for breakfast, as one grandma did, it's hard to make them eat vegetables at dinner. You can't spoil them and educate them at the same time; you only send them mixed messages.

Grandparents who overcompensate do so materially and emotionally. Not only do they try to soothe their grandchildren with presents and surprises, but they overlook setting limits. They make allowances they never would have made with their own children. For instance, one day my mother told Kevin that he couldn't watch television until he made his bed. An hour later, I found Kevin in front of the television, and my mother was making his bed. She never would have done that with us.

It is important to realize that overcompensation doesn't help a child in the long run. No matter how much you do for your grandchildren, you cannot remove the pain, repair the loss, or fill the void that is inside them. The world has taken away more than you can put back. Nor do you do your grandchildren any favors by giving in. Children need limits to know they are loved and to develop a sense of who they are. All overcompensating does is teach them to expect permissiveness; it lets them feel that the world owes them things and that they don't have to behave or work to have them. Your grandchildren need to deal with their losses in the best way they can, with support and guidance from you and the other adults in their lives. They need a combination of nurturing and discipline, and they need consistency in both. They need to know that you will do what you say you will do, even when they may not like the outcome.

You can't make up for your grandchildren's past, but with time and patience you can build a foundation of trust, love, and security in the present. Real parenting doesn't bring the immediate smiles and laughter that presents do—sometimes it brings sour looks and loud complaints —but remember that you are doing more than making your grandchildren happy in the moment. You are giving these children the necessary tools to grow and build their futures.

PARENTING 101

Beth Grafton had already raised seven children of her own, so she was insulted when the judge who granted her custody of her grandchildren sent her and her husband to parenting classes. He was, she discovered, a prudent man. "We have been sentenced back 30 to 40 years in time," says Beth when she talks about parenting today. "We have to go back to our skills of the '50s . . . in the '90s!" And, she discovered, those years do make a difference. Grandparents who become surrogate parents are often ill equipped for the job. Childrearing has changed since you raised your own children, as has the society in which you raised them. Like Beth, you may find yourself trying to use '50s skills on children of the '90s, many of whom seem to know more than their grandparents.

Children have changed. Through television and other media, this generation knows more about sex, violence, and the world around them and at an earlier age than their parents did. And if your grandchildren came from a drug-using or abusive home, they may know even more about the adult world than other kids their age. The threats of drugs, gangs, and AIDS, combined with peer pressure, create additional parenting problems you weren't faced with 30 or 40 years ago.

Standards have also changed. Many disciplinary actions you may have used in the past are no longer accepted as parenting techniques. In fact, some are considered abusive. Francis Morgan, like many parents of the old school, used a belt to discipline her own children when they were small; today that could be grounds for removing a child from her home.

Some grandparents are shy of parenting. They feel they made mistakes with their own children and don't want to repeat them with their grandchildren. Others have been away from childrearing so long that they have forgotten how kids behave. They don't have a clear perspective on what is acceptable behavior and what should be disciplined.

Like Beth Grafton's judge, I recommend that grandparents look into parenting classes. You will find them offered through child guidance clinics, family service agencies, hospitals, and even local colleges. It's not that you are necessarily doing anything wrong with your grandchildren, but parenting classes can teach you new methods for helping them learn responsibility, accountability, confidence, and self-esteem.

Grandparent support groups are also a good resource. Grandparents who have taken classes are often happy to share their new knowledge with others in the group, and you may hear techniques you haven't tried. Perhaps your group could persuade a child psychologist to hold a parenting seminar specifically for grandparents.

If you don't have access to groups or classes, you can avail yourself of the good parenting books on the market. Moreover, popular magazines like *Parenting* and *Working Mother* regularly run articles about common childrearing problems and innovative solutions.

What follows is a brief list of the principles and techniques that might be taught today in Parenting 101:

▪ *Beware of physical punishment.* There is a fine line between discipline and abuse in handling children, a fine line between evoking respect and fear. Today, hitting a child with anything other than a hand on clothing may be construed as child abuse. I don't ever advocate spanking children. When you hit children, you teach them that anger and aggression are acceptable ways to solve problems. You teach fear instead of respect. It is much better for children to learn that actions have consequences. That kind of lesson lays the groundwork for better decision making as they grow older.

▪ *Reinforce good behavior.* Your grandchildren know that bad behavior will get your attention. And that is often what they want, regardless of how they get it. Therefore, the best way to create good behavior is to *pay attention to it*—with praise and rewards. Try to catch your grandchildren in the act of being good. Be specific in your praise; let them know exactly what behavior you like. Tell them that you see they are making an effort. Behavior charts and chore charts let children keep track of the good things they've done and give them a way to measure their progress toward a reward: an allowance, an ice-cream cone, a special day at the park with Grandpa.

▪ *Try time-out.* If your grandchild does misbehave, one of the more popular techniques in modern parenting is the use of a time-out. This resembles the old scenario of a child sitting in a corner, but it is meant more as a calming technique than as a punishment.

Time-out involves removing a disruptive child from the situation in which he is misbehaving and giving him time to cool off. It doesn't have to be a long time, just long enough to give him time to think about his actions. The actual amount of time will depend on the age of the child—more than two minutes is an eternity for a two-year-old, for example—but use a timer so that he knows that the length of time is not arbitrary. When the child returns to the situation, make sure he understands which behavior warranted the time-out. Communication is important in any discipline technique.

▪ *Make your consequences logical and appropriate.* The goal of discipline is to teach children to regulate themselves, to make them responsible for their actions. Discipline works best when you can link the punishment to the behavior. If a child throws food on the wall, she must clean it up (even if you have to do it again after she goes go to bed). If she insists on wearing shoes that are too small, let her wear them. If they hurt, she won't wear them tomorrow. Of course, allowing children to learn from their own mistakes doesn't apply in situations that affect their safety or anyone else's.

▪ *Make consequences immediate.* Children, particularly young ones, have short memories and a poor sense of time. They may not remember why they can't watch television tonight if they are being disciplined for something they did in the morning. Try to make consequences as immediate as possible; it makes them more effective and teaches the concept of cause and effect.

▪ *Reinforce cause and effect.* Children also have short attention spans. For any punishment or discipline to be effective, the child must connect the cause and the effect. For instance, if you give Susie a time-out for throwing sand in her brother's face, she may need help connecting the two events. Therefore, ask her at the end of the time-out why it was used. If she can say, "Because I threw sand at Tommy instead of using my words," she will not only remember why she was disciplined but will learn responsibility for her actions. The same principle applies with older children when you take away phone or bicycle privileges.

▪ *Teach responsibility.* Children do many things to test your reactions; they also do things they don't know are wrong. Sometimes it's worth letting one misbehavior go in order to teach responsibility. For instance, if John throws food at the wall, it doesn't hurt to give him another chance, provided he understands that if he does it again, he won't get to finish dinner, he'll have to clean up the mess, or he'll have a time-out. If again he throws food at the wall, he does it knowing what will happen. Again, discipline involves teaching children to regulate themselves; that means letting them make choices and take responsibility for the consequences.

▪ *Don't make empty threats.* It is never a good idea to threaten children; simply teach them that there are consequences to their behavior. If Joan doesn't do her chores, she can't watch television. If Mark hits his brother, he may have to spend time alone in his room. But make sure that the consequences are those that you, as the voice of authority, can follow through with. Grandparents have a particularly hard time setting limits and holding to them. You feel bad, you want to be nice, you give in. Thus, you end up teaching the children that they can get whatever they want if they make you feel bad. "No television for a month" is a great threat—but an empty one if you can't keep it. Withhold television privileges for the week, or even the night, and the children will learn that their actions have consequences. (Besides, if you do ban television for a month, you may be punishing yourself as well.)

▪ *Pick your battles.* Not every misbehavior is cause for confrontation. Some things can be calmly diverted and others simply ignored. If Mary Anne is writing on the table, try giving her paper first. The problem may stop there. Did Todd leave the room cursing under his breath because you turned off the television? Try letting it go. If he is disrespectful to your face, you need to deal with it, but he is entitled to feel unhappy and resentful and to express his feelings to himself. If you make each and every improper action into a crisis, you'll only squander your energy and foster a terrible relationship with your grandchild. Weigh the pros and cons before you make an issue of something. Ask yourself, "What do I expect to gain and what do I want the child to learn from this?" Then pick your battles accordingly.

THE HYPERACTIVE GRANDCHILD

Jewell Baxter's grandsons are three and four years old, and they are out of control. They have put silverware down the toilet and painted the walls with toothpaste. They urinated in the furnace and flooded the kitchen floor when Grandpa fell asleep (the floor alone cost Jewell $750 to fix). "You can't leave them alone a second," she says. "You just can't fall asleep!" If Emily Petersen turns around for a second, four-year-old Amanda is down under the house or up in the attic. Emily isn't physically able to crawl around looking for her when she disappears and is terrified that the little girl will get seriously hurt. Six-year old Gregory can barely control himself in school. He is a smart child, but he cannot sit still long enough to complete his assignments. Now he has begun to kick and beat up other children. Even in GAP meetings he bounces off walls. "I'm going to hang that little boy!" says his grandmother in frustration.

Sound familiar? Then you could very well have a hyperactive child on your hands.

A large percentage of the grandchildren I see and hear about are hyperactive, part of a condition called *attention-deficit/hyperactivity disorder*, or ADHD (it's called *attention deficit disorder*, or ADD, when there is no hyperactivity involved).[4] ADHD affects up to five percent of children under 18, or approximately 1 in 20 kids.[5] *Time* magazine calls it "the most common behavior disorder in American children."[6] ADHD is believed to be a neurological condition caused by heredity, medical problems, or prenatal exposure to drugs and alcohol. The result is difficulty with attention, concentration, impulsiveness, and self-control.

Simply put, children with ADHD have trouble concentrating, completing a task, sitting still, and focusing. They are easily distracted, are disruptive, and may have poor relationships with other children. They have little impulse control, acting before they think about the consequences of their behavior. They may get themselves into dangerous situations and not know why or how they happened. They require constant supervision, which can be exhausting for grandparents who may not have the energy or patience they once had.

Children with ADHD may be bright and yet do poorly in school, which can lead to their believing they are failures or bad kids. Poor self-image and low self-esteem are deep issues with these children. They don't mean to drive you crazy; their bodies just seem to move faster than their brains. One little girl came crying to her grandmother after acting up in school one day. "I don't know why I did those things," she said. "I don't know what happens to me, because I didn't want to do them."

Of course, not every child who gets into trouble in school or has difficulty concentrating is hyperactive. Some children appear to be hyperactive when the problem is really an emotional disturbance or a learning disability. Sometimes a child can experience a combination of the three. On the other hand, many children with ADHD are not hyperactive but may still exhibit difficulties with attention and/or impulsive behavior (they are diagnosed as having ADD). As with any disability, the various symptoms of ADHD and ADD may range from mild to severe, depending on the individual child and even the specific situation (i.e., some children may exhibit more problems in school or social settings than at home).

If you suspect your grandchild has ADHD or ADD, have him or her evaluated by a well-trained professional—a child psychologist, child psychiatrist, or a pediatrician who has training and experience in this area. There is no simple test for ADHD; a true diagnosis is pieced together, like a puzzle, from a variety of elements, including family and medical histories, a physical exam, psychological testing, screening for learning disabilities, and interviews with the child's caregivers and teachers. You can start the evaluation process through the school or community mental health clinic; some states provide early intervention services for children as young as one or two years old (see Chapter 13). You can also have your grandchild assessed by a private doctor. Mental health clinics and parent or grandparent support groups are good sources of referrals. If your grandchild is positively diagnosed with ADHD (or ADD), he or she should be referred to a child psychiatrist or psychologist for treatment, which should include counseling and may involve medication.

Medication for ADHD

ADHD is a complex disorder. It is not easy to diagnose, and there are some disagreements about how to treat it. Perhaps one of the main issues under debate is the use of psychoactive drugs like Ritalin, a psychostimulant medication that is prescribed by doctors as treatment for clinically diagnosed hyperactive children. Other drugs that are commonly prescribed include Dexedrine and Cylert. Although these drugs are stimulants, they seem to have a calming effect on children with ADHD.

Proponents of Ritalin applaud its effectiveness in reducing restlessness and impulsive behavior and thus helping a child concentrate and focus. Properly prescribed, drugs like Ritalin have allowed a calmer existence for hyperactive children, their families, friends, and teachers and have enabled these children to improve their school and social performance and feel better about themselves.

Critics, however, feel that doctors may be overmedicating children and are concerned about the drug's side effects, which can range from moodiness and insomnia to abnormally rapid heartbeats, nervousness, and lack of appetite. Meanwhile, parents—and grandparents—of children with ADHD must work with their doctors to make informed decisions based on the individual child and his or her particular needs.

I am not, in general, an advocate of medicating children, but I have seen hyperactive kids do a complete turnaround with the right prescription and dosage. In fact, many people compare the effects of Ritalin to putting glasses on a nearsighted person; glasses don't change the physical makeup of the eye, but they do let everything come into focus. Like glasses, drugs like Ritalin can be a tool, not a

---

Could Your Grandchild Have ADHD?

If a number of the following symptoms describe your grandchild, particularly if they started before age seven, and if they have lasted at least six months, you may have reason to suspect ADHD or ADD. However, a definite diagnosis requires a full examination by a qualified doctor.[7]

- Has difficulty concentrating
- Shifts excessively from one activity to another
- Often does not seem to listen
- Has difficulty following instructions
- Often fails to finish things he or she starts
- Has difficulty organizing
- Often loses things
- Is easily distracted
- Is frequently forgetful
- Fidgets or squirms excessively
- Has difficulty staying seated
- Has difficulty playing quietly
- Often blurts out answers to questions
- Often acts before thinking
- Often talks excessively
- Has difficulty waiting
- Often engages in dangerous activities

solution. However, finding the right medication and the proper dosage may take trial and error and patience. And not every child responds well to medication.

Talk to your grandchild's doctor carefully. Ask lots of questions. Consider all your options. Above all, if you do decide to use medication, make sure your grandchild is closely monitored by doctors on a regular basis. Look for any changes or reactions to the drugs. Try to involve teachers in the monitoring process as well; they will notice changes in school that you might not see at home. Make sure the treatment program is a well-rounded one. Medication alone will not cause long term changes. Nor will it cure depression or anxiety. Your grandchild also needs a combination of therapy and behavior modification to internalize and learn to use new behaviors.

WHEN YOUR GRANDCHILD NEEDS THERAPY

My own feeling is that most children who are taken in by grandparents could use some kind of counseling to handle the adjustment. Most could benefit from therapy, even as a preventive measure. Groups are great because each child realizes that he or she is not the only one with disturbing feelings. Most of these kids have such terrible self-esteem that even short-term therapy can help them understand that none of this is their fault. Children who act out their frustrations will often come to the attention of the school, which may then refer them to counseling. Unfortunately, the children who don't act out—the quiet ones or the good students—may slip through the cracks.

Does your grandchild need therapy? Counseling is especially important if any of the following statements describe your grandchild.

- The child has been physically or sexually abused.
- The child begins to remember past abuse. Sometimes you know the child was abused; sometimes this information only becomes available when something triggers the memories and a flood of painful emotions is released.
- The child seems depressed, particularly if he or she has been abused. (Remember, even very young children get depressed; observe your grandchild closely.)
- The child has been exhibiting behavioral, psychological, emotional, medical, or academic problems for a noticeable or prolonged period of time.

- The child is experiencing extreme fear or extreme anger.
- The child is sexually acting out.
- The child is constantly fighting or exhibits cruel behavior. (Often, kids who have been abused will then abuse their siblings, peers, and pets.)
- The child exhibits a combination of bed-wetting, fire-setting, and cruelty to animals.
- The child becomes self-destructive, talks about hurting himself or shows hints of wanting to die. People think young children don't think about wanting to die, but they do. The danger signs include any potentially self-destructive behavior, from walking out in front of cars to expressing thoughts of feeling unloved or saying, "I wish I weren't here." A child who lives with you because of a death may talk about wanting to be with Mom or Dad in heaven. Behavior like this is always a cry for help. Even if your grandchild uses it as a tool to manipulate you—and if he knows it gets to you, he could use it that way—it still masks deeper issues and needs to be dealt with in counseling.

RESIDENTIAL PLACEMENT

Seven-year-old Matthew had witnessed the murder of his father by his mother and was becoming dangerously aggressive in school and at home; on one occasion he tried to smother his younger sister. Nine-year-old Jesse had been physically and sexually abused before he came to live with his grandparents; he later started to act out sexually with his younger siblings. Sally, 10, is rebellious. She refuses to listen to her grandmother and repeatedly disappears from school and home. One night she cut the window screen and slipped out of the house with her grandmother's car keys, which she gave to a stranger who then stole the car; she didn't reappear until 1:00 A.M. and would not say where she had been. Six-year-old Nicholas is destructive. He tears plaster off walls and throws things at his grandmother. He was born with drugs in his system and is severely hyperactive. He, too, would sneak out of the house at night for hours.

Unfortunately, some children need more help than a grandparent can give them. They lack the ability to express their pain in words, and their actions put them and others in jeopardy. Some, like Matthew and Jesse, have experienced such deep trauma that they cannot control their behavior. Others, like Nicholas, are driven by chemical and neurological problems. Medication for hyperactivity, weekly outpatient therapy, and a grandma's love are not enough for these children. They need the more intense therapy that a residential program can offer.

A residential program is a live-in facility where children can receive round-the-clock professional care. A social worker or school psychologist often makes the recommendation to place a child in residential treatment, but grandparents can also request placement through the proper channels. Sally's grandmother, for instance, called child protective services and told them that her granddaughter was placing herself in danger and that she, as an ailing 80-year-old, could no longer handle her. Matthew, on the other hand, was placed through the department of mental health, after a school evaluation found him to be severely emotionally disturbed.

Children who are placed through child protective services or social services become dependents of the court, and their grandparents lose control over what happens to them. This is not so for children, like Matthew, who enter residential facilities through other channels; their grandparents may retain some control over their welfare even while they are in placement.

Giving up your grandchild to a treatment center is not an easy decision to make. It practically tore Nicholas's grandmother apart. "I look at Nicholas sleeping, and I cry," she admits. "But he is getting bad. Nicholas cannot help himself, and I don't have the knowledge to help him help himself." Nor is placement always a grandparent's decision. Sometimes grandparents don't recognize that they can't provide the home or guidance a severely disturbed child needs; in these cases the social worker may recommend placement over the grandparent's objections.

Placement, for any child, is an absolute last resort. No grandparent wants to put a grandchild in a facility, but if you have done everything in your power to help a child, and if she needs more than you can provide or is a danger to herself and others, residential placement may be your only choice. It doesn't mean that you don't love your grandchild or that you are abandoning her. You can still maintain contact through letters, phone calls, and visits. What it does mean is that you are giving the child her best chance to become a healthy, happy, productive adult.

GRATITUDE VERSUS GROWTH

Children are very self-centered; they have a tough time looking outside themselves. This is particularly true of children who have suffered loss. You may want them to be grateful for your hard work and sacrifices, but it is unreasonable to expect gratitude from a child who has been traumatized and who is angry about the situation. As adults they might look back and appreciate what you did for them, but right now they are just getting by.

It's ironic that the better the job you do parenting your grandchildren, the more likely you are to be taken for granted. Don't let it upset you. It means that your grandchildren have come to expect your love and attention and that it is not a rare treat in their lives. Take heart, instead, at the good you are doing.

Many grandchildren thrive under their grandparents' care—even those who were abandoned or abused. In fact, a 1992 study of 51 grandchildren being raised by grandparents found that the majority were making normal adjustments after living in their grandparents' home for an average of four years. A smaller follow-up study two years later surveyed the grandchildren's teachers for a second opinion. The teachers agreed: The children were still adjusting well. Although both studies were limited to children whose grandparents live above the poverty level and already attend support groups, researcher Michael Jones, Ph.D., believes his results give hope to all kinds of grandparents. According to Jones, it is the quality of the grandparent–grandchild relationship that is most important in a grandchild's adjustment.[8] "These kids are at high risk for emotional problems," he told the *Orange County Register*. "The fact that they aren't suffering those problems shows how resilient kids are. And what a good job a lot of grandparents are doing raising grandchildren."[9]

CHAPTER 7

Your Grandchild and the School

The hardest thing about school was adjusting with my friends. I really didn't understand my situation—how could they understand it?
—*Kevin, age 19*

Jeffrey Campos, age six, has a hard time settling down to his studies. Alternately shutting down and acting out, easily stimulated and hyperactive, he can't function well in large classrooms. "Grandma, I can't stand the noise," he confesses when he comes home. "There's too much noise—people talking all the time!" The teachers say Jeffrey is intelligent, but he gets frustrated and overwhelmed. "For a while he didn't want to go to school at all," says his grandmother. "He thought he was stupid and couldn't do what the other kids were doing."

Heather Pierce, 10, has trouble reading; although she is in the fourth grade, she reads at a second grade level. She loves books but feels "dumb and stupid" because other children do so much better than she does. For their part, the other kids make fun of Heather.

Schoolwork is not a problem for five-year-old Bobby Franklin, but the classroom is. That is where he takes out most of his frustration, by acting out and fighting with other children. Generally, Bobby is an average kid in terms of behavior—sometimes he listens, sometimes he doesn't—but after he has had a visit with his mother, he becomes a minor terror in school.

School is rough for any kid. They get hassled about what they wear, they're expected to act a certain way, and they feel foolish if they're too different. And that's just with the other children. Strict teachers, rules and regulations, and the challenge of schoolwork itself can add new levels of stress to a child's life. But for a child being raised by grandparents, especially for a child with emotional or academic difficulties, school can be a minefield of problems, from social isolation to failing a grade.

BEING DIFFERENT: ODD CHILD OUT

Most children want to fit in, whether it is to the group playing hopscotch on the sidewalk or to the class on a school picnic. Children raised by grandparents suffer the stigma of being raised in a family that is different. And other children can be cruel about differences. Not only do they seem to have radar to seek them out, but their playground teasing can be merciless. Fourteen-year-old Tyler remembers attending a parochial school in Boston where everyone knew that he lived with his grandmother, that his mother was an addict, and that his father was dead. The teasing was mean. The other kids cursed his mother and called her foul names; they said that his father killed himself because of Tyler and that his mom took off because he was ugly. Tyler admits, "The part that got me was they said my mom left me because she didn't really want me."

Adults face peer pressure in the workplace, children find it in the school yard. Even innocent childhood jokes can take on different, and painful, meanings for children who are surviving a loss. "I'm a little more sensitive to certain things than most of my friends," says my nephew Kevin. "When I got to middle school, people would rag on each other, just with friends. It was nothing serious, but they would start telling momma jokes, and stuff like that. I would take it personally, even though I knew they were joking around." The same kind of jokes started at least one fight in high school. "I don't remember what the kid said," Kevin admits. "It didn't matter what he had said . . . just that he had said it."

Not only do your grandchild's peers make insensitive comments about the fact that you are older than their parents, but most school activities presume a parent–child relationship: from making Mother's and Father's Day cards to parent–teacher conferences. This can be troubling for the child who doesn't have a mother or doesn't know where she is.

BEHAVIOR PROBLEMS IN SCHOOL

All the emotional and behavioral problems your grandchildren experience at home may be exacerbated when they start school, and new ones may become apparent. Anxiety, fear of abandonment, and clingy behavior may take on new dimensions in a school setting. Your grandchildren face hours of not knowing where you are, how you are, and if you are coming back. Just taking them to school can be a trial if they are afraid you won't pick them up again. Some children even develop phantom health problems so you'll come and take them home.

Nor are school personnel always understanding. Ten-year-old Kirsten was tense and anxious after her grandmother had bypass surgery. Every time she heard an ambulance pass the school, she panicked. All day she asked if she could call home, just to make sure her grandma was fine, but the teachers refused her requests, believing that Kirsten was using the situation to manipulate them.

Anger, aggression, and inappropriate behavior may also find new outlets, and new triggers, in school. A little boy who has trouble with authority may defy his teachers. A little girl who is verbally or physically aggressive at home may hit or swear at other children. Your grandchildren may be bossy and have trouble making and keeping friends, which may only make them angrier. Many grandchildren only know how to get negative attention. They know how to push the buttons of their teachers and peers, just as they know how to push yours. They may get labeled as problem children, or acquire a reputation as poor students. They may skip school. Some may even fail and have to repeat grades.

On the other hand, withdrawn, depressed children may become introspective and shy at school. They seem to disappear in class. Their attitude is this: "If I sit in the back of the room and don't open my mouth, I won't get in trouble because they won't know I'm here." These children often get lost in the cracks. Loner kids may be viewed by teachers as a relief, as one less problem child to deal with. They may get good grades, but they may also slip by with Cs and Ds because they don't cause trouble; unfortunately, they may not learn anything, either.

New behavior problems in grandchildren may also appear in a classroom setting: difficulty following directions, difficulty playing with other children, difficulty waiting their turn. Many of the characteristics of attention-deficit/hyperactivity disorder (ADHD) and learning disabilities only come to the surface once a child starts school.

ADHD IN THE CLASSROOM AND SCHOOL YARD

As I mentioned in Chapter 6, many of the grandchildren I see and hear about have attention-deficit/hyperactivity disorder, which means they have trouble with attention and concentration; may be easily distracted, restless, or hyperactive; and are given to impulsive behavior. Although all children are inattentive, impulsive, and overly active from time to time, children with ADHD seem to be that way most of the time. For them such behavior is the rule, not the exception.

Children with ADHD face many challenges in school. They may have a hard time adapting to the classroom setting, performing their schoolwork, and acquiring the social skills necessary to make friends and play in groups. Children who have trouble with attention may have a hard time following directions or finishing projects. Long reading assignments and tests may be particularly difficult. If they are not hyperactive, they may be inattentive and underactive, appearing to daydream or wander off. They may be labeled "lazy" or "spacey" and accused of not trying. If they are hyperactive, they may be disruptive in class, constantly moving and unable to stay in their seats. Like Jeffrey Campos, they may be easily overstimulated and overwhelmed by a large, noisy classroom. If they are impulsive, they will act without thinking, calling out in class or blurting out answers before the questions are asked.

These traits may carry over to the playground, where children typically hone their social skills. A child with ADHD may interrupt other children's games or make jokes at the wrong moment. He may not be able to wait his turn, or he may frustrate easily and overreact. His behavior can lead to difficulty making friends, which can lower his self-esteem.

Each child with ADHD will demonstrate different symptoms and in different intensities, but the result will be a disorganized approach to learning and developing and a difficult time keeping pace with children his age. These children are not stupid. In fact, you may hear this remark from teachers: "Your grandchild! He is smart enough to do the work, if he would only *try*." It is not a question of intelligence but of attention and self-control. An informed teacher may recognize these behaviors as symptoms of ADHD. Unfortunately, an uninformed teacher may blame the child.

LEARNING DISABILITIES: THE INTERNAL STUMBLING BLOCKS

April Thomas was miserable in grade school. Reading assignments took forever, classes seemed to rush by too fast, and tests were a nightmare. She would look at words on the blackboard and not realize she was reading them backward. She would struggle with a book and come away with only bits and pieces of the story. She would listen to her teacher's instructions but not exactly understand what was required of her. Some teachers got impatient with her many questions, so she stopped asking. "I would sit in class and pretend I understood what the teacher was saying," April, now 20, recalls. "Most of the time I didn't, but I was too embarrassed to admit it."

Because she was a bright girl, April was accused of "playing dumb" and of not trying hard enough. She was actually trying very hard, but it was a struggle to understand the questions, let alone come up with answers. Eventually, April got frustrated and gave up. She didn't want to seem stupid, so she became rebellious, making wisecracks in class. And she fell further and further behind her peers.

In high school April was finally diagnosed with learning disabilities. She received a tutor, special classes, extended time to take tests and turn in papers, and other modifications. Today she is a sophomore in college. April has learned to compensate for her learning problems and to enlist the help of teachers and administrators when she needs more time for assignments or permission to tape a lecture. Still, she is shy about her disability. "It's extra embarrassing because it is an invisible disability," she says. "If I had one leg shorter than the other and couldn't run fast, it would be a reason that people could see."

People may not be able to see April's disabilities, but many other children would understand them. Approximately five to ten percent of people are affected by learning disabilities, and nearly five percent of all school-age children receive special education services to help them compensate for different problems.[1]

Children who have learning disabilities may experience problems with reading comprehension, spoken language, writing and spelling, arithmetic, reasoning, and organizational skills. They may also exhibit symptoms of ADHD. In fact, many learning disabled kids also have ADHD. Like children with ADHD, learning disabled children are not dumb. They do not lack intelligence or a desire to learn. They have a problem with how they interpret outside information, a deficit in the psychological mechanisms that process selective visual, auditory, or tactile data. Learning disabilities must not be confused with problems due to mental retardation, serious emotional disturbance, or sensory deficits like blindness or deafness, which fall into other categories of disabilities.

Just because your grandchild has trouble with math or spelling, however, does not mean she has a learning disability. Many people experience learning *difficulties*—certain subjects they don't take to easily; there are, for example, children who love reading but hate science or who just don't seem to have a head for numbers. However, if your grandchild's problems are so constant or severe that they disrupt her education or day-to-day activities (such as reading street signs or using the telephone) or if there is a significant gap between the child's academic potential and academic achievement that is not the result of environmental, cultural, or economic disadvantage, then you may suspect a learning disability.

MISSED SCHOOL DAYS AND OTHER EDUCATIONAL HAZARDS

Not every child who has problems in school has ADHD or a learning disability. Your grandson may be behind in school simply because he missed too many school days before he came to live with you. Perhaps he was constantly on the move and changing schools with his parents. Perhaps drugs were involved, and getting a child ready for school wasn't the parent's priority. Your grandchild could arrive at a new school a grade or two behind, unable to read, and convinced he is stupid. He may also resist your insistence on regular school attendance, since he never had to attend school regularly before. Here, again, routine and consistency may start to correct the problem.

Another reason a child may do badly is worry. Your granddaughter may display a lack of attention in class because she is thinking about her parents and her circumstances. It can be difficult to complete class assignments, even to listen to the teacher, when a child feels the weight of the world on her shoulders.

Of course, difficulty with schoolwork could also be an indicator of a medical problem. Maybe Tommy does badly in school because he can't see the blackboard or has trouble hearing the teacher. Glasses or a hearing aid could be the answer.

■ HOW TO COPE

• *Talk to the teachers.* Whether your grandchild is hyperactive, acting out, or grieving, I recommend creating open lines of communication with the school. Talk to the teachers, counselors, and the principal; give them insight into your situation. Let them know that if your granddaughter misbehaves when she comes to class on Monday, there may be a reason. Explain that if she had a visit with a parent on the weekend, she is probably reeling with emotions, not simply being obnoxious. Often teachers are more understanding if they know there is an explanation behind a child's problem behavior.

If his teacher understands that Johnny lives with his grandparents and doesn't know where his mother is, she might be more sensitive to his reaction to making a Mother's Day card in class. Maybe she'll have the children make cards for "someone who is special" instead, since not all children live with their mothers or fathers. Having a teacher recognize such a circumstance may give it authority in a child's eyes, and that recognition may soften the stigma of not having a parent to make a card for. The nuclear family of a mom, a dad and their child is something we can no longer take for granted. Sensitive teachers, being aware of this, have learned to reference grandparents, aunts, uncles, foster parents, and adoptive parents in their lessons or comments about family, family events, and family history.

Your grandchild's teacher may also be your ally in identifying symptoms of ADHD or a learning disability, since some traits may only appear once a child is in school. If you suspect that your grandchild has a developmental or learning problem, share your concerns with the teachers and start to compare notes. If your grandchild does have ADHD or a learning disability, ask what you can do at home to help the child progress.

Of course, many teachers are overwhelmed. They may have 40 kids in a small classroom, each with different problems, and might not be able to give out special help or consideration. Still, the more you can communicate with the teacher, principal, or school counselor, the more your grandchildren will learn about problem solving. If they are children of substance abusers, they have already learned a lot about running away from problems; this is a chance for them to learn that problems can also be worked out. I have on occasion recommended moving a child to a different classroom, but only as a last resort and never before exhausting all other possibilities.

▪ *Talk to the child.* Jeffrey's grandmother tries to reassure him before tests. "You know it," she tells him. "Just listen and think about what the teacher is asking you, and you're going to be fine. Just do the best you can; we can't ask for more than that." Heather's grandmother tries to keep her from comparing herself to other children. Your own attitudes about learning and the way you communicate them to your grandchildren can influence the way they approach the school experience.

Talk to your grandchildren. Help them emphasize and develop their strengths. Maybe your grandson has trouble with math but is good at basketball, singing, or drawing. Praise him for what he does well, and create opportunities for him to succeed. Every success will boost his self-esteem and encourage him to strive for more success. And teach him to understand his weaknesses. You can reassure him that everyone has some kind of difficulty and that there is no shame in asking for help. Remind him that everyone learns at a different pace and that having difficulty in a subject doesn't mean that he is stupid or dumb or bad. At the same time, don't be so easy on him that you give him permission to give up. His situation may create particular challenges for him in school, but it is not an excuse for him to stop trying. Tell him that he may have to work harder but that he can succeed. Encourage him to keep doing his best. Still, keep your own expectations realistic. If your grandson really does his best, you cannot ask for more.

▪ *Look into special education.* Just because some children are currently trailing behind the rest of the class does not mean they are doomed to stay behind. Free special education and related services are available to children who are somehow handicapped in the learning process. If there is a chronic problem that prevents your grandchild's schoolwork from matching her intellectual ability, whether it is a learning disability, severe emotional turmoil, or a physical handicap, the child should be eligible for special help through the school system. In fact, most states offer special services to disabled or potentially disabled children before they even enter the school system (see "Start Early," below).

The process of applying for special education will help you and your grandchild uncover the source of her academic troubles and, hopefully, find the solutions. Sometimes the solution is as simple as obtaining a hearing aid, therapy, or a tutor. It was discovered through testing that one little girl who was doing poorly in school was actually gifted; her poor grades were due to boredom and a lack of confidence.

If your grandchild is having consistent problems in school, try to address them as soon as possible. At least start documenting what you see, and if the situation continues to worsen, request an Individual Education Program, or IEP (see Chapter 13).

■ *Start early.* It is never too early to consider your grandchild's development and learning potential. Children who experience educational and developmental difficulties are often overlooked until they fall severely behind their classmates. By that time, their academic performance has already suffered and they may feel depressed, anxious, and inadequate about school.

You do not have to wait until your grandchild starts school to get the benefits of special education. Physical therapy, speech and language remediation, and other services are often available to children before they even enter kindergarten. Most states offer early intervention programs that are designed to address developmental problems in the preschool years, when children are typically most ready to learn—and at an incredible pace. These are preventive programs that assume that the earlier children get help, the more chance they have of succeeding later.

If you notice in your grandchild the absence of anything typical for a particular stage of a child's development or any delay in motor coordination, speech, or self-help skills like self-feeding—or if drug exposure or family history have you concerned that problems could develop—look into an early intervention program. Some states even provide services to infants and toddlers. (For more on early intervention, see Chapter 13.)

■ *Seek out peer activities.* There is more to a child's school years than simply sitting in a classroom. Extracurricular and recreational experiences are as important for developing social skills as a good education is for developing learning skills. Your grandchild may have taken on many caretaking responsibilities at an early age and may not know how to be just a kid. Scouting organizations, after-school clubs, summer camps, day camps and athletics provide opportunities for children to *play* with other children and learn to socialize, share, and take turns. Extracurricular activities involving sports, arts, and music also offer children who have academic problems a chance to discover other strengths and build a sense of self-esteem.

▪ *Find young role models.* Children, particularly those who don't have parents as role models, desperately need the influence of young adults. A younger person may have more energy and stamina than a grandparent. He or she may more clearly understand the choices and challenges a child faces growing up today than can older grandparents whose ideas may seem old-fashioned. My nephew Kevin often points out that his grandparents were "brought up in the old days, like in the time of World War II" (that can seem like ancient history to a child growing up in the '80s and '90s). Even kids who have youthful, active grandparents can benefit from the influence of younger adults.

Extended family can be a wonderful source of role models for a grandchild, and many grandparents successfully involve aunts and uncles in their grandchildren's lives. In my family, for example, my brother was the one who would play ball with our nephew Kevin and take him to sporting events. Beth Grafton's son and daughter-in-law take her grandchildren on vacations. However, not every grandchild has extended family members available. Some aunts and uncles may be caught up with their own families or may live far away, or they may disapprove of your raising the child and therefore keep their distance. Even if the parents were only children, you can still find young adults to interact with your grandchildren. Big Brother and Big Sister programs exist across the country to provide positive role models for children who need them. I know one little girl whose Big Sister continues to visit her even in a residential facility. Scouting programs, summer camps, and youth groups also bring together children and active young adults, as well as provide fun activities and new experiences for the children.

▪ *Aim high!* Don't let academic delays or learning disabilities stifle your hopes for your grandchildren. History is full of disabled people who succeeded in the face of tremendous challenges, and many people with learning disabilities have gone on to become scientists, lawyers, generals, even president. Consider the following examples:

> Albert Einstein didn't talk until he was four or read until he was nine; he couldn't learn math through traditional teaching

methods. His first teachers thought he was backward. Yet he grew up to win the Nobel Prize in physics and to revolutionize the way we think about space and time.

Young George Patton couldn't read or write by age 12. Still, he overcame his disabilities enough to be appointed to the U.S. Military Academy at West Point; he went on to become a general and led the Third Army in Europe during World War II.

Woodrow Wilson had learning problems as a boy. He was 8 years old before he learned his letters and 11 by the time he learned to read. His relatives considered him "dull and backwards." The only school subject he excelled in was speech. Yet he grew up to become the 28th president of the United States.[2]

Is your grandchild a future Einstein, Patton, or Woodrow Wilson? No one can really say. One of the wonders with children is that we don't know what they may become. So help them aim high. The possibilities are all ahead of them.

CHAPTER 8 | # The Drug Epidemic at Home

> Our young people—the young parents—are
> dead because so many of them are hooked on
> crack. The grandparents are trying to save the
> little ones before the same thing happens to
> them.
>
> *—Marin County social worker*[1]

J im and Fay Strassburger have watched an entire middle-class neighborhood lose child after
child to drugs. They can stand in their yard
and point to the houses. In one week in the early '70s, they attended
three funerals for kids who died of drug-related causes, bright kids
who knew the consequences of their actions. Their own son and
daughter are alive but struggling with drug and alcohol addiction; two
grandchildren live with Jim and Fay. "We've lost a whole generation,"
Jim told a reporter. "Maybe part of the next."[2]

Katherine Connor is raising five drug-exposed grandchildren, all
from the same daughter. She can frequently be seen doing her er-
rands with the infant tucked under her arm and the rest of the children
trailing after her like a line of small ducks. The mother is on the
streets and often violent. She once threw a brick through the kitchen
window, almost hitting her own son with a piece of broken glass.
When she was picked up by the police, she broke the windows and
the grill of the police car—that's how much violent strength she had
from PCP.

There is no question that we are in the midst of a national, even
an international, drug epidemic. The nightly news is full of stories
about local gangs, foreign drug lords, and the victims of drug-related

crime. But there are other victims: infants exposed to drugs before birth, young children abused and neglected by drug-abusing parents, and grandparents who turn their lives upside down to keep their families together. In the war against drugs, the front line is often at home.

Drug addiction and alcoholism are not new problems in our society. The 19th century had its morphine addicts.[3] Marijuana and LSD reached new levels of popularity in the 1960s,[4] and by the 1970s babies were being born exposed to heroin and PCP.[5] But in the mid-1980s the smokable form of cocaine powder, known as crack, first appeared in the United States, and America's drug problems intensified.[6]

Crack is a relatively cheap, fast high that is more addictive than heroin or cocaine used nasally. Unlike heroin and other drugs that have traditionally appealed mostly to men, crack is used increasingly by women,[7] many of whom are pregnant or of childbearing age. According to *Time* magazine, crack has "lured far more women into addiction than any other hard drug has."[8] It has also triggered the use of other drugs: heroin, to prolong the cocaine high, and tranquilizers and alcohol, to "come down." The result is a growing population of young people addicted to multiple drugs and infants exposed to a wide variety of drugs in the womb. Crack is also a mean drug, inducing many parents to violence. There has been a dramatic rise in reports of child abuse and neglect since the 1980s, the majority of them traceable to parental drug and alcohol addiction. In one five-year period, child abuse reports tripled in the state of Wisconsin alone.[9]

The rise of AIDS has added another frightening dimension to the drug epidemic. "AIDS is now the largest killer among young women [here]," said an East Coast health official. "We may not have to worry about [crack baby] mothers; they'll all be dead."[10]

Meanwhile, the next drug crisis has already arrived in the form of "crank" or "ice." Crank is a metamphetamine derivative that speeds up the nervous system.[11] It is more expensive than crack, but it offers its users a longer high. It is also known to produce extensive fetal damage.

These facts read like horror stories, particularly to grandparents who helplessly watch their sons and daughters sink into the terrifying reality of addiction and then try to pick up the pieces of their families. For these grandparents home is the battleground against an enemy they barely understand, and the only weapons they have are love and knowledge.

This chapter looks at some of the things you need to know in your own private war on drugs: the truth about addicts and addiction; the symptoms, risks, and needs of drug-exposed children; and suggestions for stopping the cycle of addiction in your grandchildren. Appendix A includes a list of organizations that can provide more detailed information and guidance. Remember, this is a difficult fight, and addiction is a fierce enemy; you can only take each day, and each battle, as it comes.

ABOUT THE ADDICT

There is no way to count how many addicts there are in this country. Some statistics say that 20 million Americans have tried cocaine at least once, that 5 million use it on a regular basis,[12] and that six times as many people abuse alcohol as use cocaine.[13] But those numbers don't necessarily account for the people who regularly use and abuse marijuana, heroin, PCP, or even legal prescription drugs. It probably doesn't matter. For a family struggling with the effects of addiction, even one addict is one too many.

I know grandparents who have spent thousands of dollars and all their energy trying to get their adult children into rehabilitation programs only to see them relapse and return to the streets. They witness the thoughtless abuse and neglect of their grandchildren and are often helpless to protect them. They spend sleepless nights asking the questions: "Where is my child?" "When will he recover?" "Doesn't she see what she's doing to us, to her children, to herself?" "How can we help him?" "Where did we go wrong?" If your adult child is an addict, these questions are probably not strangers to you. But before you can really answer them, you must first understand what addiction is and what it does to the addict.

What Addiction Is

Chemical dependency is not a moral weakness, bad habit, mental illness, or sign of weak character.[14] It is not a result of life's pressures or a temporary loss of control. Addiction is a disease characterized by a mental and physical dependence on a chemical substance. A person becomes chemically dependent, or addicted, when he or she develops a craving for a substance as a shortcut to feeling pleasure or avoiding pain, including the pain or discomfort of not using the substance itself.

Like many diseases, addiction is chronic, that is, it is constant and long-lasting. Addiction is also progressive in that it gets worse and worse over time, requiring more and more of the substance to achieve the good feelings and prevent the bad ones. And, for some addicts, it can be fatal.

High hopes, good intentions, and promises will not cure the disease of addiction. Intense rehabilitation, strong support, and—for some addicts—medical attention are necessary to bring an addiction under control. Few addictions are truly "cured."

What Addiction Does

Addiction takes over the addict's priorities and makes his behavior unpredictable. The high that originally seduced him gets harder and harder to achieve. It becomes the most important thing in his life—more important than family, friends, work, food, sex, anything. An addict may spend every waking hour trying to get or stay high. The disease can lie to him, making him forget the bad things that happen—the lows, the pain of withdrawal, the effects on his family. As one drug counselor put it, "If there are drugs behind you, your own son will run you over to get to them."[15] One social worker compared counseling an addict to "beating your head against a brick wall . . . because you are dealing with someone who has no control over her life. She's worried about her next hit."[16] Some young mothers have sold their baby's milk and diapers for drug money. Others sell their bodies, supporting their drug habit by becoming street prostitutes. As one former addict explained to a U.S. Senate committee, "Even though I wanted to quit, my need for the cocaine was greater than my maternal instinct."[17]

Addiction can also stunt a person's development. Pam Marshall sees it in her daughter. "It's frightening what it does to them," she says. "Once they start using the drug, they stop growing intellectually. Linda started using at 13, and her mind is still like a 13-year-old's. It's like she lost all the years in between." Another grandmother describes her adult son as "24 going on 14."

The behavior of an addict is controlled by drugs and alcohol. His behavior doesn't mean that your son doesn't love his children; her actions don't mean that your daughter is trying to hurt you. If your adult child doesn't seem at all like the child you raised, she probably isn't: drugs and alcohol have taken over her life.

▪ WHAT YOU NEED TO KNOW

▪ *It's not your fault.* Pam Marshall remembers trying to explain her daughter's addiction to herself. "It was my fault," she says. "It was her father's fault. It was her peers' fault. You blame everyone and everything except the person herself. You look for excuses. You look back and try to figure out what happened, when it happened, how it happened . . . and you don't have any answers." There is no one answer for why a person drinks or takes drugs or why one person will become an addict and another one will not. But you are not to blame. You could raise four children and have only one of them turn to drugs. You could be an alcoholic yourself yet raise a family of staunch nondrinkers. Though you may never have touched a drop of wine, your child may be an alcoholic. We each make our own choices in life. Your children made theirs.

▪ *There is little you can do to help.* One of the most frustrating things for parents to accept is the fact that there is nothing they can do to *cure* their child of a drug or alcohol addiction. Remember, an addiction is a disease. You can't make it go away. Nor can you make your addicted child seek help. Certainly, you can drive your child to a treatment center or support group, but he is the one who must enter, stay, and participate. Too many parents pay for treatment after treatment when they are the ones who are motivated, not the addict.

If you want to facilitate treatment for your adult child, you can give her a list of programs in your area. You can watch her children while she is in rehabilitation. But if she is not ready to make her own appointment and show up for treatment, then it will only be an exercise in futility. The addict must be the one to recognize the problem and commit to seeking help.

All you can do is protect yourself and your grandchildren and try not to give in to your adult child's pleas and demands. An addict will use you, and you have to understand that. If you give addicted child money, you finance his habit. You have to be strong enough both to love your child and to refuse him. It is the old rule of tough love (for more on tough love, see Chapter 5).

• *Recovery can be painfully slow.* Recovery from an alcohol or drug addiction is a long, complex process with no guaranteed results. Many people don't complete treatment programs, and the relapse rate is high. Even when addicts successfully complete a program, they are still at risk for returning to old habits. And they often can't tell you what happened or why. In 1991, several grandparent families from GAP appeared on *Donahue*.[18] Two of them were accompanied by their adult daughters, each of whom was in recovery and doing well. Unfortunately, a year later both daughters were back on the street. One was back in jail, where she gave birth to her fourth child.

Crack addicts relapse more than other drug users. According to one expert estimate, only 25 percent of crack addicts will remain drug-free for six months after treatment, compared with 50 percent for chronic alcoholics and 60 percent for heroin addicts in a methadone maintenance program.[19] "The statistics for recovery are a lot like the statistics for weight loss programs," says Jacqueline Battle of the Infants of Substance Abusing Mothers clinic at Los Angeles County–University of Southern California Medical Center. "How many people a year later have gained it back?"[20] Thus, getting into treatment is an important start, but there is still a long, frustrating fight ahead.

• *Seek emotional support.* If you have an adult child who is an addict, find a source of information and support. Al-Anon and Nar-Anon are 12-step groups for people who have relatives addicted to alcohol and drugs. Physicians, mental health professionals, and substance abuse counselors can help you understand what is happening to your child, and grandparent support groups can give you a forum where you can express feelings and frustrations and receive reassurance that your feelings and concerns are normal. Don't try to weather your child's addiction alone; find a source of emotional support and use it often.

• *Give up hope . . .* It sounds strange to say, but sometimes the kindest thing you can do for yourself is to give up hope. Hope keeps you paying for treatment after treatment, looking for the magic one. Hope keeps you and your grandchildren waiting at the door imagining that this time Mom or Dad will be sober and committed to abstinence. The truth is that your son or daughter may—or may not—recover. But the battle is not yours. You cannot make your child better; it is not in your control.

▪ . . . *but expect anything.* Despite all the doom and gloom predictions, some people do recover. Something in them is resilient enough to fight back and win. Sometimes the most unlikely candidate for success will surprise you. Take the story of Dorsey Nunn, a prisoners' rights advocate in San Francisco. A recovered addict himself, he took in his nephews when his mother died. "I'm sure Mom didn't recognize when I was serving a life sentence that I'd be the one raising the family," says Nunn. "You can look for hope in the most unlikely circumstances. Besides, if no one advocates for recovery, grandparents will be raising grandchildren for a long time to come."[21]

YOUR DRUG-EXPOSED GRANDCHILDREN

Katherine Connor hardly slept at all the first five months after her third granddaughter arrived. Because the drug-exposed baby had a tendency to stop breathing at night, Katherine slept at the foot of her own bed, propped high on pillows so she could look down into the crib. Her clothes laid out nearby, Grandma was ready to run to the hospital if she had to. As Becky got older, Katherine finally got to sleep for intervals of three to four hours.

Baby Jay was also born with drugs in his system. He could barely breathe, his body was unusually rigid, and the doctors thought he might never walk. When she first saw him, says his grandmother, "He was frantic. His little eyes darted from side to side. His tongue came out like a serpent's tongue. You knew he had problems." When he first came home from the hospital, Jay went through four months of "withdrawal," shaking and crying uncontrollably. One weekend he screamed for 52 hours straight. Sometimes his grandparents would float him in warm water to calm him down; then they would swaddle him tight in a blanket and rock him through it.

Pam Marshall feels lucky. Although her daughter Linda was a 20-year addict, her granddaughter Megan was born free of drugs in her system. "My miracle baby," Pam calls her. Still, she doesn't know what could happen 10 years down the line. There is too little information about the long-term effects of prenatal drug exposure for Pam to feel completely safe that Megan is in the clear, and she continues to watch her granddaughter closely.

Some studies estimate that one in every ten newborns is exposed in the womb to one or more illicit drugs[22] (one in five in major cities like New York and Los Angeles).[23] However, because many private and suburban hospitals do not routinely test pregnant women or newborns for the presence of drugs in their system[24] and because even positive toxicology screens only identify drug use within the previous 24 to 48 hours,[25] no one really knows how many children were exposed to drugs and alcohol during uterine development.

Whatever the statistics, the result of a pregnant woman's addiction can be heartrending: an underweight infant, shaking and crying; an underdeveloped toddler; an older child who shows a range of difficulties from learning disabilities to emotional and behavioral problems. For grandparents, unprepared to raise a second family, drug-exposed children are an exhausting challenge.

The following paragraphs discuss what you need to know about drug-exposed children: the symptoms and risks of prenatal drug exposure on children; the special demands on you as caregivers (e.g., the late-night vigils ahead of you); and recommendations from experts and other grandparents on how to handle common issues like tremors and uncontrollable crying. Understand, however, that no one can present an exact picture of how a drug-exposed child will look or act. There is no formula, no equation, to guide you. Much depends on what substances the mother took, how much of them she took, and at what point in the pregnancy she took them.

Nor does every child react to drug exposure equally. Some children may exhibit many symptoms whereas others may not experience any. Some children may have difficulties that only appear as they get older. Although the outcome of prenatal drug exposure can vary from one infant to another, all babies born to substance-abusing mothers are at risk for developmental, learning, and behavioral problems, as well as for fragile physical health.

The symptoms and risks discussed in this chapter are only generalizations. They are not included to scare you but to keep you aware of the possibilities. Try not to look for trouble, but, at the same time, keep your eyes open for the small signs that suggest that your grandchild might require extra help. The earlier you catch problems, the sooner you can address them.

Is Your Grandbaby Drug Exposed?

It is easy to tell if your grandchild was exposed to drugs in the womb if the infant tests positive for unprescribed medication or drugs in his or her system at birth. Unfortunately, toxicology screens only show drug use within the previous 24-to-48-hour period. This means that a fetus can be exposed to drugs and alcohol for months before delivery and these substances will probably not show up in his or her system if the mother abstained from chemical abuse during the week before delivery. If that was the case with your grandchild, prenatal drug exposure is a puzzle you and your doctor must piece together from a variety of clues.

The following signs may indicate prenatal drug exposure in an infant if several are present and not due to some other medical condition.[26] If you suspect your grandchild was exposed to drugs in the womb, contact a physician.

- Premature birth
- Low birth weight
- Small head
- Seemingly constant shaking or trembling
- Difficulty feeding
- High-pitched, inconsolable cry
- Difficult to comfort
- Seizures
- Is unresponsive and lethargic
- Diarrhea
- Vomiting
- Frantic sucking
- Stiff, rigid body
- Staring or unusual eye movements
- Irregular breathing pattern
- Startle response to the least sound or touch
- Easily overstimulated
- Sleeps too much
- Doesn't sleep at all
- Physical signs of fetal alcohol syndrome (FAS), such as small, widely spaced eyes, small, flat cheeks, and a short, upturned nose

Drug-Exposed Infants

The first few days after delivery can be quite an ordeal for infants born with drugs present in their systems and for the people who care for them. The babies go through a process similar to chemical withdrawal, which can include tremors, seizures, and uncontrollable crying. They can be frustrating to care for, since they do not respond to many of the cues normal infants respond to, like bouncing and cooing (in fact, some will even arch their back to get away). The stress of this period means that a drug-exposed infant can miss out on some of the early weeks of learning and bonding, which are so important to a child's emotional development. Once any actual drugs are gone from the baby's system, there can still be physical and psychological ramifications from the prenatal drug exposure, as well as possible medical risks.

Drug-Exposed Toddlers and Children

Children of substance-abusing mothers are at risk for a number of challenges as they grow up. Respiratory and neurological problems, visual and hearing deficits, birth defects, cerebral palsy, and mental retardation are not uncommon in drug-exposed children, although not every such child will have medical complications. Some of these children may have difficulty with motor development; their hands may shake when they reach for objects and they could have trouble learning to walk. Some may be slow in learning to talk or in completing toilet training. They may be easily stimulated and may show an inclination toward hyperactive and impulsive behavior. They may have difficulty paying attention, which can cause problems when they start school. In fact, many drug-exposed children exhibit symptoms of attention-deficit/hyperactivity disorder (ADHD) and various learning disabilities. However, each of these conditions has been associated with many different outcomes. Whether a condition becomes a handicap or a challenge has a lot to do with how a child is helped and how his or her needs are met.

It is important to understand that the effect of drug exposure is unpredictable. There is no typical drug-exposed infant or child. Experts do not know exactly how much prenatal exposure will affect a child's development. Not all babies exposed to drugs and alcohol suffer equally. Some children may be obviously affected by their mother's addiction: Like Becky, they may be premature and medically fragile. Like Jay, they may suffer through symptoms of withdrawal. They may have the facial characteristics often associated with fetal alcohol syndrome. Some children may not seem to be affected at all; they may look and act just like other children, but learning and/or behavioral problems may show up in preschool or kindergarten. Others, surprisingly, may completely escape harm.

How an individual child is affected can depend on what the mother used and when in the pregnancy she used it. It can depend on her health and nutrition and on whether or not she received prenatal care. It can depend on the temperament of the individual child. It might also be a question of luck. We just don't know enough yet to predict. "It's like throwing dice," says Jacqueline Battle. "You really can't tell what will happen."[27]

But while substance abuse by the mother doesn't guarantee damage to the infant, all children born to substance-abusing mothers are *at risk* for problems as they grow up.

▪ HOW TO COPE

▪ *Reduce stimulation.* Many drug-exposed infants are easily stimulated and difficult to calm. This can be particularly troublesome when you're trying to get the child to sleep. If your grandchild is an overly excitable baby, consider reducing the outside stimulation in the environment. Try to eliminate loud noises, bright lights, sudden movements. This is hard to do with other children in the house, but do as much as you can. Consider what you have on the walls and in the crib. Is it bright and distracting? Can you keep lights low? Can you turn off the television? Speak to the baby in a soft voice, or hum and rock to soothe him. Don't handle or jiggle the baby too much, and try not to do too many things at once, even soothing things. It will just rev him up all over again.

▪ *Try swaddling.* Two of the symptoms of a drug-exposed infant are a prolonged, piercing cry and uncontrollable shaking. Unlike normal babies, who cry but eventually fall asleep, drug-exposed infants are unable to calm themselves and will continue to cry and shake and flail their arms and legs. Your first instinct might be to rock the baby or to pace with or bounce her up and down as you whisper soothing sounds. Unfortunately, these things only add to the stimulation. Try swaddling instead. Wrap her snugly in a blanket and hold her close to your body. Soothing the baby in this way cuts down on her own activity and reduces the stimulation. "You wrap them close to you and let them feel your heart," says Katherine Connor. "It's like kittens with a clock."

Never swaddle a baby who has a fever or trouble breathing.

▪ *Be vigilant.* Raising any child requires you to be constantly alert to signs of illness or sounds of trouble. Drug-exposed children demand twice as much vigilance, since they may be medically fragile as infants and hyperactive as toddlers. "You need to watch these babies during the night," says Alice Sutherland, a former pediatric nurse who is raising two drug-exposed grandchildren. "They have a lot of problems in the first years. You have to stay alert. You don't sleep soundly, or you're going to lose them. You need to monitor them and go into that room and actually feel them."

Once drug-exposed children start walking, the issues change. You can't assume that the child is still in bed or that the child gate is still keeping her out of danger. The question is not "How is the child?" but "Where is the child?" "These are not dumb children," says Alice. "You have to out-think them. When it's quiet, think, 'Why is it quiet?' And find them quickly."

▪ *Learn about these children.* If you know or suspect that your grandchild is drug-exposed, educate yourself. Talk to doctors, experts, and grandparents who have been where you are now. The more you know about the effects of drug exposure, the earlier you can address any difficulties your grandchild may have, whether they involve a hearing deficit, a language delay, or poor motor control. If you suspect any kind of problem, take preventive measures. Get your grandchild a thorough physical and look into early intervention programs.

▪ *Look into early intervention.* Every state offers early intervention programs to address developmental and learning disabilities before children enter the school system. Some states even provide services to infants and toddlers. If you think your grandchild could benefit from early intervention, contact your state board of education and ask which department handles such programs. (For more on early intervention, see Chapter 13.)

▪ *Find outside support.* A drug-exposed infant can make you feel like a failure. Many of the things you did to soothe and care for your own babies may not work with this one, and you may not know why. Still, many grandparents are reluctant to admit they don't know what they're doing and are shy about asking for help. Don't suffer in silence; look for support. The National Association for Perinatal Addiction Research and Education (NAPARE) provides free information on caring for drug-exposed children. Grandparent support groups are also a wonderful source of advice and support. Not only do they offer you a forum to express your frustration, but they are a place to hear other grandparents' experiences and the solutions they found. "Drug-exposed children don't come with instructions," says Jacqueline Battle. "No kids do."[28]

▪ *Avoid the dangers of labels.* For several years now, the media has reported on the tragic stories of "drug babies" and "crack babies," painting pictures of damaged infants who will never have a chance in life, who are "born to lose," as one headline put it.[29] But just because a child was exposed to drugs does not mean that he is doomed by them. Remember, the effects of drug exposure are unpredictable. Moreover, many of the symptoms that drug-exposed infants experience are similar to those of premature infants who were not exposed to drugs or alcohol in the womb.

The trouble with these labels, besides being unfair and inaccurate, is that they can limit our understanding of an individual child. If relatives, teachers, or physicians focus too closely on the fact that a child's mother was an addict, they run the danger of assuming that all the child's problems are caused by prenatal drugs and may not consider other possibilities, such as heredity, disease, or emotional distress. One baby kept returning to the hospital with what everyone thought were seizures; now the doctors believe he was suffering from frequent ear infections. Labels can also create self-fulfilling prophecies. If you expect a child to fail, he probably will.

If your grandchild was exposed to drugs in the womb, definitely watch for related symptoms. But watch for all kinds of symptoms—just as you would with any child. Don't let anyone dismiss your grandchild as a "drug child" without asking deeper questions.

▪ *Know your grandchild's family medical history.* As more and more medical conditions are proving to be hereditary, it is difficult to overemphasize the importance of a family medical history. Respiratory problems can certainly be related to drug exposure, but they can also be inherited. Hyperactivity is also believed to be a genetic condition. Poor feeding can be signs of an allergy to milk. The more you can find out about your grandchild's family background, the better you can help your pediatrician attend to the child's needs. Even if the child is placed with you from a foster home, ask for any available medical records or medical history.

■ *Don't lose hope.* Prenatal drug exposure can be a serious medical and developmental challenge for a child, but it doesn't have to be a sentence to failure. The jury is still out on the long-term physical and psychological effects, and some early studies indicate that with proper intervention there is reason to hope for a good outcome in many cases. In fact, some experts predict that many children prenatally exposed to drugs and alcohol can develop into healthy children and responsible members of the community. "This is not a lost generation," says Dr. Evelyn Davis, a pediatrician at New York's Harlem Hospital. "These children are not monsters. They are salvageable, capable of loving, of making good attachments. Yes, they present problems that we have not dealt with before, but they can be taught."[30]

Alice Sutherland knows the truth of that statement. All three of her grandchildren were born drug exposed, and she has seen them make great strides in their development. When the oldest was struggling in public school, Alice put her in a magnet school for the performing arts, hoping the child's love of music would give her motivation. Sarah is still only an average student, but at age 13, she has already appeared in a television commercial and hopes to be an actress someday. "Success," says Alice, "all depends on the person raising the child. The drug is just a medical problem the first five or so years. Intellectually, these children are very intelligent. You watch; you'll see all individual people."

■ *Love, love, love them.* Children learn to trust the world when they have consistent and responsive caregivers who accept them as they are and who provide them with a safe environment in which to strive. The more they trust their immediate world, the more they trust themselves to try new things. If there is any medicine that is guaranteed to work wonders on your grandchild, it is your love. It's the secret ingredient every grandmother knows:

> "You're going to have to know that your life stops on a dime," says Fay Strassburger. "The only thing that exists at that time is that baby, because that baby needs all the attention, all the love and all the caring you can possibly give him."[31]

"They thrive on that," says Alice Sutherland. "That's what gets them through—knowing they are secure and that there's a lot of love."

"This is love," says Katherine Connor. "That's the key to why my babies are all surviving; they know they have a grandma who loves them."

STOPPING THE CYCLE:
RAISING THE NEXT GENERATION

Jessica Hulsey, 15, is a crusader against drugs. The daughter of addicted parents, the California teenager knows firsthand what drugs do to a family and to a child, and has spoken out against them in compositions, school assemblies, and newspaper articles. "I missed a lot," she told the *Orange County Register*. "I grew up so fast, and I had to worry about my sister and family. I will never forgive drugs for taking [normal life] away from me."[32]

Although they may not be as vocal as Jessica, many children of addicted parents harbor intense negative feelings about drugs and alcohol. They have seen what it does, and they swear they want no part of it. It's the kind of statement that fills a grandparent's heart with relief. Unfortunately, however sweet they are, declarations and promises are not guarantees. Don't let them lull you into looking the other way. The sad fact is that children of alcohol and drug abusers run a high risk of using drugs and alcohol themselves, almost 10 times the risk that children of nonaddicted parents face.[33]

The combination of peer pressure and curiosity about drugs and alcohol can be overwhelming to teenagers and children. Your challenge, then, becomes how to prevent an at-risk grandchild from becoming an at-risk teenager. While there is no foolproof way to keep a child off drugs, there are some precautions you can take:

▪ *Accept the possibility.* "Not my child." Those are the three words that get a parent, or grandparent, into the most trouble when it comes to drugs and alcohol. They keep you from watching for changed or strange behavior, they keep you from asking questions and finding help, and they offer you false hope. The truth is that any child may bend to peer pressure and curiosity. The only way to stop the cycle of drug and alcohol abuse is to understand that it is a cycle and that your grandchild may be at risk for addictive behavior. Don't bury your head in the sand. If a grandchild's behavior seems suspicious, ask questions.

▪ *Teach your grandchildren to say no to drugs.* If your grandchildren are old enough to understand, talk to them about drugs. If you have already discussed the subject in talking about their parents, continue the conversation. It is not enough to teach them to refuse drugs; they have to know why, and your best examples may be close to home. Provide them with clear, factual information. Look at your own use of alcohol and tobacco; what messages are you sending? Nurture your grandchildren's self-esteem, and discuss different ways of handling peer pressure. A child who is prepared to say no may have an easier time actually saying it.

▪ *Supervise your grandchildren.* The best way to know what is happening in your grandchildren's lives is to be actively involved in them. Know their friends and their interests. Be aware of where they go and whom they're with. Don't allow your involvement in their lives to deteriorate into an inquisition but maintain it as a normal part of your relationship. Not only will you be aware of changes in their lives, but you may build a closer, more trusting relationship with them.

▪ *Learn to recognize drug use.* Unlike childhood diseases like mumps and measles, drug abuse does not have overt physical symptoms. However, there are warning signs a grandparent can watch for, if you know enough to look. They are the same signs many grandparents innocently tossed off as "growing pains," "teenage changes," and "the flu" when they were raising their own children: changes in eating and sleeping patterns, restlessness, sudden sulking or excessive energy. The accompanying box lists the symptoms of teen drug use. Familiarize yourself with them and stay active in your grandchild's life; if the changes are there, you will then be in the best position to spot them.

Don't be paranoid, however. It can be difficult to know the difference between erratic but normal behavior in kids and behavior caused by drugs. Every change is not an alarm. The changes to be concerned about are those that seem severe or that last more than a few days. Even if they are not linked to drug use, changes could signal medical problems, depression, or trouble at home or at school. If you do suspect anything, seek professional help.

▪ *Seek outside help.* Drug information alone may not be enough to keep a child off drugs. Self-esteem, positive role models, and peer

Could Your Grandchild Be Using Drugs or Alcohol?

The Warning Signs

Although experimenting with drugs and alcohol has almost become a rite of passage with teenagers, many children don't limit themselves to curious experiments. Instead, they slip down the steep path to habit and addiction.

Has your grandchild:

- Become hostile or uncooperative?
- Become withdrawn and depressed?
- Suddenly dropped old friends?
- Become careless about his or her appearance?
- Lost interest in favorite hobbies or sports?

Is your grandchild:

- Suddenly doing poorly in school?
- Skipping classes?
- Experiencing unexplained bursts of energy?
- Experiencing a severe weight loss?
- Experiencing a change in eating or sleeping patterns?
- Unresponsive or aggressive with family members?

Does your grandchild seem:

- Constantly tired?
- Restless?
- Excessively talkative?
- Irrational?
- Drunk or spacey?

Many of these symptoms could be warning signs of excessive use of drugs or alcohol, as are dilated pupils, needle marks, and the presence of drug paraphernalia like needles, water pipes, pills, and roach clips.

Many of these symptoms are not limited to drug use; they can also indicate depression, an eating disorder, or some other psychological or medical problem. Whatever their cause, they warrant investigation.

support are also important. Many schools and youth groups sponsor antidrug programs. There are also a number of national organizations that can help you help your grandchild stay drug free: The National Institute on Drug Abuse (NIDA) runs a hotline that provides information, referrals, and emergency counseling. Mothers Against Drunk Drivers (MADD) has programs to help children develop positive self-esteem and refusal skills; the Boy Scouts of America sponsors antidrug campaigns and publishes a booklet for children; and Al-Anon runs support groups for the children of alcoholics called Alateen and Alatot. Check your yellow pages under *drug abuse* and *alcohol* for groups in your area.

A FINAL WORD

The information in this chapter has presented only some of the possible outcomes for drug-exposed children. Many of these outcomes can be frightening to consider, but they are only generalizations. They are designed to help you keep your eyes open, not to cause despair. Your grandchild's life is still being written. If anything will give them the chance to succeed, it is your love and patience in raising them.

CHAPTER 9 | # When Parents Get Their Children Back

What makes me scared is that my mom could
take me anytime she wants. I always told myself
if she does come and try to get me, I plan to run
away. I'm not going to lead that hellish life.
—*Cameron, age 15*

Grandma's house was a safe house for Marjorie Brown's two grandchildren. Jessica, age three, arrived at the age of six months with fingernail marks up and down her back and a huge bruise on one leg. Her mother, Valerie, told Marjorie to take Jessica before she hurt her. Billy came almost a year later, when child protective services removed him from his mother because of neglect. Valerie, a drug addict who had been involved with gangs since she was 14, had been in and out of jail on several counts and had only seen Billy four times in eight months. She had not complied with court-ordered counseling or drug programs and was not allowed to see her children without another adult present. Even Valerie's parole officer described her as a "walking time bomb." When the unthinkable happened and a juvenile court judge decided Valerie was ready to parent and ordered Billy back to his mother, Marjorie was floored. In her wildest imaginings, she hadn't expected this. She knew Valerie couldn't handle the baby. The social worker knew it. Even Valerie knew she wasn't ready for full-time motherhood— and said so. However, the judge, noting that Valerie had had several clean drug tests and that she wanted unmonitored visits, decided she was ready.

Today, Marjorie and Valerie have a voluntary arrangement. Billy lives with Marjorie, but Valerie can take him whenever and wherever she likes. Marjorie is scared to death. She sees Valerie driving around with gang members and dressing like one; she worries that her daughter is using drugs again. She is afraid of drive-by shootings with the baby in the car. Mostly, she is afraid of her daughter's temper. "Billy's at the point where he's walking and getting into things," she says. "Valerie has already expressed that she couldn't handle him, and she'd only had him twenty-four hours. She couldn't take the stress of his screaming. I'm afraid she's going to hurt him. If she could hurt Jessica at six months, what could she do to Billy?"

In addition to her own fears, Marjorie is having problems with Jessica. Jessica's court case is separate from her brother's, and she is not legally affected by the judge's decision. Nevertheless, the emotional toll has been heavy on the little girl. She had begun to open up and play with other children; now she is withdrawn and is having nightmares. She sees her mother taking Billy, and she is terrified that she will have to go with her, too. "She wakes up in the night screaming, 'I don't want to go with Valerie!'" says Marjorie. "I hold her and tell her she is not going, but she sees Billy come and go, and she doesn't know what to make of it. She used to love to go to McDonald's. That's our meeting place now. She won't eat at McDonald's anymore. That's pretty bad, when a child doesn't want to eat at McDonald's."

Sending children back to their parents can be a grandparent's fondest dream—and worst nightmare. The dream is that the adult children will shape up and become active, responsible parents, that the grandchildren will be safe, and that you can resume your role of occasional baby-sitter and doting grandparent. The nightmare is that the children will go back before the parents have their lives in order, before it is truly safe.

For some grandparents, dreams do come true. There are parents who hit a bad patch in their lives and come out of it. There are addicts and alcoholics who recover and resume normal lives. Unfortunately, there are also many grandparents who wake up to discover the nightmares are real: A mother who hasn't seen a child in three years shows up and wants him back; an absent father remarries and suddenly wants his children; and the court decides that the parents are ready to take their children again, although, as far as the grandparents know, they are still using drugs. Nothing can prevent the shock and heartache of sending a child back to potentially unfit parents. Even when you know it can happen, you don't want to believe that it will. But when you don't see it coming, the pain is that much deeper.

FOREWARNED AND FOREARMED

The truth is that unless you have adopted your grandchildren or the parents are dead, you are at risk of losing them. If you have the children on an informal basis, the parents have every right to take them, even after several years. If they have been placed with you through the juvenile justice system, you should be aware that the court's goal is to reunify children with their parents and that everything will be done to accomplish that. Even if you have private legal guardianship, it can be overturned if the parents prove themselves fit (although this puts the burden on the parent and is less likely). Neither you nor your grandchild is protected from the parent's ultimate right to parent, and you need to be prepared for anything, particularly when you deal with the juvenile court. Knowing these facts won't lessen the pain if you lose your grandchildren, but it can help you prepare for the worst.

Remember, you may have little control over what happens to your grandchildren tomorrow, but you have a lot of control over what happens today. You can give your grandchildren the best care you can while you have them. You can give them a foundation of love and self-esteem. If they are old enough, you can teach them skills to take care of themselves—simple things like how to call 911, how to make a peanut butter sandwich, how to call you collect. One grandmother taught her twins her phone number by inventing a song. You can also make sure they know that certain kinds of spanking and touching are not okay and that they should talk to a trusted adult if anything like that ever happens, even while they are living with you.

IF THE UNIMAGINABLE HAPPENS

If you do have to give up your grandchildren, you will feel like your heart has been torn out. Your life will be turned upside down yet again. You had traveled the road from grandparent to parent; reorganized your life around these children; and loved and nurtured them for months, if not years, and now you will be expected to give them back like any part-time baby-sitter. It's hard, and it's painful. All the complex feelings you went through when your grandchildren first arrived double back on you with a vengeance. But now there are new layers: guilty thoughts that if you had handled something differently, they might still be with you; false hopes that maybe your adult child really can get it together this time; renewed rage at the system and the parents; uncertainty over if and when you will see your grandchildren again; fear for their safety; and a feeling of deep helplessness over your inability to protect them. It can feel like there is a huge void where your heart should be. You might find yourself distancing from them, if only to protect yourself.

Your grandchildren will have their own mixed reactions to going back to their parents. They may repeat behaviors that you thought were long behind them: bed-wetting, explosions of anger, school problems. Children who don't want to leave you may feel like you're sending them away; they may regress or push you away, or they may misbehave, hoping that if they're bad enough, their parents won't want them. Children who want to be with Mom or Dad may stop listening to you once they know they're going home. They, too, might misbehave, thinking that if you've had enough, you'll send them sooner. They may be caught between conflicting feelings and may express them in angry outbursts.

Either way, your grandchildren are being uprooted again and will need help with the transition. If you are lucky, you will have time to prepare them. You can reassure them that you are not sending them away and that you'll try to keep in contact. Although you can't speak for what Mom or Dad will allow—parents may lie to their children about allowing them to see you—you can promise your grandchildren that if you can't see them, you will think about them and continue to love them. Children who start acting out behaviorally will need help putting their feelings into words. If they are in counseling, they need to focus on this change. Also, let teachers know what is happening so that they can help, too.

Sometimes, however, you don't have the luxury of transition time. The judge in Marjorie's case would have let Mom take the baby directly from the courtroom, with no transition at all, except that Valerie herself objected. If this happens, all you can do is give yourself room to grieve.

If, like Marjorie, you have other grandchildren at home, you will also have to deal with their reactions: fear that they, too, might have to leave; anger at being left behind; sorrow at being separated from their siblings; or fear for their siblings and concern that they may never see them again. All you can do is reassure them that you love them, that you understand their feelings, and that for now they are safe with you. Unfortunately, it is the man in the robe who is making the decisions.

Then there are the practical issues. What do you send with the children? Do you give Mom all the baby's things? Certainly, you want the child to have them, but will that be the case? Or will Mom sell the high chair for drug money? And what if Mom can't parent two months from now and the kids come back to you? Won't you need a high chair and car seat? My recommendation is to play it by ear. Everything depends on your individual history with the parent. Do whatever you are comfortable doing. Perhaps you can give a few things at a time and see what happens. Look at the whole picture before you decide what, and how much, to give away.

OUT OF SIGHT, OUT OF REACH

Perhaps the hardest thing for a grandparent to face in this situation is the wrath of the parent who believes you "stole" the children (even if it was the juvenile justice system that removed them in the first place). Parent–grandparent relationships will be strained at best and can escalate to outright hostility. In the worst cases, parents deny grandparents all access to the grandchildren.

A Wisconsin grandmother had to spend close to $30,000 in attorney fees just to get one monthly visit and one weekly phone call with a granddaughter she raised for nine years. A Minnesota grandfather used to go to his grandsons' school to watch them play ball, but Mom got a restraining order so that he can't even do that anymore. These grandparents send cards and gifts without knowing if they are received. Some are returned. They have lost grandchildren not only from their homes but also from their lives.

▪ HOW TO COPE

When your grandchildren go back, it can feel like the world has ended and the nightmare has begun. Nothing will take the pain away, but there are some things you can do to help yourself adjust.

▪ *Give yourself time to grieve.* Your sadness, your anger, and the huge sense of emptiness are normal. You have suffered an enormous loss, and you need to process your feelings in a safe, comfortable way. This is a time to seek out support. If friends and family are too overwhelmed, consider counseling. And definitely seek out support groups. Just because you no longer have your grandchildren doesn't mean you are barred from grandparent groups. If anything, this is a time when you most need to be with people who understand the depth of your loss.

▪ *Try to move on.* It sounds cold, but there's not much you can do once a judge has decided that a parent is rehabilitated. Whatever is going to happen will happen. Perhaps the parent *has* pulled together. If not, maybe the child will end up back in the system and they'll call you. But you can't put your life on hold until then, and it won't help your grandchild if you do.

▪ *Get busy.* Spend time with your other grandchildren; they also need you in their lives. Volunteer. Some grandparents have found it helpful to volunteer in a hospital or a school when they miss being around kids. Get involved with all the hobbies you put on hold. Spend more time with people you care about—your spouse, family, and friends.

▪ *Get politically involved.* Many grandparents at the front of the grandparents' movement have channeled their grief and anger into activism. They may not be able to help their own grandchildren, they reason, but they can fight to prevent other grandchildren and grandparents from suffering similar traumas. One of the hardest things to accept as a grandparent is how helpless you are in the system; political action offers you a chance to affect the system and empower yourself in the process (see Chapter 15).

THE NEVER-ENDING CYCLE

Two of Sandra Cobb's seven grandchildren were returned to a mother who swore she was off drugs. She tested clean, met regularly with her probation officer, had a steady job, and appeared to be ready to care for two babies. It didn't last. Several months later, Mom resumed her drug use, lost her job, and started prostituting again. When she left the boys alone in her apartment, a neighbor called the police. The children were taken into protective custody and given back to Grandma.

When you are returning your grandchildren to their parents, it is cold comfort to think that they might soon be back. It means that they will have been mistreated again and that they will return to you with emotional wounds reopened. It is rare that children go home to Mom and Dad and actually stay with them. Another truth about these adult children is that they rarely pull it together for long. They go into rehab. They get jobs. They even stay clean for one or two years—long enough to impress a judge and raise your hopes. But they walk a thin line between good intentions and immediate gratification, and they are prone to misstep.

After years of self-protection, Pam and Robert Marshall finally allowed themselves some hope. Linda had been clean nearly two years. She had a job and an apartment. She started to show more than a passing interest in her daughter, calling and visiting more often, and she started talking about a future for herself. Then something snapped. She started using drugs again. She got pregnant and hooked up with an abusive ex-boyfriend whom she tracked down in jail. Now she's back in rehab, and her parents are devastated.

Even as you grieve the new loss of your grandchildren, brace yourself for anything. This, too, could be temporary. If you are allowed to see the children, keep a close eye on them. Try to stay on the parent's good side, even if it means walking on eggshells to do it. Offer to baby-sit. Above all, continue to document. Even if you are barred from seeing your grandchildren, keep a log. Whenever you make a call or send a card, even if the parent interferes with your attempt, write it down. If you can, find some way of knowing where your grandchildren are and how they are. If they are removed again—and they very well may be—you need to know about it.

SECTION II

Through the
Red Tape

CHAPTER 10 | Grandparenting and the Law

> Never to such an extent in U.S. history has care
> of children by relatives been so interwoven
> with government.
> > —*Newsletter of the National Association*
> > *of Court-Appointed Special Advocates*
> > *for Children*

If you are a grandparent raising a grandchild, the odds are good that at some point you will end up in a courtroom. The process could be as simple as filing for guardianship with the parent's consent; it could be as heartrending as a fight to keep your grandchild from being returned to an abusive home. Either way, powerful strangers— judges, social workers, and attorneys—will be able to determine what happens to your family. Even if you are not raising grandchildren, you could find yourself rubbing shoulders with the law. The divorce rate is approximately one out of every two marriages, and some grandparents have to petition the courts just for the right to see their grandchildren.

Many grandparents have gone their entire lives without entering a court of law. They may think that law, like violence, is something that happens to other people—those in the newspapers or on television. But they do believe in justice, and they expect it to be there when they need it. Then they enter the legal system and discover that justice is confusing, impersonal, and often outrageously expensive, both financially and emotionally. The cost can attack your bank account and your spirit. The process is painfully slow. Moreover, the underlying principles are not friendly to grandparents. As one

Texas grandmother told the *Katy Times*, "The courts treat you as though you're some old busybody who just doesn't like the way your kids are raising their kids. They act as though you have no right whatsoever to care about these babies."[2]

Although this book cannot change the attitude of the legal system, it can attempt to clear up some of the confusion. This chapter and the next are designed as road maps of the key legal issues you may encounter with your grandchildren, namely, your rights as a grandparent, possible custody arrangements, and the landmarks of the juvenile dependency system. They are designed to give you enough information to ask informed questions. Knowledge is power, and the best protection you have in any battlefield is an understanding of your opponent. First, however, a few warnings:

▪ *The legal system is complex and changeable.* It is couched in gray areas and interpretations, and the interpretations are as different as the judges who make them. To quote one family court judge, "I can't say, 'This is the law, and if you connect the five following dots, you win.'" Law is never that simple.

▪ *Family law is governed by state, not federal, legislation.* This means that laws and regulations about marriage, divorce, paternity, custody, visitation, guardianship, adoption, and foster care vary from state to state, as do the legal definitions of child abuse and neglect. What is called probate court in California is surrogate's court in New York. "Visitation" in one state may be "access" or "parental contact" somewhere else. "Guardianship" may be "managing conservatorship." I have used names that are either common or self-explanatory, but you may encounter different terms, laws, and regulations in your own state or county.

▪ *Grandparent issues are uncharted waters,* not only for grandparents but for attorneys, judges, and government agencies as well. A Chicago couple seeking custody of their grandson wrote that their attorney had been in practice for 28 years and had never handled a case like theirs before. The same may be true of the judges who hear these cases. Even child welfare laws were designed with nonrelated caregivers in mind. As one attorney put it, "State legislatures are ten years behind the social phenomenon."[3]

Your case will be shaped by the specific details of your situation, by the particular laws of your state, and by the bias of the judge who hears it. If you need legal advice, talk to an attorney who specializes in your specific area of law: family law, guardianship, child welfare, and so on. He or she can advise you on the basis of the facts and circumstances of your individual case.

YOUR RIGHTS AS A GRANDPARENT

"Grandparents have all the responsibilities and none of the rights," says Barbara Kirkland, founder of Grandparents Raising Grandchildren.[4] In many ways this is true. In our society grandparenthood is a biological connection, not a legal one. The laws and regulations that protect the family presume a nuclear unit of mother, father, and child. The grandparent–grandchild relationship can be severed by adoption, divorce, and even the whim of an angry parent. In fact, until recently, relatives had no greater access to a child than nonrelatives.

Today, however, almost every state has some kind of visitation statute that allows grandparents limited rights to request visits with their grandchildren (although the court can still refuse the request). This makes the right to petition for visitation the only legal right you have *as a grandparent*. In some states or counties you may also have certain privileges, such as first preference for placement if a child is removed from a parent's custody by the juvenile court system, but these privileges relate more to government policy about the child than to your rights as a grandparent or relative.

To understand your apparent lack of clout as a grandparent in America, you must understand the power of parents.

THE PROTECTED RIGHTS OF PARENTS

Traditionally, parents have had almost exclusive authority when it comes to their children. Our government cannot dictate how people raise their children, nor can it randomly take their children away from them. Unless a child is in some kind of danger, no one, not even the court, can interfere with the parent–child relationship. Even when a child is legally removed from a mother or father's care, every effort is made to enable him to return safely home.

The idea that children belong with their parents is at the very root of our social structure.

In theory, such airtight rights are a wonderful thing. There are countries where the government easily interferes with family relationships. Our country was created on the principle of broad individual rights, and the right to privacy is one of them. Imagine a social worker, lawyer, or relative being able to come into your house to tell you how to raise your own children, and you may see why parental rights are worth protecting. Unfortunately, in practice, the children are often the losers. The laws that favor parents presume that they are able to care for their children and keep them safe. The issue of children's rights is rarely addressed because until recently few people thought about children as having individual rights and it was assumed that any rights children did have would be protected by their parents. The exploding numbers of abused and abandoned children in recent years has proven that assumption to be painfully false.

Even when the state does intervene, the rights of the mother and father seem to overshadow the right of the child to be safe from harm. That is because the legal standard commonly used in custody and visitation cases is "the best interests of the child."[5] Yet there are no legal definitions of "best interests." Judges have a lot of discretion in deciding what it means.

This unshakable belief in parents' rights is the most powerful opponent you will encounter in the legal system. If you can understand that, you have a better chance of understanding and adjusting to the battles you may fight as you try to obtain custody of your grandchild.

THE LEGAL CUSTODY OF GRANDCHILDREN

Custody is one of the main problems facing grandparents who are raising grandchildren in their homes. Without custody, you may have problems enrolling a child in school, getting medical care, or seeking government aid. Without custody, you have no control over whether your grandchild is handed back to an abusive, neglectful, or intoxicated parent. Even with some kind of custody arrangement, your power may be limited.

Custody is confusing because people use one word to mean many things. A grandfather whose grandson lives with him may call it custody. A grandmother whose granddaughters were placed with her by the court may call that custody. Grandparents who have legal guardianship of their grandchild will say they have custody. And each does have a small piece of the custody puzzle.

Custody defines a relationship of control over and responsibility for a minor child.[6] There are two kinds of custody—physical and legal—and that is where the confusion lies. If a child lives with you, she is in your *physical* custody, but you may not have *legal* custody. Physical custody means physical control over a child, including the right to have her live with you. Legal custody means legal authority to make decisions about the medical, educational, health, and welfare needs of the child. These distinctions are common in divorce settlements, where the parents may have joint custody (shared legal and physical responsibility for a child) or one parent may have full custody (legal and physical) while the other has visitation rights. But divorce is not the only circumstance that puts the custody of a child in question. The legal system can transfer the custody of a child in order to protect her from danger. This is where grandparents come into the picture.

If your grandchild lives with you, the child is physically in your custody, whether you have an informal arrangement or a formal one. The more critical questions are these: Who has legal custody? What is your legal relationship to the grandchild in your care? What are the limitations of your arrangement?

There are four types of custody situations that may affect your grandchild; each has legal and financial consequences for your family. They are informal custody, court placement (and/or foster care), guardianship, and adoption. Another issue you may be involved with as a grandparent is visitation. While this is not a matter of custody, it affects many grandparents deeply.

Informal Custody

Many grandparents who have grandchildren living with them have no legal arrangements for doing so. They start out caring for the children on a casual basis and seem to continue that way. Some grandparents don't even realize that there are legal options available to them. This makes informal custody one of the most common arrangements among grandparents. With informal custody you have, in essence, physical custody of the child while legal custody remains with the parents. Unfortunately, this situation offers the least protection for you and your grandchildren.

Informal custody can mean constant struggles over school enrollment, medical care, and financial assistance. Many school districts may not allow a nonparent to enroll a child unless he is the legal guardian, and relatives can run into difficulties obtaining medical care for a minor child. One Texas grandmother had a notarized letter from her daughter authorizing her to seek medical attention for her grandchildren, and the doctor still refused to treat them. Although the Texas Family Code allows adult relatives to seek medical care for a child, the doctor has the right to refuse treatment if the adult is not the legal guardian.[7]

On the plus side, informal custody means you don't have high court costs and attorney fees or government interference with your family. But it also means that you are at the mercy of the child's parents; they can take the child whenever they want to, and you will have no legal means to stop them. You are, in fact, little more than a glorified baby-sitter. If you only have informal custody of your grandchildren, you have no real control over their safety. In fact, your desire to protect them makes you vulnerable to emotional and financial blackmail by their parents. As long as you are without legal protection, you are open to parental manipulation.

▪ HOW TO COPE

▪ *Look into government aid.* Just because you have informal custody of your grandchildren does not mean you must shoulder the financial burden alone. Your grandchildren may be entitled to financial and medical assistance through one of several government programs (see Chapter 12 for details).

▪ *Look into guardianship.* If your grandchildren are not in the custody of the juvenile justice system, you may be able to file for guardianship. Not only is this the most stable arrangement for your grandchildren (short of adoption), but if you apply for guardianship early enough, it can keep you out of the juvenile courts and prevent interference from child protective services. If your grandchildren's situation is not so severe or life threatening that you need to involve the police or child protective services, consider private guardianship (see "Guardianship," below).

• *Consider a power of attorney.* Power of attorney gives one person the legal right to make decisions for another. For instance, a single mother could give someone power of attorney to enroll a child in school or give emergency medical consent if she is out of town. In doing so, the mother doesn't give up any parental rights; she only allows another person to make certain decisions. Power of attorney can be a useful temporary solution when a parent is incarcerated and wants a relative to care for a child or when a parent travels extensively. Of course, a document like this is only useful if officials choose to accept it, and it can always be rescinded. If you are in a situation that does not require or allow for guardianship, at least ask the parents about power of attorney.

Court Placement and Foster Care

Foster care provides temporary substitute parenting to children whose parents can not or will not take care of them. It is part of an emergency response system that is designed to protect children who are suspected of being abused or neglected or who have been abandoned. Foster care usually starts with a call to a social worker, the police, or a child abuse hotline. The children are then taken into protective custody while the juvenile justice system decides whether or not to remove them from their parents and make them "dependents of the court."

Custody of your grandchild changes when she becomes a dependent of the court. The court retains legal custody of the child, but someone is awarded physical custody. That someone has traditionally been a foster parent. Foster parents are appointed to care for a child while the court conducts a series of hearings to determine if the allegations against the parents are true and, if so, how to protect the child. These hearings are generally called "dependency hearings."

Most people associate foster care with care by strangers. However, because of a shortage of foster homes and an explosion in the number of children needing court protection, many states have begun to rely increasingly on relatives. This makes court placement the most common *legal* arrangement for grandparents, although few grandparents are licensed foster parents.

With court placement, grandparents have a limited degree of custody. You have physical custody of the child (i.e., he lives with you) and limited authority to enroll him in school and seek medical attention, but the court and child welfare agency retain legal custody. Court placement gives you more legal protection than does an informal custody arrangement—and the possibility of higher government benefits—but you also have a kind of marriage to the juvenile justice system. You will be expected to comply with court visitation, to encourage "reunification" with the parents, and to submit your family to the scrutiny of the local child welfare agency. You exchange the possibility of parental interference for the certainty of interference by social workers, attorneys, and judges (and generally without any choice in the matter).

There are differences between court placement with a relative and foster care, mainly in terms of licensing requirements and government assistance. Foster parents must be trained and licensed to have children in their homes. They may be licensed only for a fixed number of children, for certain ages, and sometimes for one sex. They must also supply separate bedrooms for girls and boys and one bed per child. Many states also limit the number of children per room. Although relatives must also be approved by social services before a child can be placed with them, they don't usually have to go through the training and licensing process. Nor are housing guidelines so specific (in most states). Few grandparents could meet the strict criteria to become official foster parents.

The other difference between court placement with a relative and foster care is one of financial aid. Federal funds are available to support children who are in the custody of the state, and foster care benefits are significantly higher than welfare benefits. Some states also provide their own programs for children who don't qualify for federal foster care. Children placed with relatives are also entitled to government support, but relatives may have a harder time meeting federal foster care requirements and few states make state programs available to them. Families often have to rely on the smaller welfare benefits. (See Chapter 12 for more information on government aid.)

If you have a grandchild in the juvenile justice system, the individual laws of your state will determine if he is placed in your custody and under what conditions. The best thing you can do is educate yourself about the dependency process and try to comply with your state regulations. (See Chapter 11 for a discussion of child protective services and the dependency system.)

Guardianship

Outside of adoption, guardianship is the safest, most stable arrangement for a grandparent raising a grandchild. In fact, guardianship *is* custody, both physical and legal. It is the legal transfer of custody to someone other than a parent when one or both of the parents are dead, missing, or unfit. The first two categories are straightforward; "unfit" is a murkier concept. Nevertheless, unfit parents are becoming a common cause of guardianship actions. As attorney Teresa de la O told the Santa Rosa *Press Democrat,* "We've always done them [guardianships], but it used to be when one parent died and the other wasn't all that interested in having the child. Now we're doing it because neither parent is parenting."[8]

Guardianship does not terminate parental rights, but it does suspend them. With guardianship, you acquire rights and responsibilities that are similar, if not equal, to those of a parent. As attorney Harold LaFlamme puts it: "You step into the shoes of the parent. You don't have a pink slip, but something close."[9]

The advantage of guardianship is control. You decide where your grandchild lives (within the state). You have legal authority to enroll her in school, consent to medical treatment, and make many of the decisions a parent can make in terms of education, sports, health care, employment, and legal actions. You also have control over when and how your grandchild sees her parents, unless there is a court-ordered visitation schedule. The parent may retain some rights, similar to joint custody in a divorce settlement, but you have legal control. And you are not at the beck and call of the juvenile court system.

What you cannot do as a guardian is make decisions about the child's religion or move the child out of state without the court's permission. Although you are not entitled to any of the child's earnings or property, you also bear no financial responsibility for your grandchild. You are only responsible for the care and safety of the child and for any damage she does while you are guardian.

The disadvantages of applying for guardianship are the cost and the risk. Filing for private guardianship can mean high attorney fees and court costs, particularly if the parents or other relatives contest your petition. If guardianship comes through the juvenile court system, it can mean, for some families, a reduction in government foster care benefits, something many grandparents cannot afford to lose.

There are also emotional risks in filing for guardianship. Unless the parents have died or disappeared, you are petitioning to suspend parental rights. This requires proving that the parent is unfit and detrimental to the child. You will have to build a case against the parent that involves more than the separation anxiety your grandchild will suffer if he is removed from your home. You will have to show things like a history of irresponsibility, drug abuse, physical or sexual abuse, or a lack of residence, as well as the effect such factors will have on the child. You will also have to prove that it is in the child's best interests to be with you. You will not endear yourself to your adult child by painting these pictures and taking custody of the child. If you win, you guarantee some security for your grandchild. But, warns attorney LaFlamme, "If you lose, you could lose big: the money and the relationship with your child and grandchild."[10]

Even at its best, guardianship is never permanent. Under normal circumstances, it lasts until the child is 18,[11] marries, becomes emancipated (recognized as an adult), or is adopted. However, you can be removed as a guardian by the court at any time if it is proven that returning your grandchild to the parents or assigning another guardian is in the child's best interests. Only adoption offers airtight custody.

Filing for Guardianship

To file for private guardianship, you or your attorney must file several legal forms, often called a "guardianship petition," in whichever branch of your civil court handles guardianship (generally either probate, juvenile, or family law). You must also notify in writing all the child's maternal and paternal relatives, particularly the parents. These family members will be notified of all hearings and given an opportunity to object to your petition and to seek custody for themselves. You will also have to pay filing and investigation fees, the cost of which can vary.

If there is an emergency situation or you believe the child is at immediate risk and in need of protection, you can often ask the court to grant you "temporary guardianship"[12] until the hearing. This is one way to keep the children safe with you while you file for custody.

Once a hearing date is set, a state or county agency will conduct an investigation to decide if the guardianship is necessary. In most states the social service agency will also run a background check on you for any arrests or involvement with child protective services. The agency may also conduct an investigation of your home and may interview your grandchild if she is old enough. At the guardianship hearing, the judge will consider the petition, the social service investigator's report, and all the available testimony before making a final decision.

If there is no opposition to your petition from parents or other relatives, seeking guardianship can be a relatively simple procedure. If, however, the parents or other relatives contest your guardianship petition, they can hire their own attorneys and confront you in a full hearing. This is where the cost of court and attorney fees can start to climb.

Guardianship through Dependency

It is possible to obtain guardianship through the juvenile justice system but only at the final stages of the dependency process. If by the final hearing the judge decides that the child cannot safely return home, he or she will order adoption, guardianship, or long-term foster care as the best plan for the child. If guardianship is granted, the court may dismiss the child's dependency status. (For more on the dependency process, see Chapter 11. See also "Foster Care and Youakim" in Chapter 12.)

Standby and Short-Term Guardianship

A "standby guardianship" is a guardianship order issued with the parent's consent for some point in the future.[13] For instance, if a single mother has cancer, she can set up a standby guardianship that takes effect upon her death (as long as there is no other parent to object and the court doesn't find it harmful to the child). Short-term guardianship is just that: a legal custody arrangement for a limited period of time. Illinois just instituted the short-term guardianship in 1994. That state's "guardianship of limited duration" allows parents to appoint guardians for their child with a predetermined termination date.[14] This allows incarcerated parents to provide legal care for their children while they serve time and still regain custody upon their release.

If you are caring for a child whose parents are sick or in jail, find out if your state offers standby or short-term guardianship arrangements.

▪ WHAT YOU NEED TO KNOW

▪ *Sometimes court costs can be waived.* In some states you can apply for a waiver of court fees and costs if you can show financial hardship. The application is sometimes called a pauper's waiver or *in forma pauperis* application.[15] If you currently receive financial assistance for yourself (not your grandchild) in the form of disability or welfare benefits, food stamps, or any other form of general relief, you may qualify for this waiver.

▪ *You may be able to "do it yourself."* Some states make it possible to apply for guardianship without an attorney, particularly if the guardianship petition is uncontested. California grandparents can find guidance in *The Guardianship Book: How to Become a Child's Guardian in California* (Nolo Press)[16]; there may be manuals and booklets explaining the process in other states as well. If you don't need or cannot afford an attorney, find out if you can apply for guardianship without one. Contact your local Legal Aid office for information.

▪ *You must prove that it is harmful to the child to continue in the parent's custody.* Just because you are currently raising your grandchild is not enough reason for a judge to make you a guardian. Parents have a right to ask someone else to care for a child, particularly when they are in and out of the picture, without it being considered abandonment. If, on the other hand, the parent has disappeared for a significant amount of time, you may have a better chance for guardianship to be granted.

▪ *You must also show that the child is better off with you.* Be careful when you do this; reasons like better income can backfire. Says Pamela Mohr, attorney and executive director of the Alliance for Children's Rights, "It can work against you if it appears that you are wealthy and are trying to get the child for that reason. It makes the court protective of the parent. We don't want to take custody from poor people just because they are poor."[17] What kind of information is the court looking for? Information about the physical and emotional health of the child; how the child behaves after visits with the parent;

proof of your ability to provide a stable home environment if the parents cannot.

▪ *Parents will often be granted visitation rights.* A parent who doesn't have custody is entitled to reasonable visitation in a guardianship situation, unless the court decides that visitation poses a danger to the child's physical, mental, or emotional health. Even jailed parents may be granted visits if the court believes that they are in the best interests of the child. If either parent is granted visitation, be prepared to cooperate.

▪ *You can protect your grandchildren.* As a legal guardian you can determine where and when an unstable parent sees your grandchild. You can even get a restraining order, if necessary. But you must be able to show the court that the parent is a threat to you or to your grandchild's safety. Many grandparents won't get restraining orders against their adult children in fear of retaliation. It can also be difficult to call the police on your own son or daughter. But if you do have to call the police, a restraining order gives you more credibility.

▪ *Guardianship is always temporary.* Even if your grandchild has lived with you since birth, the court can revoke your guardianship status. Remember, the prevailing belief is that children belong with their parents. However, while parents can request the court to overturn a guardianship arrangement, they must prove that they can care for the child and that continued guardianship is no longer necessary. This is rarely accomplished when the problem is substance abuse.

Pam and Robert Marshall clearly understand this. They filed for custody of their granddaughter when the drug-addicted mother, Linda, was in jail (the father is unknown). "I know that guardianship can be overturned," says Pam, "but what it does is temporarily protect Megan. Linda would have to go into court and prove she has a home, a job, stability and could take care of her. As of yesterday, I doubt that."

▪ *Don't give up.* People will tell you many things. For instance, several attorneys told Pam Marshall that no court would allow her to take custody of a granddaughter. While it is possible that your state laws may prevent you from filing for guardianship, don't just take anyone's word for it. "No matter what anyone tells you, do it anyway," says one grandmother. "I was told I could not win. And you know what? I have three healthy, happy grandchildren."

Adoption

In many states you can adopt your own grandchildren under certain circumstances: for example, when the child is orphaned or legally abandoned, when the parents consent to the adoption, or when their parental rights are terminated by trial or the juvenile court system.

Adoption is the most secure custody arrangement available to nonparents. It permanently dissolves all legal ties between parent and child and creates a new parent–child relationship in the eyes of the law. In effect, you would no longer be grandparents to your grandchild but new parents, with all the rights and responsibilities of a biological parent. To quote one child welfare agency, "When you adopt a child, your legal relationship with that child is the same as with a child born to you."[18]

Adoption gives you full legal custody. It means the end of continual court appearances, and it means that the parent can never again contest or interfere. As an adoptive parent you can now put your grandchild on your health plan and allow her to inherit directly from you. You also acquire the full legal and financial responsibility for parenting the child. Unlike guardianship, adoption means that your relationship is permanent, extending past the child's 18th birthday, just as with your own children.

Adoption also means peace of mind, not only for you but for your grandchildren, who don't have to worry about ever being taken away again. Nancy Harper's granddaughter Marissa was thrilled when her grandmother adopted her. She thought it was wonderful that the judge said that she could stay with Grandma for the rest of her life and never leave. I heard about a little boy who took his stuffed bear to court with him. When the judge asked about it, he replied, "Well, he's always been at my Grandma's too, and he wants to know if he can be adopted, too, because he never wants to leave Grandma's house, either." Today, both boy and bear are legally adopted.

If adoption is such an airtight solution to the custody nightmares, you might ask, "why don't more grandparents pursue it?" There are several reasons.

▪ *Grandparents don't easily give up on their adult children, and adoption means terminating the rights of the parent.* It can be a difficult emotional choice to make. On one hand, adopting a grandchild is a relief: It validates the fact that you are raising your grandchild and ends your dealings with social workers and the courts. On the other hand, it means admitting defeat where your adult child is concerned. Says attorney Robert Walmsley, "In terms of the grandparents, adoption is generally the last resort, when they see no hope of the adult child ever being responsible. Parenthood is precious. You hoped your child would shape up. By this point, you've lost all hope."[19]

▪ *Many grandparents believe that adoption is unnecessary because they and the children are already family.* They may also hesitate to adopt because the parents are still in the picture. The fact that the birth parents may continue to interact with the children can make grandparent adoption confusing and complicated. Because ties are not severed, children may be confused about whom to listen to and may be prevented from making a clean start with Grandma and Grandpa as a new family.

▪ *It is difficult to terminate a parent's rights.* Unless the parents consent to the adoption, have already lost custody, or are completely out of the picture, you may need to prove that your own child is unfit to raise his or her own children. This can involve a full trial with witnesses; everything about your family will be open to scrutiny.

▪ *Adoption is costly.* Not only do you have court costs, but unless your grandchildren are eligible for adoption assistance, you can also lose access to government aid. Many grandparents don't adopt their grandchildren because they live on a fixed income and can't afford to raise children without welfare benefits.

▪ *Your age can become a negative factor if the adoption is contested.* One New Hampshire couple had legal guardianship of their son's two children for two years before filing for adoption. Fourteen months into the trial, a young couple on the mother's side contested the adoption and won.

If you are considering adopting your grandchild, here are some things you might want to consider:

▪ You will be a full legal parent again. Are you ready for that?
▪ Will the parents continue to interact with the child? How will you handle that?
▪ Does the child have a relationship with the parents? How will adoption affect that relationship?
▪ How is your health? Do you have the stamina and good health to commit to raising another set of children?

- What is your financial situation? If you are getting government aid, can you afford to give it up? Are you eligible for Adoption Assistance (see Chapter 12)?

If you decide to go ahead with the adoption, consult a good adoption attorney—as well as a therapist about the impact this move could have on your grandchild and your family. If the child is old enough, listen closely to what he or she has to say about it. Some children are eager to cut their ties to their parents, others will object.

VISITATION

Legal visitation is not a form of custody, but it is an important issue when the custody of a child changes. In a divorce, for instance, the mother may get legal custody and the father may receive visitation privileges. The grandparents can sometimes be left out in the cold. However, divorce is not the only situation in which grandparents are prevented from seeing their grandchildren. Grandparents may also be denied visitation in the following circumstances:

- A daughter dies and the husband remarries.
- An unmarried son fathers a child and the mother moves away.
- A stepparent adopts the grandchildren.
- A grandchild is placed in foster care.
- A married daughter simply refuses to let her parents see their grandchildren.

Even grandparents who have raised a child for years can lose total access to that child if the parents reappear or regain custody. One Ohio grandmother provided day care for her married daughter for 50 hours a week for four years; after a family argument, the parents refused her even occasional visitation. In situations like these, many grandparents turn to the law for help.

Grandparent Visitation and State Laws

Nearly every state in the United States has some kind of grandparent visitation statute, although they are barely 30 years old and narrow in scope.[20] These statutes do not give grandparents a legal right to visit a grandchild but a right to *petition* for visitation. The court reserves the right to refuse any petition based on the merits of the case. Each statute defines who may petition for visitation, when, and under what circumstances. Some states also outline what standard the court should apply in awarding visitation, usually "the best interests of the child."

▪ *Who may petition.* While most states only allow grandparents to petition for visitation, a number of states extend the privilege to great-grandparents, siblings, and other relatives.

▪ *When you may petition.* The majority of states limit the right to petition to specific circumstances, such as the divorce or death of a parent. However, some states include additional circumstances, such as incarceration of the parent; abuse, neglect, or abandonment of the child; juvenile delinquency; and when custody has been given to a third party or when the child has been placed in foster care. Others even allow grandparents to seek visitation when the parents are still married or when the parents are unmarried. Although adoption usually cuts all ties between a child and his or her biological family, a few states allow grandparents to petition for visitation in instances when a grandchild has been adopted by a stepparent or other relative.[21]

Visitation statutes, however, are relatively new in U.S. law. Many have not yet been tested at the court level and have no case law to back them up. Even those that have been upheld by the courts have little in the way of legislation or procedures to enforce them, and because there is no uniformity from state to state, a parent who really wants to prevent visitation can always move.

Visitation in Dependency

If a child is removed from the parents by child protective services and is not placed with you, the court may consider whether it is in his best interests to have visits with you. Many factors can influence this decision, including your prior relationship with the child and whether such visitation might interfere with parental reunification.

If the parents' rights are terminated by the court, your relationship with your grandchild could terminate as well. Some states do allow grandparents to petition for visitation when a child is adopted by a stepparent or relative but not when the adoptive parents are unrelated.

▪ HOW TO COPE

▪ *Know the law.* Visitation laws vary. Find out the parameters of your own state's visitation laws and proceed accordingly.

▪ *Consider alternatives to legal action.* Litigation is not only expensive but also time-consuming, and it can permanently damage already fragile family relationships. Once a lawsuit starts, people cling to their own side of the story and stop listening. Animosity grows. The children are the ones who get caught in the cross fire. Furthermore, while people's feelings constantly change and evolve, court decisions are fixed and inflexible. Is there anything you can do to keep your family out of the courtroom? Would family counseling address the parent's unwillingness to allow visitation? Is mediation a possibility? Some states have informal dispute resolution or mediation services to help settle visitation problems. If you must battle in court to see your grandchild, it can certainly be worth the fight, but first try to seek other alternatives.

▪ *Take heart.* Although the law once gave complete weight to the rights of the parent, public opinion concerning the rights and well-being of the child has influenced the courts. Increasingly, the courts are recognizing that a child's well-being involves a stable relationship with grandparents. As one New Jersey Supreme Court jurist put it, "It is a biological fact that grandparents are bound to their grandchildren by the unbreakable link of heredity. Visits with a grandparent are often a precious part of a child's experience."[22]

WHEN YOU NEED AN ATTORNEY

At some point in this second parenthood you may need to consult an attorney. Perhaps your grandchild has ended up as a dependent of the court and you risk losing her to the system. Perhaps you are trying for guardianship. Maybe you don't have your grandchild, but you are petitioning for visitation rights. Each of these can be an overwhelming legal battle, and you may want an expert on your side. Even if you are settled in a comfortable custody situation, there are other wars to fight on behalf of your grandchild—with various agencies for proper government aid; with your school district for proper educational services; even with hospitals and Medicaid for medical coverage. Although you are your grandchild's best advocate, sometimes even the sharpest advocate needs help.

Do You Need Legal Counsel?

Whether or not you need an attorney depends on what it is you are trying to accomplish. If everything is going smoothly or you are filing an uncontested visitation and guardianship agreement, you may not need an attorney. Much will depend on the laws of your state.

On the other hand, you do want to hire an attorney whenever the parent or parents hire one first; it keeps the playing field level. You may also need an attorney if you are contesting a judicial proceeding, petitioning to become part of a proceeding, filing a contested visitation or guardianship petition, adopting a child, or appealing an administrative decision.

If you have a question you can't answer, you may need to consult with an attorney, but you may not need to hire one to represent you. Consultation fees vary. Each state has its own laws about when you can and cannot legally represent yourself, but one thing is certain: If you feel you need an attorney, you should consider hiring one.

What to Look For

Attorneys, like doctors, have different specialties. This is true even within the field of family law. If you petition for guardianship, you don't want an attorney who specializes in divorce or dependency. And if a dependency hearing is imminent, you need an attorney who really knows the juvenile justice system. "People buy a car and read *Consumer Reports* and investigate," says attorney Michael Salazar. "But when it comes to picking a lawyer, they assume the first lawyer they find will be an expert. This is an exact specialty, like brain surgery."[23] In other words, know what you're looking for, and do your research.

When you look for legal counsel, you also want to make sure your case is not the first grandparent case your attorney has ever handled. Although this is, indeed, a new area of law, you don't want to be someone's maiden voyage if you can help it. This is where knowledge is power. Learn the terms. Then make sure your attorney knows them. Does he understand the ins and outs of the dependency process? Can he discuss changes in visitation law? If not, find someone who can.

It is just as important to make sure your attorney believes in your case. When a South Carolina couple wanted to mount a legal battle for their grandson, they were discouraged by an attorney who told them, "He's got parents."[24] This is not an attorney you want working for you.

Where to Look

Where you look for an attorney or an advocate depends on your resources and circumstances. Attorneys charge by the hour, and their rates vary according to your location, the size of their firm, and the difficulty of the case. Your total cost will also depend on what needs to be accomplished; filing a document will cost considerably less than a protracted fight in court. One grandmother's attorney told her that her custody battle with the child's mother would cost her "a room addition and a trip to Europe" before they were finished, and he wasn't far off. On the other hand, some cases can be simple and straightforward.

Your best source for legal referrals are other grandparents and grandparent support groups. Which attorneys have other people worked with? What were their experiences? They know which ones are effective and which ones are not. Also, if you are involved in a dependency case, you might consider asking the court clerks which lawyers they recommend. "Everyone knows who they'd hire if they were in trouble, and the ones they'd stay away from," says attorney Michael Salazar.[25]

If you are on a fixed income, you will have a smaller pool to choose from, but you still have options. Ask your state or local bar association if any family law attorneys work "pro bono" (i.e., donate legal assistance) or at reduced rates. Contact your local Legal Aid society or legal services office to find out about free or low-cost representation for people who are income eligible. A law school or law clinic might even provide voluntary services to people on fixed or limited incomes. These organizations may be shy about helping you because of the newness of grandparent litigation and their own inexperience with the issues, but don't be afraid to ask. Every day and with every case, grandparent issues lose their novelty, and organizations like Legal Aid are sure to recognize the growing need for legal assistance.

Court-Appointed Attorneys

Many states offer court-appointed attorneys to key parties in a dependency case who cannot afford their own attorneys, namely, parents who have been accused of abusing or neglecting their children and, sometimes, the children themselves. A court-appointed attorney has the same obligations as a private attorney in terms of representing her clients in court. Occasionally, a grandparent or relative will be eligible for a court-appointed attorney. Some states allow relatives and foster parents who have acted as day-to-day parents in a child's life to petition for "de facto parent"[26] status and become a party in a case, which gives them the right to legal representation. If these de facto parents cannot afford an attorney, the court may be able to appoint one for them.

While a court-appointed attorney can be a financial help, this method of acquiring legal counsel can be a game of Russian roulette in terms of an attorney's sensitivity. You could get a compassionate, caring individual who truly supports your case or one of those who are just doing their job. One grandmother's court-appointed attorney, speaking to me on behalf of her client, told me she was "dumb as dirt" and "too emotional." The risk is even greater when the only attorney in the picture is a court-appointed attorney for the child. In this case, he is only bound to represent the child. Whether or not your view is ever heard will depend on the attorney and how sympathetic that individual is to grandparents.

If your court-appointed attorney is wonderful, treasure her. Unfortunately, there isn't much you can do if you're unhappy with your attorney. You can request a replacement, but you may not get one.

▪ HOW TO COPE

▪ *Be persistent.* If your attorney doesn't return your calls in a timely fashion, keep calling back. Attorneys have busy schedules and busy office staffs; sometimes messages fall through the cracks.

▪ *Tell your attorney the whole truth.* Tell the negative as well as the positive. Don't hide anything. Withholding information because you fear it could hurt your case can do more damage than telling the truth. If you have something in your past that could cause trouble—for instance, a jail record from your youth—let your attorney know. He can address the problem in a way that could minimize damage to your case. If you don't tell him, and the other side finds out, they could have a field day in court.

"Every lawyer assumes his client has not told him all the things that he would like to know," says attorney Charles Ollinger. "Sometimes it's intentional. Sometimes it doesn't occur to a client to mention [something]. It is surprising how important those [facts] can be upon occasion."[27]

<table>
<tr><td>CHAPTER 11</td><td></td></tr>
</table>

| CHAPTER 11 | Child Protection and the Dependency System |

You have to have an understanding of what the
dependency law is, for a grandparent, to
understand what kind of Pandora's box you are
opening when you make that one call to CPS
[Child Protective Services].
—*Ted Youmans, attorney*[1]

laire and Evan Powers basically raised their
granddaughter, Sarah, until she was 10 years
old. Sarah had arrived in the world with the
deck stacked against her: a father who drank, a mother on drugs,
and an abusive relationship between the two. Claire and Evan, her
father's parents, were her ace in the hole; they often let her mother
stay the night or agreed to keep the baby with them when violence
broke out at home. Almost from the beginning, Sarah was in and out
of Grandma's house.

Then, when Sarah was 18 months old, her parents split up. Dad
wanted the baby off the streets, so Mom and Sarah moved in with
Evan and Claire. In a few months Mom disappeared without warning,
and with Sarah. When the father found her in a crack house six months
later, he sued for custody. One day while the case was still pending,
Mom showed up with Sarah. "I can't take care of her anymore; I'll be
back in three months," she told Claire, and took off. Dad got custody
of two-year-old Sarah, but Grandma and Grandpa got the bulk of the
responsibility. For the next four years they bought her clothes, took
her to the day-care center, and baby-sat, sometimes for a week at a
time. Sarah was spending more and more time at Grandma's house,
and eventually father and daughter moved in with Evan and Claire.

By this time, however, Dad was also using drugs and was increasingly abusive to his parents and his daughter. He moved into a motel near a crack house. One day he decided he didn't want his parents to have Sarah; he packed her up and took her down to the crack house with him. Claire called the sheriff. She had called child abuse hotlines three times before because of her son's drug use and child abuse, but each time she was told there was not enough evidence. This time there was. Sarah's father was arrested at the crack house; Sarah was taken into protective custody, then placed back with Claire. Finally, Claire thought, her problems were over. Little did she know they were just beginning.

When Claire called the sheriff, she started the wheels of justice turning. The wheels of justice, she discovered, sometimes run over the very people they are meant to help. The social services agency not only started dependency court proceedings against the father but went out looking for Mom, who had not been seen in several years.

Sarah's mother had been a heavy drug user for most of the eight years of Sarah's life. She knew where her daughter was, but she never had contact with her. She didn't send her letters, and she didn't offer support. She had no parental relationship with the child, who barely knew her. She was living on the streets when they found her. Still, the system offered her a free lawyer, reunification services, a drug rehabilitation program, and, eventually, Sarah. Even though she had essentially abandoned the child. Even though she had been investigated for child abuse three times before Sarah was six months old. Even though the child told everyone—the social worker, the judge, the attorney, her grandparents and her mother—that she didn't want to go with her mother, that the only home she had was with Grandma and Grandpa. "Sarah jumped up on my lap in court and hugged me; I was crying," Claire recalls. "She thought she was going home with me because she had told the judge that she wanted to."

Today Sarah is 12 years old. She has lost weight, has trouble sleeping, and is developing behavioral problems. Claire and Evan can only see her for one weekend each month, and achieving that right cost them $35,000 in legal fees. The mother doesn't make it easy, either: Visits are never hassle free, and she sends Sarah to her grandparents for three days with only the clothes on her back. "She would like people to believe she's clean, but I don't think she is," says Claire. "Even the judge said, at the time, that the mother has unresolved drug problems and the boyfriend is an alcoholic, but he had to protect the mother's visitation rights. These were visitation rights she'd had for years and never used."

Claire and Evan Powers lost their granddaughter by calling a system they thought would help them. Claire says that call was "the biggest mistake ever." The system protects the parents. It gives them attorneys and it gives them services. "They follow them around with a pillow so if they fall down they don't get bruised," she says bitterly.

"The system." Grandparents shudder when they talk about it. Two words that seem to stand for everything impersonal, overbearing, and bureaucratic in government. Power gone out of control. When grandparents talk about "the system," they mean the dependency system, the combination of child protection agencies and juvenile court proceedings that are designed to protect and aid children in crisis.

Many grandparents have never dealt with the system before now, having raised their own children without contact with courts and social workers. Even those who are familiar with the juvenile courts find that involvement as a grandparent is completely different from involvement as a parent. In any case, the dependency process can be an overwhelming and frustrating experience. Every grandparent needs to know about this process—not only to protect themselves if they find themselves in the system but to learn when and how to avoid it. And why.

WHAT IS THE DEPENDENCY SYSTEM?

The dependency system is part of the government's emergency response to protect minor children who are suspected of being abused, neglected, or abandoned. Every state has at least one part of its child welfare agency that is dedicated to investigating reports of children in crisis—often called child protective services (CPS)—and at least one court, typically, the juvenile court, responsible for deciding these cases.

The dependency process is a series of hearings in which a judge decides whether or not allegations against the parents* are true and,

---

* For simplicity, we are using the plural "parents" throughout this discussion. It is understood that in many cases only one parent may be involved.

if so, how to protect the child while the parents try to solve their problems. Among the issues considered in the various dependency hearings are the following:

- Whether the child should be removed from the home
- Where the child should be placed during the dependency process
- What measures, such as drug rehabilitation and counseling, the parents must take to regain custody of the child
- What the court can do to help the parents reunite with the child (for example, devise a visitation schedule or order parenting classes)
- What services, such as counseling, the court can recommend for the child
- How the family is progressing
- If and when the child can safely return home
- What permanent custody arrangement can be made if the child cannot return home (permanent plans are generally a choice of adoption, guardianship, or long-term foster care)

During the course of these hearings the child is considered a "dependent of the court" (thus the term "dependency hearings"). This means that legal custody of the child transfers from the parents to the state (whereas physical custody will be awarded to someone who can care for the child). The dependency system is, for many children, the entrance door into foster care, although a number of states give preference to placing children with relatives.

Dependency hearings are the most powerful court proceedings connected with a child. Once CPS intervenes and juvenile court takes jurisdiction, you and your grandchild are locked into the system for a defined period of time. Decisions are taken out of the hands of your family and placed in the hands of the court; parents and grandparents lose control of the situation. In most states the dependency system has exclusive jurisdiction; it overrules all other courts, including family law and guardianship.[2] This means that while the case is active in the dependency process, no other court can make decisions about the child. In other words, once your grandchild goes into the system, you are married to the courts for as long as the process lasts. For a grandparent, this can pose serious problems:

- *Dependency is a nightmare of bureaucracy.* Everyone in the system seems to work against each other. Caseloads are high. Communication within the system is poor. Sometimes critical information never reaches the attending judge. One child welfare agency director describes dependency as "a mass custody suit where six to eight different interests are represented." Often, the ones who lose are the children.

■ *The dependency process is a mystery because it is confidential.* Most cases are closed except to the parties involved—generally, the child, the parents, and the child welfare department. This means that the public and the press cannot come into these courtrooms the way they may come into criminal and civil courts. You may not be allowed to speak on behalf of your grandchildren, even if you are raising them, unless you have "standing" (see "How to Cope," below).

■ *Dependency is relentless.* Although there are state and federal time lines for when certain hearings must take place, attorneys often waive these deadlines, and the process can drag on—sometimes for years.

■ *Dependency splinters families.* When you are in the dependency process, you are at the mercy of strangers. I have seen social workers decide that Grandma is too old, too overbearing, or too possessive to have a child (or, in one case, not "grieving properly"). They pull children out of the grandparents' home and place them in foster care or a group home; the grandparents might not even get visitation rights. If this happens and if the parents' rights are terminated, your role as grandparent will also end.

■ *Dependency favors parents.* The dependency system does not worry about grandparents. When social workers and judges talk about keeping families together, they mean biological parents and children. Grandparents don't count as "legal" family and have little credibility in court. "In court, you are not seen as reliable people speaking for the child; you are looked upon as meddlers," says attorney Ted Youmans. "It's terrifying to get involved with the system and realize someone else has control over a member of your family."[3]

The catchphrase in the dependency system is "family reunification." This means that, except in very limited circumstances, the social service agency will work to enable parents to regain custody of their children. Toward that end, the system will offer parents all kinds of services to help them correct the problems that led to their losing custody and to help them "reunify" with their children. The presumption is that children belong with their parents and parents should have every opportunity to raise their own children. Says Judge Lawrence L. Koontz, Jr., of Virginia, "The goal of the court is to restore custody to one of the natural parents whenever possible."[4]

Meanwhile, you, as a relative caregiver, must encourage this parent–child relationship if the child is to be placed with you. The court will place a child with strangers rather than let family members interfere with reunification. This can be devastating, particularly if you are prevented from seeing or contacting your grandchild. Grandparents repeatedly get lost and overwhelmed in the maze of steps and hearings that make up the dependency process. Here, as everywhere, knowledge is your best defense.

DEPENDENCY: STEP BY STEP

Dependency law is extensive and complex. This discussion is only a general blueprint of the process; it is designed as a tool to help you ask questions about the laws and regulations in your own state. Although each stage of the dependency process has various possible outcomes, each stage explained below assumes, for simplicity's sake, that the child has been removed from the home and placed with relatives. The schedule used in this discussion reflects Los Angeles County procedures. Your own state laws may outline more steps, different names, and a different time line.

The Call

A parent is arrested or injured, and no one is around to take the children. A child is left alone in an apartment for hours. A teacher suspects a student is being abused at home. The dependency process starts with a call to child protective services about a child who is suspected of being abandoned, neglected, or abused. CPS then sends out an emergency response social worker to investigate the situation.

Anyone can call CPS about a child at risk, including clergy, neighbors, and family members. Some states also have a list of "mandated reporters," that is, individuals who are required by law to report any suspicion of child abuse or neglect (e.g., teachers, doctors, therapists, and child care providers.) When the investigation takes place depends on the nature of the allegation. A call about suspected abuse generally receives more immediate attention than a call about neglect. Even if the caller can provide an address but no name, CPS must respond.

Depending on what the social worker finds, one of several things can happen:

- The case can be dismissed for lack of evidence.
- The parents may agree to seek counseling, rehabilitation, or other services to correct the problem, and the child remains in the home. The court may or may not get involved.
- The child may be considered to be "at risk" and removed from parental custody.

Of course, what social workers actually find during an investigation often depends on when they visit and how thorough they are. A worker who makes an immediate unannounced visit, for instance, will often see a different picture than one who makes an appointment. Even a day's notice can give neglectful parents time to clean the house, stock the refrigerator, and generally make a better appearance.

The Pickup

If a social worker (or police officer) finds enough evidence to indicate that a child is in danger of abuse or neglect at home, the child will be taken into protective custody. Some states may release a child into the care of a relative if one shows up with proof of relationship and a clean background check. At this point the case can either be dismissed or referred to the juvenile court through a "petition of dependency" (see below). However, if no one comes to take the child or if for some reason CPS won't release him, the social worker must refer the case to the juvenile court for a hearing. During this time the child could be inaccessible to the family.

What You Need to Know

Keep track of your grandchildren. If you know they have been picked up by CPS, be persistent in locating them. Be sure to take birth certificates or something that proves your relationship to the children, especially if their last name is different from yours. Your actions may not prevent the dependency process from kicking into gear, but if CPS will release the children to you, it may make it easier for you to get placement down the line. At the very least, let the social worker know you are interested in placement or future visitation.

The Petition

A petition of dependency is the legal document that tells a judge why the social worker thinks the court should intervene to protect a child. In essence, it is the state's formal allegation against the parents for the abuse and neglect of a minor, and it formally requests that the child be made a dependent of the court. The petition must be filed within *48 court hours* (i.e., two working days) after the child is taken into protective custody.[5] It includes whatever facts the child welfare agency believes will support its claims and identifies the sections of the law under which the parents are accused; these accusations are important because they determine which programs the parents will have to complete in order to regain custody of the child. For instance, if the petition claims the child has been physically abused but there are no allegations of drug use, the court cannot send the parents to drug treatment.

The Detention Hearing

The detection hearing (sometimes known as "arraignment and detection," "shelter care hearing," or "temporary custody hearing") is the first judicial proceeding in a dependency case, the hearing that sets the case in motion. It is a quick hearing, without much investigation beforehand and with just a brief report from the emergency response worker.

At the detention hearing the parents are formally informed of the reason the child was taken into temporary custody and the allegations against them. This is also the stage where parents are informed of their right to an attorney. If they cannot afford one, some states will appoint one free of charge. Some states also appoint an attorney for the child; others use the same attorney who represents the child welfare agency (often called the Department of Social Services, or DSS).

Two issues are decided at the detention hearing stage: how the parents will respond to the allegations and whether there is enough evidence to detain the child in temporary custody until the court determines whether the allegations in the petition are true. If the parents do not dispute the charges, the case will go on to a disposition hearing. If the parents deny the charges, the case will move on to mediation or trial. The judge can also schedule another hearing to provide more information.

Courts are typically reluctant to take children from their parents, and this includes the child who has been taken into protective custody. If the judge can safely release a child to the parents, with DSS supervision, he or she usually will. However, if the child cannot be returned to the parents, she may be placed in a temporary foster home or with a relative until the case is resolved. It is also possible that the case could be dismissed at this point, with or without continued supervision by social services.

What You Need to Know

The detention hearing is a critical hearing. If you are aware of it, try to show up. You probably won't be able to attend—these hearings are confidential—but you can let the court officers, social workers, or child's attorney know, for the record, that you are a grandparent and want to be a resource. Many state laws give preference to placing children with relatives, but they have to know you exist. Social services will run a background and criminal check on you before you can take your grandchild home.

If the court won't consider you for placement, you might be able to request visitation while your grandchild is in the care of another relative or in foster care. The best-case scenario is that the child is placed with you. At worst, the child is taken from the parents and placed in a foster home and you don't find out about it for months. This is particularly common when grandparents live in another state.

Mediation and/or Trial

The decision-making phase of the dependency process involves mediation and/or trial. This is the stage where the court decides whether or not the allegations against the parents are true and, if so, whether or not the state will assume legal custody of the child. These determinations are generally made in a "jurisdictional hearing" (or trial), but some states try to avoid the need for a trial by settling the case through mediation.

Mediation Stage

Some states insert a mediation stage (sometimes called a "pretrial hearing" or a "pretrial resolution conference") between the detention and jurisdictional hearings. This is the state's attempt to settle a case without going to trial. Sometimes the allegations in the petition can be proven untrue and the case is dismissed. Sometimes a parent is willing to admit to the charges in the petition, or the petition can be amended to reflect charges a parent *will* admit to. For instance, Dad may have earlier denied the allegations of drug abuse but by the mediation stage may admit to occasional cocaine use. If a settlement is reached, the case could go directly to a "disposition hearing" (see below), sometimes even the same day. If, however, the parents continue to deny all allegations, the case goes to a jurisdictional hearing, or trial.

Trial Stage

If a settlement is not reached through mediation or if a state does not provide mediation services, the case goes into the trial phase of the dependency process. (This trial is also known as the adjudication or jurisdictional hearing.) DSS presents evidence that the child has been abused or neglected. The attorney for the parents questions the evidence and presents counterevidence. Witnesses may be called. Finally, the judge decides if the charges in the petition against the parents are true, which charges are true, and whether or not to make the child a dependent of the court. If the court finds the petition is not true, the case is dismissed and the child returned to the home. If the court finds the petition is true, the case is set for a disposition hearing.

What You Need to Know

It is important to understand which charges are proven or admitted at the trial stage; they will be important at the disposition hearing, when the court decides what plan the parents must follow to regain custody of the child. For instance, if a petition claims a parent has a drug problem and is physically abusive but the judge doesn't see enough evidence to prove drug abuse, the case plan cannot include drug rehabilitation services. However, if additional proof appears later on, DSS can often make new allegations or amend the petition, so make your grandchild's social worker aware of what you know— and can prove—as the case goes along.

The Disposition Hearing

If the allegations against the parents are judged to be true, the case goes to a disposition hearing. This is where the court decides what to do to both protect the child and help the parents regain custody. At or before the disposition hearing the child's social worker submits a report on the status of the case and a case plan recommending where the child should live, how often the parents should visit or call, and what services should be offered to the children and to the parents to improve conditions in the home and facilitate the return of the child to the parents.

The judge considers the social worker's report and recommendations, as well as evidence and arguments from other parties, before making a decision on the case. Final court orders typically include a "reunification plan," which stipulates what conditions the parents must fulfill in order to regain custody of the child, a visitation schedule, and a decision on placement for the child. The placement plan occasionally sends the child home with a parent under DSS supervision; more often, the child is placed in the home of a relative, a foster home, or a group home.

Periodic Reviews

Once the child has been placed with a relative or foster parents and reunification services have been offered to the parents, there will be periodic hearings (also known as "administrative case reviews," "judicial reviews," and "dependency status reviews") to review the family's progress. These reviews are conducted every six months by either the court or the child welfare agency and consider both the case and the case plan. The following questions are addressed: Is the case plan being followed? How are the parents progressing? Does the child need additional services? When might the child return to parental custody? If by the second review it seems unlikely that the child will return home, a permanent plan may be established. If the parents are doing well but are not quite ready to resume custody, the court can grant a six-month extension before deciding on the permanent plan.

What You Need to Know

Although relative caregivers may be entitled to receive notification of each review hearing in advance, they are rarely notified in time, if at all. Since you know these reviews are every six months, try to keep track of when they are scheduled. Let the judge, the child's lawyer, and the social worker know that you want to be informed of these hearings, and try to attend. Be prepared to talk about how you are complying with the reunification plan if you are asked and to provide comments and observations about the child's reactions to parental visits. This is another place careful documentation can be helpful. Also, keep records of all legal documents, bills, correspondence, and contacts with the lawyer, the social worker, the court, and the parents. If you write letters to the court, copy them to all the attorneys involved to make sure everyone reads them.

Permanency Planning Hearing

Federal law requires that a permanent plan for each child who enters the dependency system be established no later than 18 months from the date of the original placement.[6] At this point the child must either be safely returned to the parents or assigned to a permanent plan by the court. In either case, reunification services end. If a child cannot be returned home, the court has three options, in order of preference: adoption, guardianship, and long-term foster care. Adoption has the highest priority because it is the most permanent solution. Guardianship only lasts until the child is 18 years old, and it can be terminated before then. Long-term foster care is the least stable option.

What You Need to Know

Some social workers may try to pressure you into adopting your grandchild. Not only is it a more permanent plan for the child, but because it may end government benefits, it is less costly to the system. They are not supposed to pressure you. Although the courts do look at adoption as a first choice, there are reasons grandparents may not want to adopt, or even seek guardianship, of a grandchild: They may not be ready to give up on their adult children. They may be under financial stress and need the government aid. They may feel that their age or medical condition might rule out adoption.

"The truth is that the court looks at the relative caretaker very differently than they look at a nonrelated caretaker," says attorney Pamela Mohr. "They realize there is a familial obligation. Even if the kid is not legally your kid, the kid is your grandkid and will be your grandkid for the rest of your life. They aren't worried about your just abandoning the child."[7] (See "Adoption" in Chapter 10 and "Adoption Assistance Program" in Chapter 12.)

▪ HOW TO COPE

▪ *Find out about relative placement.* Federal law encourages state agencies to place children in the "least restrictive" environment.[8] This is often interpreted to mean placing children with family, when possible. Moreover, because of the shrinking number of available foster homes and the increasing number of children needing care, many states now have formal regulations and guidelines that give preference to placing children with relatives—often grandparents—before nonrelatives. If your grandchild is in the system—or runs a risk of ending up in the system—find out your state's policy on relative placement.

Of course, a state's preference for placing children with relatives doesn't guarantee that placement. The court must first evaluate your ability to provide a secure and stable home for the child. It will also consider your willingness to support visitation and reunification with the parent and whether or not you have a criminal record.

If your state does not support relative placement or if the child is not placed with you, you can still try to get visitation privileges. Stay as connected with your grandchild as you can, and let the social workers know if you are interested in permanent placement if the parent and child cannot reunify.

▪ *Start early!* It is critical that you express your concern for your grandchild as early in the dependency process as possible, especially if you want the child placed with you. Although many states require DSS to identify family resources, this is not always fully accomplished. There may not be enough time to look for family. Parents may be uncooperative about supplying names and phone numbers. Some social workers may simply neglect to interview relatives. Unfortunately, if too much time passes, the court may rule out relative placement altogether; the child may have bonded with foster parents, who may be considering adoption, and the court may be unwilling to disrupt the situation. "It's really a heartrending situation," says attorney Pamela Mohr. "There's no answer for those cases and, unfortunately, they're fairly common."[9] If you cannot locate your grandchild but suspect that she is in the system, contact child welfare in the child's last known location and let them know that you are a resource.

Even if you can't get placement early on, you can ask for visitation. This at least would allow you to continue your involvement in your grandchild's life, a fact that could be important if you later seek placement or custody. In fact, don't hesitate to let the social worker and the court know if you are willing to take your grandchild on a permanent basis in the event that the parents cannot fulfill the reunification requirements. The sooner you express your interest, the more likelihood you have of being considered.

▪ *Attend hearings!* Once your grandchild is in the system, attend every hearing that you can. You may not be permitted into the courtroom, but let the bailiff or the court clerk know, for the record, that you are there, that you are a grandparent, and that you are interested in placement or visitation. The fact that there exists a real person who is willing to take a child can sometimes affect a judge's decision. You can also write a letter to the judge. If you do, send copies to all the attorneys involved and keep it simple.

▪ *Ask about standing.* "Standing" is the right to participate in a case as a party, which means you are entitled to receive notice of hearings, to be represented by an attorney, and to present evidence. Although rules of the court often change from county to county in terms of who may speak in court, when they may do so, and under what circumstances, the parties who have standing in a dependency case are generally the parents, the child, and the child welfare agency. Grandparents and other relatives typically do not have standing in a dependency case; they may not even be permitted in the courtroom. However, some states will allow a person who has raised and provided for a child for some time to qualify as a *de facto* parent, that is, a parent "in actuality" or a substitute parent.[10] This person, whether related to the child or not, may be entitled to standing and in some cases to a court-appointed attorney. However, you may have to hire a private attorney in order to prove de facto parent status.

Some states allow relatives limited participation in a dependency case without full standing.[11] Judges also have the authority to let you in the courtroom if they want to hear what you have to say. Keep asking questions until you know exactly what kind of involvement you are entitled to in your court system.

▪ *Behave yourself in court.* Grandparents have an image problem in court. In their fury to protect their grandchildren (and their frustration with the system) they often argue with court clerks, attorneys, and even judges attempting to clarify the danger of the situation and the need to move quickly. Despite their best intentions this approach often backfires, and the grandparents become known as rabble-rousers and troublemakers. Social workers may forget to return their phone calls, court clerks may claim to have misplaced documents, and the court may turn a deaf ear to their concerns.[12] You will have more success if you follow two rules:

1. Be gracious with court officials. Remember that you are asking for help when you deal with the court system; you don't score points by making demands. "Clerks are in charge of what happens to papers," notes attorney Charles Ollinger. "The judge is in charge of what happens in the courtroom. When you go in there, you're playing in their ballpark, by their rules."[13]

2. Be polite in court. Don't interrupt or blurt out comments. Try to stay calm; avoid arguing with the parents in front of the judge. Cooperate with your attorney, if you have one. Above all, don't argue with the judge. (For more on court behavior see "A Word About Judges," below.)

▪ *Support reunification.* If you wish to have your grandchild placed with you, you have to not only keep your feelings about the parents private but actively work toward reuniting the parents with the child—even if you've seen them abuse your grandchild and even if you think reunification is the most horrible thing that could happen to your grandchild. If you cannot support reunification, the court may not place the child with you. It may not be able to. And if you speak or act against the parents while the child is living with you, social services can remove him. Of course, that doesn't mean you must let a parent see a child when he or she shows up intoxicated on your doorstep, but it does mean you must do everything else to actively encourage reunification.

▪ *Be prepared for delays.* From the moment the child is removed, a clock starts ticking. According to federal law, a permanent plan must be established for a child no later than 18 months from the date of the original placement. However, it rarely happens that way. Marjorie Brown's granddaughter was six months old when she was placed with Marjorie and was three by the time a permanent plan was established. Sue Ellen Rice's grandson entered the system three years ago; he and his family have been in permanency planning hearings for almost a year now, as his mother continues to fight for custody.

Various factors contribute to these delays. Rising caseloads make scheduling difficult at every stage. Hearings may be continued over several dates to allow for further investigation or psychological evaluations. Attorneys may waive the time line on a client's case. Sympathetic judges may refrain from enforcing the time line, thus giving parents an additional chance to complete their requirements and prove themselves. There may also be discrepancies in when the court starts the clock. The phrase *original placement* leaves room for interpretation. According to attorney Michael Salazar, some cases can be in the system for two years without even going to trial.[14]

There may also be a conflict in the law itself, says attorney Pamela Mohr. Although federal law sets an 18-month time line on dependency cases, some states require that parents be offered at least 12 months of family reunification services. If those services only start at Month 16, there is a problem. Mohr encourages relatives to make sure services are really offered to parents from the beginning. "Even if the parents are hopeless," says Mohr, "if you really offer 12 months of reunification, the court will have less qualms about [letting you take the kids]."[15] It is difficult to really pressure the court in this instance. At least make sure your attorney really knows how to maneuver in the dependency system, and then find a support group where you can vent your frustrations with other grandparents.

HOTLINES ARE NOT ALWAYS HELP LINES

Claire Powers called a hotline to help her granddaughter; in the end she lost her. The system went out, found Mom, and pulled her back into the picture. And Mom came running. To quote one family law judge, "The most disinterested parent in the world becomes the most interested when someone tries to interfere with their God-given, constitutionally protected right to parent."

But this is not the only reason to avoid hotlines. If you call a child abuse hotline on your adult child and he or she finds out, you can bury yourself in the system. If your grandchild is removed from a parent, he or she may do everything possible to keep the child out of your home. Some parents will even lie; they may say that you were an abusive parent, an alcoholic—anything to make you pay for making the call. "It's like calling the cops on your daughter or son," explains attorney Ted Youmans. "You're probably not going to be befriending the kid. You'll be alienating yourself right from the start, and the system will probably treat you with alienation as the one who complained."[16]

Remember, anything that interferes with reunification is suspect, and a bad relationship between parent and grandparent is a red flag to social workers and to the courts. Judges are wary of grandparents whose children say, "I hate them. I can't get along with them. I can't visit my kids at their house; they interfere." Those grandparents may not get placement.

HOW TO AVOID INVOLVEMENT WITH THE SYSTEM

Most grandparents involved with the dependency system had no choice in the matter—a social worker showed up on their doorstep with their grandchildren in tow or the hospital held a drug-exposed infant in protective custody. In other words, the system arrived with the child. Some grandparents, however, have many chances to bypass government involvement if they realize there is a problem and know enough to think ahead.

▪ *Keep track of your grandchildren.* Do so especially when parents have problems. Offer to watch your grandchildren occasionally. Visit and call often, if the parents will let you. If there has been a problem in the past, let schools and local hospitals know that you are available as an emergency contact. Once children are in the foster care system, it can be not only difficult but heartbreaking to try to get them out.

▪ *Keep track of your adult children.* Do so even with those who don't have children yet. I have talked to grandparents from various states who tell me that they didn't even know they had a grandchild until the child was four or five years old and already in foster care. If a parent is arrested without someone available to take the child, children's services will probably take over. Keep the lines of communication open and active, especially when you're in another state. If your adult child has any responsible friends, give them your telephone number in case of emergency. Because my parents lived nearby, they were immediately able to take in my nephew when my sister died. However, had Nikki died in another city, Kevin might have gone into a foster home before anyone in the family knew it. Furthermore, since Nikki didn't have a will, child welfare might not even have known that Kevin had grandparents who could take him. The bottom line is that keeping track of the parent is the only way to keep track of the child.

▪ *Think ahead.* In case of emergency, how could you prove your relationship to your grandchild? Do you have your adult child's birth certificate? Do you have your grandchild's birth certificate? If your own child is the father, is he acknowledged on the birth certificate? If you are on good terms with the parents, in case of illness or accident, could you get a signed statement proving your relationship? Unless a grandchild is old enough to identify you, proving your relationship can be complicated, particularly if the child has a different last name from yours. Planning ahead can save time and heartache in the event of an emergency.

▪ *Consider guardianship.* If the grandchildren are with you and their parents have vanished, consider becoming their guardian. The dependency system will make you jump through legal hoops, will conduct visits once a month, and will put a social worker on your back, adding to the stress and tension you are already experiencing. But, says attorney Michael Salazar, "If you go into probate, you're on your own."[17] In other words, you're in control, not the system. (For more on guardianship, see Chapter 10.)

WHEN YOU MIGHT WANT THE SYSTEM INVOLVED

In spite of all the disadvantages, there are actually reasons you might want the system involved in your grandchild's case: the child's safety and your own peace of mind. Perhaps you cannot afford to apply for guardianship. Perhaps your family situation or personal history would prevent a judge from giving you custody. Perhaps your grandchild isn't with you, and the situation is too dangerous to wait for a guardianship hearing. This is a time when you may actually want to call child protective services. Sometimes *anything*—even foster care—is better than leaving a grandchild in an abusive home. It's not a perfect solution, but it can be the lesser evil.

Understand, however, that if you are the one to call the police or CPS, there is a possibility the child will not be placed with you. A lot depends on your background check, what your son or daughter says about you, and whether or not you live in the same state. Still, sometimes it is worth involving the system to protect a child who is at risk.

WHEN THE SYSTEM WON'T GET INVOLVED

It may seem to you that social workers and judges are just hovering in the doorways ready to snatch up any child who may be in danger, that after one call the child will be whisked away to safety. At least that is the belief of hopeful grandparents who call child abuse hotlines. Actually, it's not true. A great source of anger and frustration for many grandparents is when the system won't get involved in a case.

There are times when calling CPS won't do anything. Allegations of child abuse and neglect require witnesses and physical proof. This can infuriate grandparents who know of the kind of abuse that doesn't leave marks. Emotional abuse may not show on a child's body, but the scars are often more difficult to heal. Moreover, the legal definitions of abuse and neglect not only vary from state to state but are interpreted differently from social worker to social worker and from one judge to the next. Furthermore, leaving children with grandparents, family, or friends is rarely considered desertion or abandonment. Child welfare agencies regularly turn away children who are living with relatives without parental interference; their reasoning is that the child is not in danger.

Generally, a grandparent in this situation has three choices: continue to care for the child informally, return the child to the parents and wait until she is abused or neglected, or file for private guardianship. As we saw in Chapter 10, guardianship offers greater protection.

A WORD ABOUT SOCIAL WORKERS

In the field of social work, as in most professions, there are good workers and bad ones. Which kind you get is the luck of the draw, but the difference is often immediately clear. Good social workers are thorough. When they investigate a case, they really investigate. They talk to the children, they look for bruises and ask for explanations, they study a home for things that signal neglect. When I worked for CPS, I was sent out on a child abuse case with a social worker who never even entered the house. When Mom came to the door, he told her we had received a report of suspected child abuse. Mom said everything was fine. The social worker saw that the baby had a bottle, said okay, and left. He never looked at the other children or talked to them. This was not a good social worker.

Good social workers are supportive. They listen to your concerns, return phone calls, link you up with resources and information. They let you know what kind of financial assistance is available to your grandchild and how you can apply for it. Some will even refer you to a support group. A number of the GAP grandmothers come to me through social worker referrals.

Bad social workers are a nightmare. They range from the poorly informed to the actively heartless, from the ones who give you incorrect information about department regulations and government benefits to the ones who have a fixed prejudice against grandparents. One case worker, who didn't know me, talked to me about a grandmother I know. "She's ruining everyone's life," she told me. "I can't deal with her." She also called her "crazy" and "invasive." This attitude is a common problem for grandparents. Many social workers see them as picking fights with their children out of vengeance—"hollerin' wolf" as one grandmother calls it.[18] In fact, the war stories are legendary. I received a letter from a woman whose daughter died, leaving her with three small children to care for. Like many grandparents, she discovered that it is difficult to feed and clothe growing children on a fixed income. Her social worker told her she was expected to "cut coupons and shop at Goodwill, just like everyone else on welfare." When one young woman placed her two children with her mother, social services removed them because the grandmother was "too old." Beth and Alan Grafton had a fight on their hands to get custody of their grandchildren after their son-in-law murdered their daughter. The reason? Beth would cry when she discussed her daughter's death. The worker assigned to the case decided that Grandma "wasn't grieving properly" and recommended against custody. "The courts seem to think grandparents just love taking grandchildren from their children," says a Texas grandmother. "It's the hardest thing to do in the world. Grandparents raising grandchildren—they're not doing it because they want to, they're doing it because they have to."[19]

If you are raising your grandchildren, you will, most likely, have to work with social workers. They're like a force of nature; you can't get around them. You find them at each stage of the game, from intake workers to long-term case workers. Moreover, sometimes everything can depend on the decision of a social worker. As one young woman admitted to Claire Powers, "I look at 30 minutes in this child's life and play God." So, some words of advice . . .

▪ *Be nice to social workers.* After all, you want them on your side. Social workers have great power: They present information to judges; sometimes they're also your only source of information. Endear yourself to them, if you can. Don't make demands. "Once you attack a social worker, the likelihood of your getting satisfaction from that system is less than five percent," says attorney Michael Salazar.[20] In other words, use kid gloves and don't get them angry.

▪ *Use understanding.* It is easier to work with people if you understand what obstacles they are fighting. Social workers are as much at the mercy of an unfeeling system as are children and grandparents. Social workers in some large cities oversee as many as 125 child abuse cases.[21] They are undertrained and underpaid—and they burn out quickly. An official in one city reported that half his staff had been working less than a year.[22] Between being new on the job and having case overload, many social workers don't have time to keep up with changes in the law. Says grandparent activisit Ethel Dunn, "You go into social services [and] they are in chaos, not because everyone in the social service system is a poor social worker but it's simply that they don't have the wherewithal to do the job they're given."[23]

▪ *Tell specific facts.* Tell your grandchild's social worker what you saw with your own eyes, not what you heard from other people. If you can, offer witnesses; they may be viewed as less biased.

▪ *Consider whose case it is.* You may, as a grandparent, talk about "my case" and "my social worker," and it can certainly feel that way. You are trying to protect your grandchild from parents and a system that seem to have anything but your grandchild's best interests at heart. Grandparents have a lot riding on their social worker and their case. A good social worker may understand this, but he won't see it the same way. He can't. He is your grandchild's social worker, handling your grandchild's case. His job is to protect the child's interests and, if possible, return her to the custody of her parents.

Remember, not every social worker who disagrees with a grandparent is a bad social worker. Not every child who cannot be with his parents should be with his grandparents. There are grandparents who really should not have their grandchildren because of health, medical, or psychological problems. Some children may be better off in a foster home if there is no other relative to take them.

A WORD ABOUT JUDGES

The judge is the wild card in any legal situation. Judges don't write laws, but they interpret them. Judges don't investigate cases, but they rule on them. In a limited time frame and with selective information a judge makes binding decisions about a child's future, and each decision is as individual as the judge who made it. Judges get reputations among grandparents. Some judges are rule-bound. "They're lawyers," says attorney Charles Ollinger. "They are taught to think unemotionally, to think about 'best interest' in legal terms. The good ones listen to people who understand emotional realities—psychologists, child care professionals—but there aren't many judges like that."[24]

Some judges can seem terribly unfair and inconsistent. Like the one who let nine-year-old Travis Jackson testify against his father for killing his mother but wouldn't let him choose to live with his grandparents. Or the judge who sent Esther Smith's grandsons back to an alcoholic mother who had not complied with her case plan because he felt the case had been in the system "long enough." Others are plainly insensitive. "Some grandparents have a need to steal their grandchildren," one judge told a grandmother. "Is that the case here?" I have even heard about a probate judge who turned to an attorney and barked, "What's all this about 'bonding?' We're not talking about real estate here!"

Every once in a while we hear about a judge who not only is sensitive to grandparents' and grandchildren's interests but understands what is at stake. One unorthodox judge in Arizona settled a dispute in which everyone in a large family was fighting bitterly over two grandchildren. The judge had every person involved in the case come into the courtroom and forbade anyone to speak. Then she had the children brought in. She watched to see whom they ran to—it turned out to be the grandparents—and awarded them custody.[25]

For the most part, however, few judges even think about grandparent concerns, let alone support them. Part of the reason is that they often cannot. Judges interpret the laws but they are limited by them, and according to the law, reunification of child and parent has the highest priority. "I can't take a child from a parent because I'd like to," says California Judge John C. Woolley. "I can't even take a child from a parent because down deep in my heart I really want to. I can only interfere in a parent–child relationship if to continue that relationship would be a detriment to the child and further to place the child with a nonparent is in the child's best interest. It's not a balancing act; it's a dual-focus question."[26]

Another problem, however, is that judges, like social workers, have impossible caseloads. They may not have time to read all the critical documents involved in a case, and they may come to court unprepared. Their decisions can reflect that.

If you find yourself in the dependency system or if you apply for guardianship or adoption or even if you appeal an administrative decision about government aid, you may find yourself facing a judge. If you do and you are given the opportunity to speak in court, there are a few principles you may want to keep in mind:

- *Be respectful.*
- *Be clear.* Make your statements short and to the point. Stick to facts. Ask the judge if he or she has any questions.
- *Be informed.* There are some situations in which grandparents may represent themselves in court, such as in visitation or guardianship hearings in certain states. If you are in such a situation, you are

expected to be as familiar with the laws and procedures that affect your case as an attorney is. If you represent yourself, educate yourself.

▪ *Don't argue with the judge.* It is particularly critical to follow this rule before a decision is reached. "It is," says Ollinger, "like arguing with a waiter before the waiter brings the soup. You don't know what is going to happen!"[27]

No two courtrooms are the same. Everything that happens in a particular courtroom is filtered through the perpective of the presiding judge. Which judge you get is often the luck of the draw. Unfortunately, it can set the tone for your granchild's entire case.

CHAPTER 12

Government Aid and Public Assistance

Just when you think you should be living the life of Riley, you've got a whole new family. I spend at least $80 every week on groceries; if it was just the two of us, it would be half of that.
—*Grandmother in North Carolina*[1]

Raising a grandchild is not only an emotional and legal challenge but a financial one as well. Some grandparents deplete their savings, take out second mortgages on their homes, and even do without their own necessities in order to provide for their grandchildren. Few think about government aid. Many grandparents simply don't know that financial assistance is available to them; often this is because they have their grandchildren on an informal basis. However, even when children are placed by child protective services or the court, many social workers neglect to tell grandparents and relatives that they are entitled to aid for a child.

Remember Leah Croft? She was already raising her daughter's six-year-old twins when another grandchild, Josh, arrived at her house—late at night, unexpected, and in the arms of a social worker. Leah was a single, working grandmother on a moderate salary. The twins had lived with her for four years, and she had stretched her limited budget to accommodate them. She didn't know the twins were entitled to welfare benefits, so she had never asked for them. Then the new baby arrived, and the expenses nearly took her over the financial edge. Although Josh was placed with her by child protective services, no one from the agency told her that he might be eligible for foster care. Furthermore, after Leah found out and applied for foster care, no one told her she could get welfare assistance for the baby while she waited. For five months she put diapers and baby supplies on her credit card, because that was all she had. Leah eventually received retroactive benefits for the months she waited, but she is still paying the interest those credit card charges incurred.

Lack of information is the toughest financial problem you may face as a grandparent; it keeps you out of the game entirely. If you don't know you can't ask, and if you can't ask you may not get the help you need and deserve. The good news is that government assistance is available to you, primarily through programs that support dependent children. Just because you are caring for your grandchildren does not mean you have an obligation to support them—even if you are their legal guardian. Only parents (biological or adoptive) have that responsibility. The government recognizes this, which is why programs like foster care were developed. Although grandparents fall into a gray area between parents and foster parents, there are a number of assistance programs that may apply to you and your grandchildren, from welfare and foster care benefits to social security and adoption assistance.

THE DIFFICULTIES OF WORKING WITH THE GOVERNMENT

Government aid means working with the government. You may find yourself fighting a maze of bureaucracy, poor information, and seemingly unfair rules. You may also struggle with the social stigma of welfare or the inequalities of the foster care system. The very agencies designed to support your grandchildren can seem like more of a hindrance than a help. Be aware of the pitfalls. Advanced knowledge can often prevent problems, and it will always prepare you to face them.

Misinformation

After lack of information, the most common problem grandparents face in dealing with government agencies is poor information. You may ask the right questions, but the answers you get are either half true or completely wrong. The reason is that many social and welfare workers just don't know the right answers. They may be undertrained or unaware of changes in the law. Perhaps they don't understand how a particular program applies to grandparent families. For instance, you yourself may not be eligible for welfare, but your grandchild may be. But if no one tells you, you won't know.

Government employees are rarely malicious but may be ill informed. Unfortunately, some of them will swear their poor information is the gospel truth. Be cautious when you deal with social workers and eligibility workers. Ask questions to clarify what they tell you. Learn what you can about local rules and regulations, and contact other grandparents and support groups to compare notes. Accurate information is your key to government assistance.

Bureaucracy

Dealing with government agencies is rarely a cut-and-dry experience. It can mean long lines, extensive paperwork, and bureaucratic mistakes. You may wait in three different lines at the welfare office just to get a packet of forms, then wait in another line to schedule an appointment. If you work, you may have to take the day off in order to attend an interview. If your grandchildren have to be there, you'll need to cart toys and lunch along for them. It could turn into a whole day affair. This is particularly difficult for grandparents who are disabled and cannot sit for long periods of time. Calling isn't better. Because some eligibility workers have restricted telephone hours, it can take days to connect with them.

If you are having a difficult time reaching an eligibility worker, you may want to talk to her supervisor. First, document the times you try to call and the names of people you speak with. Write letters when you can (and keep copies for yourself). Then, if you do have to go over the worker's head, you have proof of what occurred.

Long lines and mistakes are an inevitable part of dealing with the government. All you can do is be alert for errors and be patient with the rest—and try to do something nice for yourself when you get home!

Unequal Benefits

There are two key assistance programs that grandparents and relatives get involved with: welfare (Aid to Families with Dependent Children, or AFDC) and foster care. Both provide cash and medical assistance to needy children, but foster care offers substantially higher benefits. In one year the average (national) welfare payment to a grandparent who was the sole caregiver for a grandchild was $109 per child per month, compared to $371 per child per month to foster parents.[2] Foster care also increases with the child's age and may include respite care and clothing vouchers. Grandparents may receive foster care benefits for a grandchild but only if that child is a dependent of the juvenile court system and meets selected criteria (see "Foster Care," below). This means that of children who are abused and abandoned by their parents and living with grandparents, only those placed by court order may be eligible for the higher benefits.

In many states, unrelated foster parents are also entitled to additional benefits and services that may not be available to family members.

One reason for the inequality, according to children's rights advocates, is that society expects families to take care of their children. Foster care benefits only provide for children who become the responsibility of the state. However, notes the *Washington Post*," Child welfare laws were written before the crack epidemic, which made the extended family a critical response to lack of care by parents."[3]

It is a sad fact that government programs designed to help children who have been abused or abandoned by their parents don't always support keeping those children in families. Some grandparents live at the poverty level and can barely afford to raise grandchildren even with help from welfare. They may find themselves sliding into debt or even surrendering their grandchildren to the dependency system and the care of unrelated foster parents.

One couple in Missouri took in five grandchildren when their son and daughter-in-law lost custody. The grandfather makes $23,000 per year, and Grandma stays home with the kids. Each month they receive only $384 in welfare benefits for the care and feeding of five growing children. They cannot get food stamps because Grandpa makes too much money. "We are now behind in our bills," he writes. "Our utilities are about to get cut off, and we can't seem to make ends meet. We don't want to send these children to a foster home, but with these financial problems, we are almost forced to send them to one." Had these children qualified for foster care, the family would have received at least $900 a month, an average of $180 per child.[4] To quote one grandmother in Cleveland, "No one can tell you you're raising your grandchild for money!"

Social Stigma

Perhaps the hardest thing about asking for help is the social stigma. Too many people think welfare is synonymous with being lazy instead of needy, and that attitude can be reflected by many state employees. Grandparents often receive scorn rather than sympathy when they take in a grandchild and need to seek aid. Some grandparents don't look like they need assistance and are made to feel guilty about asking for it. There are eligibility workers who act as if they're pulling money out of their own pockets. "You do walk on eggshells when you deal with social services," says Ada MacKenzie. "Those people talk to you like they talk to a dog."

Grandparents who get foster care benefits have it slightly easier. They don't have to sit in line at the welfare office to talk to eligibility workers. Because they are taking over for the state, they are treated more like Good Samaritans than welfare recipients—although the only difference between the two might be a call to child protective services.

This kind of prejudice, like bureaucracy, is a frustrating reality of government assistance. You can try to ignore it. You can air out your feelings in a support group or with other grandparents. But try not to let it eat away at you; it will only drain you of the energy you need to raise your grandchildren. The truth is, every grandparent who takes a child is doing something wonderful for society. If these kids went to the state, the state would be putting out a lot more money and resources to care for them.

Don't be discouraged. These programs exist to help children in need. If your grandchildren qualify for them, they deserve the assistance. And you deserve the financial relief. Even if what you get from welfare isn't enough to raise a child, it still helps, and every bit of help counts. A few hundred dollars can make a great difference to a grandparent struggling on a fixed income, and the medical assistance can be a lifesaver if you cannot put your grandchildren on your insurance policy.

The rest of this chapter looks at federal assistance programs one by one. It discusses what they are, what you get, what you need to qualify for them, and what you as a grandparent need to know to receive the most help. Each program description is only a blueprint of what you may encounter. Although these are federally sponsored programs, they are administered by state, county, and local governments, and their regulations and benefits often vary. Also, many of these programs are subject to change whenever welfare and health care reforms take effect. So, consider this chapter a primer; it offers enough information to spark questions. Then check local resources for current, detailed information about the implementation of federal assistance programs in your state. Remember, the more information you have, the better armed you are to work the system—instead of being worked over by the system.

AID TO FAMILIES WITH DEPENDENT CHILDREN (AFDC)

What It Is

AFDC is the major child welfare program in the United States. It is designed to provide needy children and their families with monthly cash assistance to help pay for basic needs like food, clothing, and rent. Although the federal government sets general AFDC guidelines, each state sets its own definition of neediness, establishes its own income limits and benefit levels, and administers the program. The actual funds for AFDC come from a combination of federal, state, and, occasionally, county sources. A majority of AFDC recipients are single women with children, but the program applies to any close family member who cares for low-income children.

Who Is Eligible

In order to qualify for AFDC a child must fulfill three major requirements: He must be a (1) deprived of parental support, (2) living with a relative caretaker, and (3) poor or financially needy. In most instances, if you are raising your grandchild, he is eligible for AFDC benefits. But let's look at the requirements one at a time:

Deprived of Parental Support

The government considers children deprived, or dependent, if they are living without the support of one parent because that parent is dead, missing, disabled, or unemployed. Most children who live with their grandparents are deprived of parental support.

Living with a Relative Caretaker

If you are a grandparent and your grandchild is living in your home, you are by definition a relative caretaker.

Poor or Financially Needy

In order to be financially eligible for AFDC, the income and resources of the child's "family unit" must be below certain federal and state limits. An AFDC family unit is basically the parent(s) of a dependent child, the child, and any dependent brothers or sisters in the home.

Only the income of the child, the parents, and the siblings can be used to determine financial need and only if they live in the same house. The income of parents who do not live with or help support a child does not count toward the child's AFDC grant (although the government may go after the parents for reimbursement or child support). Nor can your income affect your grandchild's application. Unless your grandchildren have their own regular source of income, they will probably qualify as needy.

Relative caretakers, even guardians, have no legal responsibility to financially support a child, and your finances cannot be considered. The exception is if you yourself are in financial need and want to apply for aid *with* your grandchild; in that case, your income and resources will be taken into consideration (although your home, furniture, and most personal possessions will not be).

Miscellaneous Requirements

There are also several additional requirements your grandchild must satisfy before she can receive AFDC. The child must be a U.S. citizen or legal permanent resident of the United States and a legal resident of your state. She must also be under 18 (under 19 if a full-time student) and have a valid Social Security number. If there are any other rules that apply to your family, your grandchild's case-worker should be able to explain them to you.

What You Get

Those who receive AFDC get monthly cash benefits, medical assistance, and, occasionally, food stamps. The amount of money a family can receive depends on the number of people in the family unit and on the amount and source of income. Benefits vary from state to state and sometimes from county to county. For example, in 1990 a two-person family (presumably parent and child) could have received $88 a month in Alabama, $274 in Ohio, $560 in California, and as much as $752 in Alaska. The national median that year was $294 for a family of two.[5]

Medical assistance is the second part of AFDC benefits. Families receiving AFDC are automatically entitled to Medicaid or to their state's equivalent. However, many children who don't qualify for AFDC may still qualify for Medicaid; make sure you ask about it for your grandchild (see "Medicaid," later in this chapter).

Many AFDC families are also eligible to receive food stamps. While a grandparent's income cannot be considered for AFDC eligibility, it is counted for food stamps. Thus, it is possible that you could receive AFDC for your grandchildren but not qualify for food stamps. Even so, it is worth a try. (See "Food Stamps," below.)

The Application Process

How It Should Work

You can apply for AFDC at your state or local welfare office. Call ahead to confirm office hours and make sure you have the right office for your area. Find out if you need an appointment or if you can just come in. (See "What You Need to Bring," below.)

To apply for AFDC you must file a written application and pass income and resources tests. The welfare office has a responsibility to help you with your application and to help you get the documentation you need.[6] My experience has been that they don't often do this, but they should. If you run into problems, contact your Legal Aid office.

Your application should be processed within 45 days. If aid is denied, the denial must be in writing. If you feel this decision was unfair, you can request a "fair hearing." The written denial usually explains how to do this.

Once you begin to receive AFDC, you must make monthly reports about your grandchild's income (and about yours if you applied with your grandchild). The amount of the benefits will be determined month to month, based on each month's circumstances. You will also face a periodic "redetermination," a process in which the welfare department reviews each family's eligibility as if it were a new application.

What You Need to Bring

When you go for your intake interview, try to take as many records as possible to prove your grandchild's eligibility (and yours, if you are applying with your grandchild). Make sure you have photocopies for the application. Never give away your originals. Don't panic if you can't put your hands on everything; it is the responsibility of the welfare office to reasonably help you get all the required documentation.

To apply for AFDC for your grandchild, you will need the following:

- Proof of the child's age and identity, for example, a birth certificate (few grandparents actually have their grandchild's birth certificate, but you can request a copy from the county where your grandchild was born).
- Proof of the child's residence, for example, school records or a letter to the address.
- The child's Social Security number.
- Proof of your tie to the child (the parent's birth certificate, along with the child's birth certificate, should establish your relationship).
- Proof of income of the child.
- Proof of the child's citizenship or immigration status.

The welfare office cannot limit you to a particular form of identification or proof. For instance, if you cannot find a birth certificate, you should be able to use another proof of age or identity.

▪ WHAT YOU NEED TO KNOW

There is great confusion out there about how grandparents apply for aid for their grandchildren and how aid is determined. Many eligibility workers are used to dealing with regular parent–child applications. They just don't know how the laws and regulations affect grandparents, and they often give out information that is simply *wrong*. The following paragraphs discuss some critical issues grandparents need to understand:

▪ *Your income doesn't count.* One of the biggest problems a grandparent faces with an AFDC application is answering the questions about income. These are equally baffling to eligibility workers, who may give out the wrong information and often count Grandma's income when they shouldn't.

I cannot emphasize this enough: Unless you are applying for AFDC *with* your grandchild or you have adopted your grandchild, your income does not count. You are considered a "non-needy care-taker" and you are filling out the application for your grandchild, not for yourself.[7] Despite what they tell you, fill out the form *as if you were the child.* For instance, if the question is "Do you own a home?," the answer is no (you may own a home, but the child does not). If the question is "Do you have a bank account?," the answer is no if the child does not have a bank account. It doesn't matter what your income and circumstances are; your grandchild is eligible for AFDC. This is true even if you become a legal guardian. If you fill out the forms based on *your* income, the application will be denied. That is exactly what happened to Janet Baker when she was given the wrong information at the welfare office. Not only did they turn her down, but they made her feel awful for even daring to ask for help. "It was three months before I finally got some assistance for the children," says Janet. "By that time, our financial situation was even worse. I felt really battered. The process of finding out just how to do that was a major step for me. I felt degraded."

According to Yolanda Vera, staff attorney for the National Health Law Program, there are only three situations in which your income can be counted in the AFDC application: If you have adopted your grandchild, if you are applying for aid *with* your grandchild, or if you are reaching into your pockets and giving the child money every month. But, says Vera, "If you say, 'I love my grandchild, but I don't expect to support her,' then they cannot count your resources or income, even if you are a Rockefeller."[8]

▪ *You can apply for AFDC for yourself.* If you are raising an AFDC-eligible child and you yourself meet the criteria for welfare benefits, you may apply with your grandchild as a family unit. Even if your grandchild receives Supplemental Security Income (SSI) or foster care (see below), he may still qualify your family for AFDC, although he won't count toward the amount of assistance you receive.[9]

▪ *Immediate aid is possible.* Families who don't have enough to meet their basic living needs may be eligible for "AFDC Immediate Need Cash," a program that is partially funded by the federal government. If you qualify, the agency should speed up your AFDC application and advance your first AFDC check within a few days. You can apply for Immediate Need Cash when you apply for AFDC, but you may have to push for information about it. Although Immediate Need Cash (or its equivalent) is available in some states, it is not often discussed, at least not with grandparents. Try to take as many documents as possible to show that you qualify.

▪ *You should keep records.* Papers get lost and conversations forgotten. Remember to keep copies of all the documents you turn in to any welfare office. Also, keep track of all conversations you have and all attempted contacts with agency personnel. If you can, send letters that confirm any information you receive, and keep copies of those letters. If your information is incorrect, the agency should write back and correct it. If not, you have it confirmed in writing.[10] This could be useful if you ever have to appeal.

▪ *You can appeal.* If your application is denied or your benefits are discontinued, you must be notified in writing. If you feel that your benefits have been denied or discontinued unfairly or that you are not receiving the correct amount of benefits or that you are being mistreated by a welfare worker, you have the right to request a state hearing. Although this can be done by filling out a hearing request form or making a phone call, the most efficient way to request a hearing is to fill out the form on the back of your denial notice. Photocopy both sides of the notice for your records before you return it.

▪ *You may want to get legal representation.* If you do appeal, it can be helpful to have an advocate or an attorney handle your case. Grandparents who cannot afford counsel can sometimes find pro bono or discounted help through organizations like Legal Aid or welfare rights groups. The Legal Aid Foundation of Los Angeles has helped some of our grandparents appeal government decisions and receive aid they could not get on their own.

▪ *You might lose AFDC to unscrupulous parents.* Many parents are manipulative and know how to use the system to their advantage. I can't begin to tell you how many cases I know of in which parents continue to receive AFDC although they are no longer supporting their children. This is illegal. AFDC money is there for the care of needy children. If Mom or Dad continues to take the checks when you are raising the child, they may be guilty of fraud.

However, grandparents who lack legal custody often won't make waves about AFDC; they are too fearful that Mom or Dad will turn around and take the child back in order to get the benefits. Even when grandparents do make waves, not much may happen. I know grandparents who have repeatedly reported the parents for fraud, and nothing has changed; they still have their grandchildren, and the parents continue to receive AFDC.

FOSTER CARE AND YOUAKIM

What It Is

Foster care benefits—properly known as federal IV-E (four-E) foster care—are a type of AFDC benefits for children who have been removed from their homes by child protective services and are living somewhere else.[11] "Youakim" (pronounced "yo-kim") benefits are federal foster care benefits in cases where a child has been placed with a relative. Some areas also have state and county foster care programs, which may not apply to relatives.

The name Youakim refers to a 1979 lawsuit, *Miller v. Youakim*, in which the U.S. Supreme Court ruled that children who are placed by court order cannot be denied foster care benefits because they had been placed in the home of a relative.[12] Before 1979 only nonrelatives could get foster care benefits. Every state participating in the federal program should offer these benefits, although not every state refers to federal relative foster care assistance as Youakim. (If your state child welfare agency does not recognize the term *Youakim*, ask for federal relative or family foster care. For simplicity's sake, in this chapter we will use the term *Youakim*.)

Who Is Eligible

For your grandchild to qualify for federal foster care or Youakim, she must fulfill three general requirements: she must be (1) a dependent of the court, (2) AFDC-eligible and AFDC-linked, and (3) in an approved placement. These requirements get confusing, particularly since states vary on their interpretations of the law, so let's look at them one at a time:

Dependent of the Court

To be a dependent of the court your grandchild must have been removed from her parents, other relatives, or legal guardian and placed with you by a juvenile court order. If you have taken your grandchild into your home or if child welfare placed the child with you without a court order, she will not be eligible for Youakim.

AFDC-Eligible and AFDC-Linked

AFDC-eligible simply means that your grandchild fulfills the major requirements for AFDC eligibility—that is, he is deprived of parental support, needy, and living with a relative—as well as the additional requirements of age, residence, citizenship, and a social security number.

AFDC-linked is more complicated. This is the requirement that is most open to interpretation and confusion. According to federal law, AFDC linkage means any one of the following three things:

1. The child was receiving AFDC in the month the child welfare agency petitioned for his removal.
2. The child could have received AFDC if the parent had applied in the month of the court petition.
3. The child was living with a relative for six months before the petition was filed and could have received AFDC with that relative.

The question of whether a child *could have* received AFDC centers on the child's financial situation in the month he was removed. If the child was removed from his parent's home, the parent's income should count toward AFDC eligibility. The difficulty with this requirement is that in order to determine if the child was eligible you often need to talk to the parent who had custody if you need information about the parent's finances. Unfortunately, the parent may not be around or may be too angry or too high to be helpful. If the parent is available and cooperative, getting this information is not a problem. If the parent was receiving welfare at that time, it is also not a problem, since the welfare office has access to those records. But if he or she is missing or uncooperative, you could have a tough time meeting this requirement.

Another problem with linkage is that while federal law says one thing, states often pass regulations that say something else, sometimes creating policies that are more restrictive than federal requirements. This means that children who are eligible for family foster care under federal law could still be denied federal benefits because of individual state regulations.[13] If your grandchild meets your state requirements for AFDC linkage, you don't have a problem. If he doesn't meet state requirements, but meets federal requirements you can request a hearing.

Approved Placement

The last requirement for federal foster care assistance, and for Youakim, is that the child be in an approved placement. That means the child is placed in the home of a relative approved by the child welfare agency or in a licensed foster care facility.

What You Get

Foster care benefits include monthly cash benefits, health care services through Medicaid, and some additional social services. Foster care benefits are higher than AFDC because foster children are presumed to have greater needs than children on welfare. Unlike AFDC, where benefits are determined by family size, foster care and Youakim are based on the age and needs of each child. In many areas, special needs children—those who are developmentally delayed, physically challenged, prenatally drug exposed, and so on—may also be entitled to additional benefits called "specialized care rates." These rates increase the amount of a child's foster care grant. However, states vary according to the specialized rates they provide and the eligibility requirements for them. If you think your grandchild qualifies for specialized care rates, talk to the social worker. If the child qualifies, you may be required to attend a short training course about handling those special needs.

Foster children automatically qualify for Medicaid and may also be eligible for certain social services, including a clothing allowance, free school breakfast and lunch, and, occasionally, respite care. However, both the dollar amount of Youakim benefits and the scope of health care coverage and services vary state by state, and sometimes even within individual states.

Youakim continues until a child's 18th birthday. In some states benefits can continue until the child is 19 as long as the child remains in foster care; continues to meet financial eligibility requirements; and continues to attend a high school, vocational, or technical school full-time and expects to finish by her 19th birthday.

Although Youakim benefits only address the needs of the dependent child, you may be able to apply for AFDC for yourself while you receive foster care benefits for your grandchild if you are financially needy.

The Application Process

How It Should Work

The children's services worker should be the one to start the application process for you. Once the child has been removed by child protection and placed with you by court order, the children's services worker is supposed to explain your benefit choices, which in most cases is either AFDC or Youakim (if the child qualifies).

For many grandparents, choosing between AFDC and foster care benefits (Youakim) can be something of a gamble. It is easier to qualify for AFDC, but Youakim benefits are higher. If you go with AFDC but your grandchild was eligible for Youakim, you lose the higher benefits. On the other hand, if you choose Youakim and a month later discover that your grandchild doesn't qualify, you will have lost a month of AFDC benefits. You can apply for AFDC while you are waiting for a foster care decision (see "What You Need to Know," below.)

Once you decide, the worker should either help you collect the information you need to establish the child's eligibility for Youakim or, if you choose AFDC, process your grandchild's AFDC application. He should also explain your foster care rights and responsibilities and immediately obtain a Medicaid card for your grandchild.

How It Often Works

Unfortunately, social workers often neglect to explain government benefits to relative caregivers. I have had grandparents call me months, and even years, after a child was placed with them by the court, and they hadn't even known the child was eligible for benefits and Medicaid.

▪ WHAT YOU NEED TO KNOW

- *Youakim is a court-related program.* To be eligible for Youakim your grandchildren must be placed in your home by a court order. If the parents just leave them with you or if you take them in informally, they will not be eligible for these benefits: If for example, your grand-daughter calls and tells you that Mom has been sleeping for two days and there is no food in the house. If you simply pick her up and never involve the courts, she will not qualify for Youakim. If, on the other hand, you call a social worker and make a referral of neglect *and* if child protective services removes the child *and* if Mom was eligible for AFDC and signs the necessary papers, or was already receiving it, then the child should be eligible for federal foster care benefits.

The problem is that most grandparents won't leave children in a neglectful situation in the hopes that a social worker will get there in time. They will rush in to rescue their grandchildren—and end up paying for it in the pocket. Foster care is related to court placement, and the courts only get involved when a child is in danger. If you have the child and the parent is not an immediate threat to her safety, the child welfare system may consider the child well protected and refuse to open a case. One social worker told a grandmother that the only way to become a foster parent would be to abandon her grandchildren, have them placed in foster care, and then apply for custody. Of course, Grandma knew that there was no guarantee that she would actually get the children and that in the meantime they ran the risk of being further traumatized. Grandma stayed with lower benefits.[14]

- *You can apply for AFDC and foster care assistance at the same time.* Relatives are sometimes told they can apply for either AFDC or foster care, but not both. They are also told that once they make a choice and benefits start, they cannot change their minds. Neither of these statements is true. While you cannot receive duplicate aid for the same child in the same period, nothing in the law prevents you from applying for both, especially if there is a chance that the child might not qualify for Youakim. You can also start on AFDC and then switch to Youakim, if your grandchild qualifies.

Unfortunately, each approach has its disadvantages: If you only apply for Youakim and are approved, your grandchild will receive the higher benefits dating back to the day you applied. If, instead, you apply for both and receive AFDC while you wait for Youakim approval, you will lose those retroactive benefits. On the other hand, if you only apply for Youakim and are eventually denied, your grandchild will have gone several months without any benefits at all. This is particularly hard on lower-income grandparents who not only need the higher benefits but also need immediate help.

▪ *You can appeal.* If your grandchild does not qualify for Youakim benefits and if you dispute that decision, you can request a state hearing.

▪ *Guardianship generally eliminates Youakim.* Social workers often encourage grandparents to become the legal guardians of their grandchildren without explaining the full economic impact of this decision. But becoming a guardian can sharply affect your financial situation, especially if you are raising your grandchild on a limited income. To receive foster care payments, a child must be a dependent of the court. Once you become your grandchild's guardian, that dependency ends and so does the child's eligibility for the higher Youakim benefits. He may still qualify for AFDC, but it will mean less money and, possibly, fewer services.

Rebecca Tybor is a grandmother who has her grandchildren with her in long-term foster care. Applying for guardianship would give her much more control in her granddaughters' lives. Right now, if she wants to take the kids on a trip, she may have to consult the courts; as guardian, she would have free rein. But she can't afford to lose the benefits she has with Youakim, so she stays "married" to the child welfare system. There is one exception to this dilemma: If the judge who rules on your guardianship states in her order that "the placement and care of the child remain the responsibility of the Department of Social Services" (42 U.S.C. Section 672), you may still be eligible for foster care benefits.[15] If you cannot do without the child's foster care benefits, ask the judge to insert this language into the guardianship order. However, you will continue to have child welfare involved in your grandchild's case.

SUPPLEMENTAL SECURITY INCOME (SSI) FOR CHILDREN

What It Is

Like AFDC, SSI is a federal cash assistance program for people in need. But while AFDC is designed to help children who are poor and deprived, SSI assists those who are poor and blind or disabled. Also,

SSI typically offers higher benefits than AFDC and does not automatically end at 18. Children who continue to meet SSI financial and disability requirements may continue to receive benefits into adulthood.

Who Is Eligible

Two factors determine SSI eligibility for children under 18: financial need and disability. Your grandchild must fill both requirements to qualify for SSI benefits.

Financial Need

With SSI, as with AFDC, financial need is based on the income and assets of the child, not the guardian. Your financial situation should not affect your grandchild's application. However, SSI will count any AFDC, Youakim, or adoption assistance benefits your grandchild receives, as well as Social Security Survivors Benefits (see below). Each state sets its own eligibility limits, within federal guidelines, for income and resources.

Disability

For SSI purposes, children are considered disabled if they have a physical or mental condition that is as severe as one that would prevent an adult from working. In other words, the condition keeps them from doing things and behaving in ways that are normal for other children of the same age, such as holding their head steady at three months or walking by 20 months. This disability must also be one that is expected to last at least 12 months or result in the child's death. Social Security regulations include a specific list of conditions that qualify as disabilities. If your grandchild's condition is not on that list or not equal to a condition on that list, eligibility will be determined by her ability to function in everyday life.

What You Get

Children who qualify for SSI receive cash assistance and health care services through Medicaid and Children with Special Health Care Needs (CSHCN) programs.

Monthly Cash Benefits

How much cash assistance your grandchild receives depends on where you live, since many states supplement the federal program with state funding.

Health Care Services

In addition to Medicaid, SSI children are entitled to additional health care services under the Children with Special Health Care Needs (CSHCN) provisions of the Social Security Act. CSHCN programs are usually administered by state health agencies. The names and regulations of these programs vary from state to state, but most offer specialized services through private doctors, clinics, hospitals, and community agencies. A child who is not eligible for cash assistance through SSI may still be eligible for medical assistance through a local CSHCN program. Check with your local health department, social services office, or hospital for more information.

The Application Process

How It Should Work

You can apply for SSI by calling the Social Security Administration (SSA) and scheduling an interview with your local Social Security office. The SSA will then send you forms to be completed before the interview and to be filed with your application.

Once you apply, the local Social Security office will decide whether your grandchild's income and assets/resources are within federal and state SSI limits. Then all the information about your grandchild's medical condition will be sent to a state agency, usually called the Disability Determination Service (DDS), for review by a disability evaluation specialist and a doctor. The DDS team will look at how your grandchild's condition affects her functioning in everyday life to decide if she meets the SSI criteria for disability. To do this, they will consider both medical evidence and nonmedical evidence (i.e., letters from teachers, doctors, child care providers, etc.). If your grandchild does not have thorough medical records, you may be asked to take the child for a special exam that Social Security will pay for.[16]

How It Often Works

It is not uncommon for the Social Security Administration to take more than six months to decide SSI eligibility, and even then many cases are incorrectly denied, often owing to a lack of medical or psychiatric documentation. However, many denials are overturned on appeal. If your grandchild is denied, you have a legal right to appeal the decision. If the appeal is successful, he may even receive retroactive benefits based upon the date of the original application.

What You Need to Bring

The more information you bring to your SSI appointment, the easier it will be for Social Security to process your grandchild's application. You will need two kinds of documentation for your grandchild's SSI application: records that show income eligibility and those that confirm the child's disability.

To show your grandchild's income eligibility, you will need to bring the child's

- Social Security number
- Birth certificate or other proof of age
- Financial records and other information about the child's income and resources
- Proof of citizenship or immigration status (birth certificate, green card, visa, passport, immigration papers, etc.)

To prove your grandchild's disability, you must describe, in as much detail as possible, how the disability prevents him from doing things that other children of the same age can normally do. Just because a child is born drug exposed, for instance, is not enough to qualify him as disabled. While some children are indeed severely disabled from prenatal drug exposure, others seem to function normally. DDS needs thorough, detailed information. Records that can help include:

- *Medical records.* Bring information on *all* medical problems, past and present, that the child has experienced. Even problems that seem unrelated to the disability could be important. In fact, to avoid forgetting anything in the interview, you might consider making a list of all the reasons you think your grandchild is disabled.

■ *List of medical personnel.* Bring the names, addresses, and phone numbers of all doctors, hospitals, clinics, and specialists who have treated the child. Be as specific as possible. If you can, provide dates of visits and medical account numbers to help get records as soon as possible.

■ *Nonmedical records.* Social Security doesn't just use medical evidence to decide a child's eligibility for SSI. The agency also considers evidence that shows whether a child can do "age-appropriate activities." Since the disability examiner is not able to see the child, he has to rely on reports from nonmedical sources about what the child can and cannot do and how she manages everyday tasks. Helpful nonmedical records include school records; special education or early intervention plans, if the child has one (see Chapter 13); the names and addresses of teachers, therapists, social workers, child care providers, clergy, relatives, and neighbors who can describe the child's ability to perform everyday activities.

■ *Letters with specific examples.* If possible, ask all your medical and nonmedical sources to provide you with written reports about your grandchild in addition to their standard records. Ask them—as well as family members and clergy—to describe in detail how the disability interferes with the child's everyday activities and to give specific examples. Write down your own observations about your grandchild's disability as well.

Don't wait to have all your paperwork together before you apply. Although it can take months to decide whether your grandchild qualifies for SSI, the payments will go back to the date of your initial visit or phone call as long as the application is filed within the following 60 days.[17] The Social Security staff is supposed to help you find missing documents or suggest substitutes, and many communities have special arrangements between medical providers, social service agencies, and schools.

■ WHAT YOU NEED TO KNOW

■ *You don't have to mail original documents.* Although the Social Security Administration requires original documents to process your application, you can take them into your local Social Security office in person and they can make the copies they need and immediately return your originals.

▪ *It's important to get things in writing.* Anything government workers tell you about your case—instructions or changes—ask them to put it in writing. Also, keep copies of anything you send to government offices. On the copy, mark the date you mailed the letter.

▪ *Your grandchild's doctor can do the evaluation.* SSI decides most cases on the basis of medical assessments. A child has a right to have evidence submitted by her own doctor and to have that individual conduct the follow-up assessments as well. If there is a need for additional testing, Social Security should pay for it, whether the agency uses your grandchild's physician or its own.[18]

▪ *There are special cases.* Although Social Security can take several months to evaluate whether a child is disabled, there are exceptions. Individuals whose condition is so severe that they are automatically presumed to be disabled can receive SSI benefits for up to six months while the formal disability decision is being made. These conditions include, but are not limited to, HIV infection; blindness; Down syndrome; and some cases of deafness, cerebral palsy, and muscular dystrophy.[19]

▪ *Cash gifts to your grandchild will count against the SSI benefits.* According to attorney Pamela Mohr, if you want to give the child a gift or start a college fund, do it as a "blocked trust" account that he or she cannot access; otherwise, it may count as income.

▪ *SSA must be notified about changes.* Once your grandchild gets SSI, you must notify SSA about any change in his address, income, medical condition, living arrangements, and school attendance. The agency must be notified if he leaves the United States. If you do not report these changes on time, your grandchild could lose his SSI eligibility.

▪ *It is important to keep receipts.* SSI is only for the daily support of the eligible child, and you must account for this money every year. If you spend it on anything else, such as a college fund, Social Security could require you to pay it back.[20]

▪ *SSA can send SSI checks to your bank.* In some cases it is possible to have SSI checks deposited directly to your bank account, if you have one. If you can do this, it is the safest way to handle your grandchild's benefits. However, it is still important to keep detailed records of how this money is spent.

• *During the appeal process, your grandchild may still be eligible for AFDC and Medicaid.* Appealing an SSI denial can be a long process, and you won't receive benefits for your grandchild during the course of it. If you do appeal an SSI denial, see if you can apply for AFDC and Medicaid in the meantime.

• *You may want to get legal assistance.* The appeal process can be long and complicated. It can be helpful to have an attorney or advocate in your camp. If you can't afford an attorney, your local Legal Aid office may be able to help you. If your grandchild is developmentally delayed or mentally ill, you may be able to get legal assistance through a Protection and Advocacy office in your state (see Appendix A). Some private attorneys also take selected cases on a contingency fee, meaning that they get paid only if you win your appeal. Talk to your state or local bar association for referrals.

SOCIAL SECURITY SURVIVORS BENEFITS

What It Is

Social Security Survivors Benefits are monthly insurance payments to children under 18 whose parents have died. When most people think of Social Security, they think of retirement benefits, but Social Security taxes also pay into survivors' insurance for certain family members, including children.

Who Is Eligible

To be eligible for Social Security Survivors Benefits, a child must be under 18 (full-time students under 19 and older disabled children are also eligible), unmarried, and the dependent of a parent who has died. The parent in question must have worked, paid Social Security taxes, and earned enough credits to generate benefits. Because my sister didn't earn enough Social Security credits before she died, my nephew Kevin wasn't eligible for survivor's benefits; he received only AFDC and Medicaid.

A child's disability is not relevant for Social Security Survivors Benefits; only the parent's work history is. According to the Social

Security Administration, 98 percent of children are eligible for benefits if a working parent should die.[21]

What You Get

Children who qualify for Social Security Survivors Benefits receive monthly cash benefits. These benefits are based on the average lifetime earnings of the parent and on how much the parent paid into Social Security. A child can receive both SSI and Social Security if she is eligible for both.

The Application Process

How It Should Work

Apply promptly by phone or at any Social Security office since in most cases benefits will only be retroactive to the date of application. Even if you don't have all your paperwork together, apply anyway. The Social Security office should help you collect any documentation you need.

What You Need to Bring

You will need original documents or certified copies of the child's Social Security card and birth certificate, the parent's Social Security number, the parent's death certificate, and the deceased parent's W-2 forms or federal tax return (if self-employed) for the most recent year. You should also bring a checkbook or savings passbook if you want the benefits deposited directly to an account each month.

ADOPTION ASSISTANCE PROGRAM (AAP)

What It Is

AAP is a federal cash assistance program that provides monthly benefits to children whose adoption may depend on financial aid. Some states also have state-run programs for children who may not be eligible for federal adoption assistance.

Foster children are eligible for financial, social, and medical assistance, including Medicaid, all of which they typically lose when they are adopted. Most adoptive parents willingly shoulder the financial responsibility for these children in exchange for the security of adoption. With respect to some children, however, there are circumstances that place added burdens on their caregivers: They may suffer from a physical disability or an emotional disorder, or they may be part of a sibling group that must be placed together. Relatives or foster parents who care for these children may depend on the government assistance they receive; it may be that they simply cannot afford to adopt the child without it. AAP is designed to provide the financial assistance to encourage the adoption of these "special needs" children.

Adoption assistance lasts until the child is 18 years old. It can be discontinued earlier if the adoptive parent is no longer legally responsible for the support of the child, and states can extend eligibility to age 21 if the child is physically or mentally disabled.

Who Is Eligible

Special needs children are children who have situations or conditions that make it difficult to find an adoptive home for them without assistance. These might include age, race, or ethnicity; a background of severe neglect or abuse; inclusion in a sibling group; a family history of mental illness; or a disability (physical, medical, mental, or emotional). Exactly which situations and conditions create "special needs" may change from state to state. While AAP is funded by the federal government, each state defines its own eligibility requirements.

Before he can be considered a special needs child, the state must verify that a child cannot or should not be returned to his family, that he is free for adoption, and that reasonable efforts have been made to place him in a family without financial aid.

There are also financial requirements for AAP, which serves children who would have received federal assistance if they had not been adopted. Therefore, federal AAP benefits are available only to children who (1) are getting federal foster care payments at the time of adoption, (2) are receiving or are eligible to receive SSI at the time of adoption, or (3) can show AFDC eligibility at the time they were removed from their parents and at the time of adoption. As is true for AFDC, your income should not affect your grandchild's eligibility for AAP, although it will affect the amount of monthly aid he receives. A state-run AAP program may have financial qualifications that differ from those of the federal program.

What You Get

Children who are eligible receive monthly cash payments, medical assistance, and, occasionally, additional social services. Adoptive parents may also be eligible for reimbursement for one-time, or "nonrecurring," adoption expenses, which may include adoption fees, court costs, and attorney fees.

AAP cash benefits are negotiated between the administering agency and your family and are based on your financial circumstances and the particular needs of the child you are adopting. Actual rates vary from state to state, but they cannot be more than the family foster care (Youakim) benefits for which your grandchild would be eligible.

Medical assistance is available to children who have special medical needs that are already present or that may appear later on. Children who qualify for the federal program automatically receive Medicaid. Medicaid coverage varies from state to state, and some states cover children who are not federally eligible.

Some AAP agreements also include services like respite care, specialized day care, counseling, and other social services that might be provided to foster parents.

The Application Process

How It Should Work

The Adoption Assistance Agreement is a legal document that is negotiated between the adoptive parent and the state or county adoption agency. Each agreement is based on the needs of the particular child. The agreement specifies the amount of the payments; the eligibility requirements for Medicaid and social services; and the other payments, services, and assistance programs that are available. The agreement includes wording that guarantees that it will be in effect regardless of what state you live in, and it includes provisions to protect the child's interests if you move to a new state.

You can apply for adoption assistance when you begin the adoption process. Sometimes an adoption worker will deliver a proposed AAP agreement when she comes to assess your home. Otherwise, make sure you ask about it. Once you do apply, look at the initial agreement carefully. If it is not acceptable, negotiate it *before* the adoption goes through. Afterward, you must report any change in your family circumstances, and you must recertify the agreement on a regular schedule set by your state.

■ WHAT YOU NEED TO KNOW

- *Adoption assistance isn't a favor.* If your grandchild qualifies for AAP, he is entitled to it. Find out what your state's criteria for AAP are, and don't be afraid to ask.
- *Negotiation should precede adoption.* Negotiate and sign the AAP agreement before you adopt your grandchild. Once the adoption is final, the state has no incentive to negotiate with you.
- *Even negotiation for AAP benefits for at-risk children should precede adoption.* Think ahead. Your grandchild may not appear to have serious problems, but certain circumstances like prenatal drug exposure or a mentally ill parent could make her vulnerable to problems in the future. According to attorney Pamela Mohr,[22] if you have reason to believe that your grandchild is at risk for future problems, some states allow you to apply for AAP; the agreement you sign will say that your grandchild does not qualify for AAP now but that her eligibility can be addressed again if problems arise in the future. However, you must negotiate this agreement and complete the paperwork before you adopt your grandchild.
- *It's a good idea to talk to a legal expert.* An attorney or an advocate can help you understand the various services and assistance to which your grandchild may be entitled. He can also identify which services are most important to the child, negotiate modifications of the agreement, enforce the agreement, or appeal decisions. If you have an attorney handling your adoption, talk to him about AAP. If not, consider talking to someone. I know a grandmother in Pittsburgh who adopted her grandchild. When she asked about assistance, the social worker asked her why she wasn't happy enough to get her grandchild and why she needed to apply for money, too. Sometimes it's easier to have a professional handle these issues for you.

HEALTH CARE AND NUTRITION ASSISTANCE

Any parent knows that children run up a small fortune in health care costs. They need vaccinations and school physicals. They get colds, scrapes, and a collection of childhood diseases. The more adventuresome ones sprain and break things as they test their limits and endurance. Moreover, the cost of doctors and medicine is exorbitant. If you add the health risks of prenatal drug exposure or the cost of psychiatric care for traumatized children, your health care costs can run sky-high.

Unlike parents, who can get insurance for their children, most grandparents cannot put grandchildren on their insurance policies. A few rare employers have allowed grandkids to be included when a grandparent has guardianship, but most grandparents must adopt their grandchildren in order to get private health insurance for them. This is where government benefits become very important. Even middle-class grandparents, who may be able to financially support their grandchildren, need the medical benefits that come with AFDC, SSI, and Youakim.

MEDICAID

What It Is

Medicaid is a health care program for people with low income and limited assets; it helps pay doctor and hospital bills and some medications. However, Medicaid is not so much one program as 50 individual programs, with each state providing a different combination of benefits. Although the states all function within the same federal guidelines, there is significant variety in eligibility criteria, as well as in the conditions and treatments covered. What follows is a brief and broad explanation of Medicaid benefits. This information always needs to be confirmed by someone at your state level.

Who Is Eligible

Although Medicaid varies from state to state, children who qualify for AFDC, Youakim, and SSI automatically qualify for Medicaid. Additionally, many poor children who don't qualify for financial assistance through AFDC or SSI may still be eligible for Medicaid coverage. Check with your local office to find out if your grandchild is eligible.

What You Get

Medicaid coverage can vary greatly from state to state. However, all participating states must provide children with medically necessary doctor and hospital services, lab work and X rays, and early screening. In many cases, additional medical services, like prescription drugs, eyeglasses, dental care, counseling, and inpatient psychiatric care for individuals under 21, are also provided. (See "Early Periodic Screening, Diagnosis, and Treatment," below.)

The Application Process

How It Should Work

In many states Medicaid comes automatically with AFDC, SSI, and Youakim eligibility; the forms might even come together. In other states you will have to sign up for it separately. Be sure to ask. Medicaid coverage is supposed to take effect within 45 days of your application and be retroactive to the day you applied. Additionally, states must provide Medicaid to the child for the three months before the application was filed, if he or she would have been eligible at that time.

How It Often Works

Unfortunately, processing a Medicaid application often takes much longer than 45 days, and a medically needy grandchild could exhaust your resources while you wait. Don't let it happen. If you have a problem or an emergency, call your eligibility or welfare worker.

▪ WHAT YOU NEED TO KNOW

Once your grandchild's benefits begin, you will need to find doctors who accept payment through Medicaid. Because of lower reimbursement rates and the paperwork involved, many doctors are reluctant to accept it. If you run into problems, remember that most county hospitals, county clinics, and free clinics are good resources.

EARLY PERIODIC SCREENING, DIAGNOSIS, AND TREATMENT (EPSDT)

What It Is

EPSDT is a provision of the federal Medicaid program that specifically addresses the needs of children. It is designed to provide financially needy children with preventive health care by detecting and treating early signs of disease or disability and by connecting them with ongoing, comprehensive medical assistance. Federal policy defines the parameters of EPSDT programs, but they are administered by individual state programs whose names and regulations may vary. In California, for instance, EPSDT is handled through a program called Child Health and Disability Prevention (CHDP). It may have another name in your state. EPSDT is a critical program for your grandchildren because it provides many services that may not be available to adult Medicaid recipients.

Who Is Eligible

Every child who is eligible for Medicaid is eligible for federally funded EPSDT services. (See "Medicaid," above.) Some states also provide early screening and prevention services to low-income children who are not eligible for Medicaid. If your grandchildren are not eligible for Medicaid, ask state resources if there is a state-funded program that applies to them.

What You Get

Services include free childhood screening and free medically necessary follow-up diagnosis and treatment for conditions found during the EPSDT screens.

Screening

Regular well-baby and well-child checkups are the foundation of the EPSDT program. These typically include a full unclothed physical exam; assessment of physical and mental health development; vision, hearing, and dental screening; health education; a nutrition check; age-appropriate vaccinations and booster shots; and appropriate or necessary lab tests, including tests for lead poisoning. However, states vary in how well they carry out these requirements.

Diagnosis and Treatment

Your grandchild is entitled to a broad range of free diagnosis and treatment services through EPSDT. Your state should provide "medically necessary" corrective treatment for any physical or mental illness or condition that is suspected or detected during an EPSDT screen, as long as it is covered by federal Medicaid. This means that EPSDT may require your state to provide certain services to children even though it may not provide those same services to adult Medicaid recipients. These services can include assessment for and provision of glasses, hearing aids, and medical equipment; dental care to relieve pain and infection; dental health maintenance and teeth restoration; rehabilitation; respiratory care; home health services; and inpatient or outpatient services to evaluate physical or mental illness.

Although each state may have its own definition for "medically necessary," federal law requires every state to provide diagnostic and treatment services "to correct or ameliorate defects and physical and mental illnesses and conditions discovered by the screening services."[23]

Additional Help and Information

State agencies are obligated to inform the caregivers of all eligible children about EPSDT and to make those services available to them. To this end, you should be provided with a list of specific EPSDT providers near you, as well as their addresses. You should also be offered scheduling and transportation assistance, if you need it, for your grandchildren's regularly scheduled checkups.

The Application Process

How It Should Work

You should be offered information on EPSDT services when you apply for AFDC, Youakim, SSI, or Medicaid for your grandchildren. If your grandchild is eligible (and most GAP grandchildren should be), you can schedule an appointment through whichever state or county agency administers the program.

Your grandchild's periodic checkups should be scheduled on a regular basis determined by your state. However, you are entitled to request additional screens whenever these are needed to determine the existence of a new disease or condition or whenever an existing condition seems to change or worsen. For instance, if your granddaughter starts to squint in school, you may request a vision screening even if her next scheduled appointment is several months away.

How It Often Works

Grandparents are rarely informed about EPSDT services, and while federal guidelines require states to use broader standards when providing services to children, many states still apply the stricter adult Medicaid standards. Thus, states frequently deny services to children even though the services are covered by EPSDT.[24]

▪ WHAT YOU NEED TO KNOW

▪ *EPSDT is an important resource for your grandchildren.* If it is offered to you, take it. If it is not offered, ask for it. Many people turn down these services because they think they are unnecessary if they have Medicaid. Whereas Medicaid is designed to treat illness, EPSDT is designed for early detection and prevention. Without early intervention, many conditions, including mental health problems and learning disabilities, can become more difficult and costly to treat.

▪ *Not all Medicaid providers handle EPSDT services.* Make sure you get a specific list of those who do.

▪ *Many providers are poorly informed.* There are a number of private EPSDT providers and personnel in county facilities who are not aware of the full extent of early screening and treatment benefits. They may not be aware that additional (interperiodic) screens and checkups are allowed, or they may be reluctant to provide them because reimbursement is slow. They may also mistakenly bill you for services that should be paid for by the state. If this happens, photocopy the bill and send it back to the doctor with a letter of explanation. Always keep a copy for yourself.

▪ *Many states don't fully implement federal EPSDT regulations.* As with many government programs, there can be a discrepancy between federal EPSDT ideals and state practice. For instance, while mental health assessment and dental care follow-ups are both required by federal law, some state programs may not offer them. If you have problems receiving EPSDT services for your grandchild, you can ask for a hearing. Contact your local Legal Aid or Protection and Advocacy chapters for help (see Appendix A).

FOOD STAMPS

What It Is

Food stamps are checks or coupons that can be used in the grocery store like money. You can use food stamps to buy food or seeds to grow food. You cannot use them to purchase items like diapers, toilet paper, tobacco, alcohol, or pet food.

Who Is Eligible

Many families who receive AFDC are entitled to food stamps. However, your grandchild's eligibility for food stamps, unlike AFDC, will be affected by your income and the income of everyone in your household. For purposes of food stamp eligibility, a household is a family or group of individuals who live in the same place and prepare food together. If you and your grandchild are *both* receiving AFDC, it is likely that you are both entitled to food stamps. However, if your grandchild is getting AFDC and you are not, he may not be eligible because your income would be counted on his application.

What You Get

The amount of food stamps you can receive depends on a number of factors, including your income, your resources, how many people are in your household, and the cost of your living expenses. Your eligibility worker should be able to tell you which resources can be counted against your eligibility.

The Application Process

How It Should Work

You can apply for food stamps through your state or local welfare office at the same time you apply for AFDC. In some states the application form for food stamps comes as part of the same application package.

■ WHAT YOU NEED TO KNOW

▪ *It always pays to apply.* Many grandparents either are too embarrassed to apply for food stamps or believe they won't qualify. If there is any possibility that you and your grandchildren may be eligible for food stamps, apply for them. Raising children is an expensive proposition; you deserve any help you can get.

▪ *You have a right to a "fair hearing."* Request one if you do not qualify for food stamps, and you feel you were unfairly denied or if you need to address mistakes or unfair treatment.

▪ *Keeping records is necessary.* If you do qualify, keep receipts and bills for all your purchases. You will have to report changes in your income and expenses on a regular basis, and you may need receipts to verify your records.

SPECIAL SUPPLEMENTAL FOOD PROGRAM FOR WOMEN, INFANTS AND CHILDREN (WIC)

What It Is

WIC is a nutrition education and supplemental food program for low-income mothers, infants, and children who are at health risk. WIC originates in the U.S. Department of Agriculture and is administered by either a health or human services agency in each state.

Who Is Eligible

Low-income mothers, infants, and children who are at health risk are eligible for WIC. It can continue from birth to two to five years of age, depending on the state. Although grandparents are not eligible for these benefits, grandchildren may qualify. Eligibility is determined by your income and the health needs of the child (a drug-exposed infant, for instance, is definitely at a health risk).

What You Get

WIC is similar to food stamps in that you get checks or vouchers to be used at the grocery store like money. However, WIC vouchers are earmarked for specific foods that support the nutritional needs of the child. For instance, one voucher may be for a dozen eggs, another for a quart of milk or for infant formula. Those who are eligible also receive educational information about nutrition and child development through a class or a counselor. Finally, you can use WIC as a referral center for other appropriate health care services for your grandchild.

The Application Process

How It Should Work

You can start your application for WIC by calling your county health department or your state social services or welfare office. If they don't handle the WIC program in your area, they can refer you to the agency that does. Once you call, a WIC worker may be able to do a preliminary screening by phone, asking you questions about your income. If you meet these first requirements, the worker will schedule an interview for you and your grandchild.

Three things happen in the interview at the clinic or office. First, you are given a second, more in-depth, screening for income. If you meet this requirement, your grandchild will be screened for "health risk" criteria: An assessment of her diet is made on the basis of what the child ate in the last 24 hours, she is tested for anemia by means of a finger-stick blood test and is weighed and measured, and a health questionnaire on the child is filled out. This package determines whether the child is eligible.

WIC determines eligibility on the spot; you won't have to wait days to find out. In most states you get your first vouchers before you leave the office. However, as with all benefits, delivery varies from state to state. Once you qualify for WIC, you are certified for six months. You will then be recertified every six months until the child is no longer eligible.

How It Often Works

Applying for WIC vouchers involves another appointment, another meeting, another place to haul your grandchild, and more forms to fill out. None of this is made easy for you. Moreover, because WIC is not fully funded, not every child who is technically eligible gets covered. When states cut back, they do so by age, dropping the upper age limit from five years to four or three or even younger.

▪ WHAT YOU NEED TO KNOW

If you have a child under the age of five, apply for this! Many grandparents hear about the income qualification and assume they won't qualify. Since WIC allows income levels higher than AFDC, Medicaid, or food stamps, you may still meet the WIC criteria even if you have a retirement income.[25] Even if your grandchild doesn't qualify for this program, WIC can be a good first line of referral to other health care services.

WHERE TO LOOK FOR ADDITIONAL SERVICES IN YOUR STATE

This chapter has only reviewed basic federal assistance that may be available to your grandchildren. You might also look into government-funded Head Start programs as a source of day care as well as early childhood education and socialization for very young grandchildren.

Many states and communities have independent programs and organizations that support children and families in need. Survivors of crime victims can often receive financial assistance for funerals or counseling through programs developed to assist this population. State or local public health offices and community health centers may provide free or low-cost health care for children. Religious and charitable organizations like Catholic Charities, Jewish Family Services, and Family Service America may offer help with food, clothing, and transportation. Churches, synagogues, and community centers may sponsor child care and after-school activities, as well as camp scholarships for fixed-income children.

Ask your grandchild's teacher or doctor about additional local resources. Find out if your area has an information and referral line. And don't forget grandparent support groups. In addition to providing emotional support, some grandparent groups help with general assistance, and they are a wonderful source of information.

CHAPTER 13

Special Education
and Early Intervention

If you've told a child a thousand times and he
still does not understand, then it is not the child
who is a slow learner.
—*Walter Barbee*[1]

Ever since 1954, when the U.S. Supreme Court ruled to desegregate schools in *Brown v. Board of Education*, American children have enjoyed the right to equal education.[2] But if your grandchild cannot see the blackboard, read the alphabet, remember instructions, or stay in her seat, she cannot take advantage of the education she is entitled to, no matter how good that education may be.

Fortunately, the civil rights movement of the 1960s also drew attention to the rights of the handicapped, including the need of disabled children for equal access to their equal education. Congress therefore passed laws that gave states a financial incentive to offer special resources to kids with disabilities.[3]

Children having serious difficulties in school are entitled to a number of special education programs and services to help them make the most of their public education. Two particular federal laws, or parts of them, apply to children with special education needs:

Section 504 of the Rehabilitation Act of 1973 prohibits discrimination against the disabled in any program that receives federal funds, including schools.[4] If your grandchild has a disability that limits certain activities but does not affect his academic performance, he may be entitled to modifications in the classroom and curriculum through Section 504.

IDEA (Individuals with Disabilities Education Act, formerly Public Law 94-142) requires all states and territories to provide a "free appropriate public education" (FAPE) to all children with disabilities and defines the rights of those children and their parents or guardians.[5] "Appropriate" means that the curriculum meets the special education needs of each child's disability. If your grandchild's disabilities seriously hinder his academic achievement, he may be eligible for special education services through IDEA.

A "free appropriate public education" is a right and an entitlement, not a privilege. It is implemented through a procedure called an IEP, or Individualized Education Program. This is a detailed plan of special services, tailored to the needs of each child, which the school must provide to ensure that the child's education is indeed "appropriate."

The IEP is considered the centerpiece of special education law, and each stage of the special education process is a stepping stone toward completing it: the assessment of the child through a battery of tests, observations, and reports; meetings of teachers, professionals, and parents (or, in this case, grandparents) to evaluate whether the child qualifies for services and which services would help him; and the IEP itself, which must be carried out by the school or school district.

This process helps determine whether the problems a child is exhibiting are due to a physical, emotional, or learning disability and suggests how an environment might be created that would enable him to benefit from his public school education. This can mean individual tutoring, putting the child in a special class in the current school, or transferring to another school, whether public or private, that can better handle the disability.

"Free appropriate public education. Those are the buzz words," warns attorney Larry Hanna, special education commissioner for the Los Angeles Unified School District. "You get a compact VW, not a Rolls Royce or a Mercedes. You don't get services that are going to make you an Einstein; you get the services that will get you through, give you an even playing field." Even so, an even playing field can mean the difference between getting an education and slipping through the cracks for a child with ADHD or a learning disability.

According to the U.S. Department of Education, approximately five percent of all school children get special education services. However, nearly one-fourth of them eventually drop out.[7] The more you can learn about the special education process and the IEP, the better you can use it as a tool to provide your grandchild with an education that will allow him to learn.

THE SPECIAL EDUCATION PROCESS

The Request

The special education process begins with a written request to your local school. Anyone—a teacher, a therapist, a pediatrician, a parent or guardian, or, in your case, a grandparent—can request a special education evaluation for a child. No matter how small your town is, the school should know about the IEP. Your grandchild may have to go to another school or district for the evaluation—some areas have created a consortium among several schools to handle this—but you must still start the process with a written request to your local school. Date the letter and keep a copy for your files. This request will start a clock ticking; the school district is required to process eligibility for special education within a prescribed time frame. That time frame is dictated by state law, and many school districts fall behind their prescribed schedules. (The schedule in this chapter represents *California* law. Your own state's time frame may be different, so find out what it is. Don't let the school drag the process out so that your grandchild falls further behind.)

The Evaluation or Assessment Plan

Once the school receives your request, it has *15 days* (in California) to send you a plan for how it will evaluate your grandchild. This is a key step; don't take it lightly. The kind of testing done in the assessment will determine the kinds of services your grandchild is eligible to receive. If the child needs psychological counseling or speech therapy but those tests are not included in the assessment plan, they won't be considered in the IEP.

What testing do you want the school to do? If you don't know, take the plan to someone who can help you. You need to make sure the school is offering the right assessment for this child at this age and with these particular needs. Assessments are expensive; with budgets tight, school districts do try to cut corners where they can. You have to be the child's best advocate. Persistence and perseverance do pay off. If the assessment plan is adequate, sign and return it. If not, write in the additional tests you want before you send it back.

The Actual Assessment or Evaluation

Once you return the signed plan, the school district has *50 calendar days* (in California) to complete the assessment, which is a multidisciplinary evaluation usually conducted by a school psychologist, educational diagnostician, social worker, and other evaluators. This evaluation includes medical, educational, psychological, and sociological components. Try to get as much input into this process as possible. If you think the school's assessment is inadequate, and if you can afford it, you can have your own assessment done privately. If the final IEP reflects issues raised in your assessment, but not in the school's, the district may have to repay your costs.[8]

The Eligibility Meeting

Once the assessment is complete, the school district will schedule a meeting to determine if the child is eligible for special education services. However, some state and local agencies combine the eligibility meeting and the IEP meeting (see below) into a single conference.

What Determines Eligibility?

According to federal regulations, all "children with disabilities" are eligible for special education and related services. This includes children who have been evaluated as being mentally retarded, physically handicapped, health-impaired, or seriously emotionally disturbed, or as having specific learning disabilities. However, terms like "emotionally disturbed" and "learning disabled" are hard to define, and the final criteria for special education eligibility varies from state to state.

You might think your grandchild is learning disabled—and by many standards she may be—but the child must fit your state's criteria to be eligible for services. For instance, if your state defines a learning disabled child as one of normal intelligence who is two years behind her age-group but your dyslexic granddaughter is only one year behind, she may not qualify for special education in that state.

Even if your grandchild is not eligible for an IEP through the Individuals with Disabilities Evaluation Act, she should be able to get certain classroom modifications through Section 504. These might include having your grandchild placed at the front of the classroom, allowing her to use a tape recorder in class, or giving her more time to complete certain tests and assignments.

If it is determined that your grandchild does have a disability that makes her eligible for an IEP, the school district or public agency has up to 30 days to hold an IEP meeting.

The IEP Meeting

The IEP meeting itself can take place in any number of places—a district office, a hospital, your home—but it is most commonly held in your grandchild's own school. It should be held at a time and place that is mutually agreeable to school personnel and you, as the child's guardian.

The IEP is based on a team concept: A group of professionals work with the parents (or grandparents) and, if appropriate, the child to determine what services his special education will include. The team players are the school administrator or principal, the child's teacher, the school nurse, and a psychologist.

During the IEP meeting this team will examine your grandchild's test results, profiles, class work, teacher reports, nurse's reports, and any other material that is presented as pertinent. If a psychologist or a doctor needs to present information in person, this is where it happens. If a medical doctor is scheduled to be present, try to have your grandchild's own doctor there as well. Remember, you are an important part of this team. As primary caregiver, you are the one who knows your grandchild best, and no services can be provided without your consent.

Several things are decided at the IEP meeting: goals and objectives, placement, related services, and, for some children, transition services. The IEP form will be filled out on the basis of these decisions, and the IEP will become the blueprint or game plan for your grandchild's education.

Goals and Objectives

If your grandchild is found eligible for special education services, the next thing to decide is what kind of program and services are needed. What are your grandchild's specific disabilities? What does he need to learn to catch up to other children his age? These are the questions that must be addressed at the IEP meeting. These questions should be answered with specific goals and objectives and a schedule for measuring whether or not they are being achieved. For instance, if Carrie is a bright fifth grader who tests at a second grade reading level, she clearly needs help with reading comprehension. But her IEP should say more than "Carrie will get help with reading." Instead, Carrie's IEP goals might state that "Carrie will be able to read at a third grade level by the end of the first semester. By the end of the year, Carrie will be reading on a fourth grade level." The goals should also state which test will measure this progress.

Goals and objectives are critical in deciding which kind of placement and services your grandchild is eligible for in the coming year. Make sure they can be measured objectively. A teacher's observation or opinion is not an objective measurement.

Placement

The law requires that each child be placed in the "least restrictive environment." That means having the child in as much of a regular school program as possible while accommodating his special needs. Special options can range from extra help in a mainstream class to residential placement. Other possibilities include special day classes, a resource specialist for tutoring, state school, or, occasionally, a private school paid for by the school district. If your grandchild does need a special school and there are none in your area, he may be sent out of the district.

Related Services

If a child qualifies for special education, school districts are also supposed to provide certain additional services to help her come up to speed. "Related services" can include speech and language services, psychological counseling, special readers, tutoring, medical services in school, parent training, physical and occupational therapy, adaptive physical education, and even transportation if you live far from a special education program.

Transition Services

The IEP is designed not only to help disabled children graduate but to help older children with disabilities make the transition to life after school. Thus, an IEP could include not only special instruction but employment or college counseling, certain community experiences, and even instruction in specific daily living skills like filling out applications, handling money, and finding living arrangements. Starting at no later than 16 years old (and sometimes at 14 or younger) your grandchild's IEP should include a plan for the transition services he will need to move on in life.

Remember, although the IEP works on a team concept, it is also a negotiation session. Your concern is your grandchild's needs, but the school must focus on hundreds of children and must do so with dwindling funds. Since it is expensive to put kids in special classes and nonpublic schools, a school district does resist. "The school district is battling the budget," says education commissioner Hanna. "So the less they give you, the more they have and the happier they are."[9] On the other hand, the more prepared you are, the more you can get out of the system.

The IEP

The product of the IEP process is the actual IEP, the written Individual Education Program that you as the child's guardian must approve and sign before services can take effect. Read the IEP carefully before you sign it. Make sure it does what it is meant to do. Ask yourself the following questions:

> Is it comprehensive? A good IEP should cover every area of your grandchild's development, including behavior, socialization, communication, self-help, academic, and motor skills.

Is it specific? Are goals and objectives clearly stated in terms of objective, observable, and measurable behavior?

Is it sequential? Does it offer a solid step-by-step plan to teach your grandchild what she needs to learn?

Is it realistic and appropriate? Does it match your grandchild's current abilities? Does it encourage growth at a reasonable rate?

Is it understandable? Is it written in language that you can comfortably follow and discuss?

Was it mutually developed? In other words, were you an active part of the IEP team and does the final plan reflect your concerns?

Is it designed to close the gap between the child's ability and her achievement?

Remember, the IEP is key to your grandchild's education; you want to make sure the door it opens is the right one.

Don't Do This Yourself

Even the most sophisticated, resourceful grandparent can find the IEP process to be overwhelming. You have to tell strangers how badly off your grandchild is, and that can be hard to do without getting emotionally involved. The forms can be confusing, and the process can drag on until you run out of patience. It is good to learn the terminology and the process, but you have enough to do already without having to learn all the detailed procedures of educational law and the difference between various types of assessment plans.

The individual who helps you negotiate an IEP with your grandchild's school could be an attorney or advocate, a therapist or social worker, even another grandparent or a friend. A local education attorney or advocate knows the ropes: whom to ask, what to ask, and what to ask for. She may have even worked with this IEP team before. An educational therapist, a psychologist, or a social worker can evaluate the assessment plan and help fill out the IEP form with your wish list. These professionals have a better grasp of what are reasonable goals for your grandchild at his age and with his particular psychological and educational background. If you can't find or afford an advocate, look for another grandparent or parent who has been through this before; ask that parent to go to the IEP meeting with you. At the very least, take a friend or relative for support. Despite what anyone may tell you, you do have the right to have someone there.

Preparing for the IEP Meeting

The more information you have before your first IEP, the fewer problems you are likely to encounter. Here are some things you can do to prepare yourself for the IEP meeting:

▪ *Learn about your and your grandchild's rights.* Your grandchild has rights and so do you, as the primary caregiver or guardian. Get copies of federal rules and regulations (IDEA and Section 504), your state rules and regulations for special education, and the policies in effect in your school district. Remember, the only interpretation that ultimately counts is the federal one.

▪ *Find out the chain of command in your school district.* If you are not satisfied with the outcome of the IEP meeting and need to go higher up, you will already know whom to go to.

▪ *Keep records.* Write down the names and numbers of everyone you talk to. They could be helpful later on.

▪ *Review your grandchild's school records.* Go to the school and photocopy everything that is in the child's cumulative and confidential reports. You may have to check in different departments to get all of them. If the child has ever been in any kind of facility, get their records as well. Copy everything: handwritten notes, notes scribbled on the folder or jacket, any work the child has done. You are arming yourself on all fronts.

▪ *Speak with the psychologist.* Find out who the psychologist is and get her reports on your grandchild. Be nice about this; presume that the psychologist is doing the best job she can for the child. If you are using an advocate, he will know how to ask the right questions.

▪ *Request your own copy of the assessment report.*

▪ *If you have had an outside assessment done, plan to bring it.* Or, if possible, bring along the expert who did the assessment; he or she may be able to provide additional information.

▪ *Gather outside information.* Collect medical records and any school or test records the school district may not have. Because reports don't tell you everything about a child, be sure to bring in real-life examples of your grandchild's abilities and disabilities in different areas. Talk to other adults who come into contact with your grandchild—doctors, social workers, clergy members, even family and neighbors. Ask them to put their comments and observations in writing. Submit this information for the assessment.

▪ *Set your own goals for your grandchild.* If you let the school district define all of your grandchild's goals and objectives, it may only offer minimal services and will probably not address all your grandchild's needs. Make a list of what things your grandchild can do and what you think he should learn during the school year. Get blank copies of the IEP forms, photocopy them, and fill them in. Focus on your goals for your grandchild and how you want them to be accomplished. Does he have problems hopping or jumping? Ask for adaptive physical education. This is your wish list.

▪ *Think about placement.* What do you want for your grandchild? Talk to someone who knows your school district and ask the following questions: What special classrooms are available? What do they offer? Where are there special schools? Inspect any classroom or school where you think they might place your grandchild. Interview the teacher. If you're not happy with the placement, take in your own plan. You may have a fight on your hands, but it could be worth it. You might even be able to get your grandchild placed in a private school, but that is a difficult proposition.

▪ *Ask for therapy.* One important goal that is often overlooked is psychological counseling. Being in a special education classroom, as helpful as it is, has a stigma that is hard on children. Their self-esteem is low. Other children may tease. Always try to get mental health testing and psychological counseling into your grandchild's IEP, and make sure that it is with a trained therapist. The school may view sessions with a guidance counselor as therapy, but many guidance counselors may not be qualified to deal with the issues your grandchild may be experiencing.

▪ *Consider nonacademic activities.* Lunch, recess, physical education, and activities like art and music are important parts of the school day. Make sure your grandchild's IEP lets her take advantage of the nonacademic part of school as well.

▪ *Carefully consider having your grandchild at the meeting.* Despite what anyone may tell you, you are entitled to have the child present. The question is, Do you want to? The IEP process can be devastating. Personally, I don't recommend that a young child be present at an IEP meeting. Perhaps a high school student may be confident enough to provide some input, but I can't think of a good reason to have an elementary school child present. These children have such fragile self-esteem that they can't help but be affected by everyone talking about their problems. However, your grandchild must eventually learn to become his own advocate.

▪ *Be vigilant.* In so many arenas you have had to step gingerly with bureacracy; this is one place you must be willing to push. Just because public schools have a duty to identify children who need special education doesn't mean they always do so. Children get lost in the school system. The ones who are quiet and nice may get Cs or Ds and yet be passed along without services. One little girl was denied special education services because the school blamed her problems on her "dysfunctional family" (she lived with her grandparents). Only after a long legal fight did her grandfather manage to place her in a residential program for the learning disabled.[10]

Don't back down. "The people I see who are the noisiest, who go down to the schools and bug them, they're the ones who get the services they need," says Hanna.[11] So, even if you have an advocate, be vigilant.

During the IEP Meeting

▪ *Be confident.* Your image may affect how school personnel respond to you. Bring your own set of rules, regulations, and supporting material. Have your grandchild's file organized neatly and in chronological order; keep state and federal regulations in a separate folder. This way you also look prepared. Speak clearly and maintain eye contact. And remember, this committee is paid to work *for* you and your grandchild; they are not dispensing favors. Special education is a right, not a privilege.

▪ *Have people sign in.* Pass around a sign-in sheet at the beginning of the meeting. This will let you address everyone by name.

▪ *Ask questions.* Especially when you don't understand something, ask about it. You have a right to simple explanations of anything that is unclear to you.

▪ *Repeat what you are asking for.* Do this as often as necessary. To quote the Coordinating Council for Handicapped Children: "You are not at the IEP to discuss the limitations of the school budget. You are there to determine what your child needs to have an appropriate education."[12]

▪ *If necessary, request another meeting.* If you cannot come to an agreement, are running out of time or need more time to think, you have the right to request another meeting. You do not have to make a decision at that moment.

▪ *Don't sign the IEP until you understand and accept it.* Remember, you do not have to sign an unsatisfactory IEP. If you do not agree with the school's evaluation, you can get an independent evaluation and request a new meeting based on it. You can also file an appeal through a mediation process or a "due process hearing" (see below).

After the IEP Meeting

▪ *Request your own copy of the final IEP.*

▪ *Follow your grandchild's progress closely.* Periodically ask the teachers for a progress report. Remember, you can initiate changes or a review if your grandchild is not improving. You can also request another IEP meeting.

▪ *Ask teachers what you can do at home to help.* Many skills your grandchild will be learning at school can be practiced at home.

▪ *Keep records.* Record all questions and comments you want to discuss with the school, meetings and phone conversations you want to remember, and any information that may be useful in future reviews and evaluations. It is easy to forget what you don't write down.

▪ *Try to resolve any problems you have with the school within the school district.* On the other hand, if you cannot come to an agreement with school officials and your grandchild is not being properly supported, you can file an appeal.

The Appeal Process

If the final IEP is not acceptable to you and you cannot resolve the issue with the school district, you can appeal. Some states offer a mediation process first, but any issues that cannot be resolved in mediation will be taken to a due process hearing. Likewise, if the

IEP is not being followed, you can file a formal complaint with your state board of education, the U.S. Department of Education, or the Office of Civil Rights and start an investigation. You are entitled to be present when your complaint comes before the board of education. Sometimes, if the school district thinks you will fight them all the way to a hearing, they may give you what you want—it's cheaper. If the due process hearing is not satisfactory, the appeal process can go on to a U.S. district court and, in some cases, up to the U.S. Supreme Court.

If you do start the appeal process, you may want to consult an attorney or advocate. Most states have Protection and Advocacy agencies that can provide you with guidance. So look around before you decide you can't afford representation. And don't be afraid to "rock the boat." A free *appropriate* public education is a right that belongs to your grandchild; you have a right to make sure that what is provided is appropriate.

The Review Process

Once your grandchild has started the IEP process, she will be reviewed annually and reassessed at a minimum of every three years to see if her needs are being met and progress is being made and to determine what changes are needed as the child gets older. The IEP may also be revised anytime you see a need for revision and make a request.

EARLY INTERVENTION AND SPECIAL EDUCATION SERVICES FOR INFANTS, TODDLERS, AND PRESCHOOLERS WITH DISABILITIES

One of the wonderful things about IDEA is the possibility of early intervention, that is, of addressing the needs of disabled children before they enter the school system and start to fall behind. Federal law extends special education assistance to preschool children as young as three years, and, in some states, to infants and toddlers (birth to two years).[13] Children who are at risk for developing disabilities, such as drug-exposed infants, are also eligible in a number of places.

The goal of early intervention is to identify and treat problems and delays in children as soon as possible. This can be as simple as prescribing glasses for a three-year-old or as intensive as complete physical therapy for an infant with cerebral palsy. The theory is that the more special assistance a child receives early on, when the rate of learning is fastest, the fewer the special education services he may need later in life.

The process of applying for early intervention is similar to applying for the IEP and involves the following stages:

The Request

Make a request, in writing, for an evaluation and assessment of your grandchild's eligibility and needs. Start the process at your local school, just as you would if the child were already enrolled there; speak to the principal or someone in charge of special education. If you have any problems, call your state's department of education and ask who in your area is responsible for special education programs for preschoolers with disabilities. If your grandchild is under three, ask about early intervention services for infants and toddlers; they are not offered in every state.

The Assessment

Your grandchild will be evaluated by a team of professionals, which may include a psychologist and an occupational or a physical therapist as well as other experts, depending on the rules and regulations of your state. You are an important part of this team and should participate as much as you can in this process. Many of the preparation suggestions for the IEP apply here (see above).

The Plan

If your grandchild is eligible for special education programs or early intervention, the assessment team will create an IFSP (Individualized Family Service Plan). Like the IEP, this plan describes the child's developmental level, the goals to be achieved, which services the child will receive, where and when she will receive these services, and what steps will be taken to ease the child's transition into school or another program.

Unlike the IEP, which focuses on the individual student, the IFSP addresses the whole family. The philosophy is that the best way to meet the needs of a small child is to work with the family. This can include family counseling, respite care, and educational services to help everyone understand and cope with your grandchild's disability.

The Services

The special education programs developed for preschoolers are free programs in public schools and are specifically designed to help children with disabilities. Early intervention services may be offered through public or private agencies in a variety of settings: clinics, hospitals, neighborhood day-care centers, the local health department, even your home. Although there is no cost for evaluation and assessment, not all early intervention services are free. However, some services may be covered under Medicaid.

Again, each state develops its own policies for carrying out the IDEA. You will need to find out about the specific policies in your state. The National Information Center for Children and Youth with Disabilities (NICHCY) publishes free resource sheets listing agencies and contact people in each state (see Appendix A for more information).

AND IT'S ANOTHER NOTEBOOK!

Lots of paperwork is generated with special needs children: assessment reports, IFSPs, IEPs, medical forms, phone numbers, conferences, growth milestones, immunizations, therapy reports, and so on. The more organized you are, the better you can protect your grandchild's right to a free and equal education.

What to Keep in Your Child's Home File

- ▪ A copy of IDEA (formerly Public Law 94-142) and its regulations.

- A copy of your state's rules and regulations on special education.
- A copy of the school's IEP procedures.
- A "chain of command" list. Keep a list or chart of the chain of command within the school system, beginning at the local level and ending with state and federal agencies. Include addresses and telephone numbers for easy reference.
- A list of school and IEP players. Every year, list your grandchild's teacher, school, principal, and psychologist, as well as any related services personnel, special education teachers, the school district superintendent, school board members, and the special education administrator.
- Copies of all school records. These may come from the child's cumulative records, psychological reports, and any other papers the school district might have about your grandchild. Keep them chronologically, with the most recent year on top.
- Report cards.
- Copies of test results and recommendations from independent assessments.
- All written (including handwritten) letters and notes to and from school personnel.
- All written communication with outside professionals regarding your grandchild's unique needs.
- Dated notes on parent–teacher conferences.
- Dated notes you have taken during conversations with the child's physician and other professionals who see your grandchild.
- Dated notes on all telephone conversations with school personnel or others regarding your grandchild.
- A list of any medications being given to your grandchild at home and at school as authorized by the child's physician. Include the kind of medicine and dosage information. In addition, note prescription numbers and any changes in dosage or reactions.

ADDITIONAL RESOURCES

There are many kinds of support and information services out there for families with disabled children, from public agencies to support groups for families of children with disabilities. Also, many states have published manuals that explain their special education and related services for children with disabilities. Contact your state Department of Education or any of the groups or organizations listed in Appendix A for more information.

ONE LAST WORD: AIM HIGH

A disability does not have to be a sentence to failure. It's not that these children can't learn—many are very smart—but they need to learn differently. Give them goals and aim high. The IEP offers transition services for adjusting to life after high school, and Section 504 of the Rehabilitation Act of 1973 prohibits discrimination against disabled applicants or students at schools that receive federal funds. There is financial aid and special programming even at many top colleges and universities. Taped textbooks, extended time for testing, tape recorders, computers, and interpreters for students with hearing problems are just a few of the modifications that are helping disabled teenagers participate and succeed on American campuses.

"Go for doctor, lawyer, not secretary," says special education commissioner Hanna, who is himself dyslexic. "The [school] will want to put them into bricklaying, truck driving. Don't let it happen."[14]

Strength
in Numbers

CHAPTER 14 | Their Arms about Us:
Finding and Forming
Support Groups

"GAP is a place where I can go as a grandmother and let my hair down and scream and holler and say what I feel. It is a shoulder to cry on."

"GAP is a place you come to when you reach the end of your rope. Three years in court keeps you from talking about things, and you need to vent. This was the first place we were allowed to sit and cry and tell our story."

"It doesn't matter here whether you're poor or rich, black or white. We become a family here. They have become my family."

"There is no place like this. I lived in constant fear of snapping. I come here and all these mothers start picking me up and, next thing you know, I'm whole again."

"I came in here and I was a beat person. I was a rug. I'm not a rug anymore. I'm a strong person now because of GAP. I'm a human being."

"Instead of aging, I've become younger. I don't look younger, but inside I feel like a very young person. I can cope with anything now—and I am."

There are many reasons why I urge grandparents to seek out support groups, as I have repeatedly done throughout this book. Each of these reasons comes back to the same root: While you are sacrificing everything to help your grandchildren, you need someone to help you. A GAP group lets you look out for one another.

A group is a fallout shelter, a place for people to come together when everything seems to be raining down on their heads and exploding around them. It is the best antidote to the overwhelming feelings of loneliness. It cuts isolation. You can cry and yell in a group and not be judged. You can make friends who understand you because they have been there. You can go to a meeting and sit next to a another grandfather who is angry at a son who won't parent or another grandmother who is frustrated with her granddaughter for disrupting her life. You can unload your concerns without criticism. It lets you see how normal your feelings are.

A group is a living library. You can find guidance from the experiences other people have had in similar situations. Someone who has already raised a grandchild to age 15 can give you specific feedback on your five-year-old. This is also a source for practical information, like phone numbers of attorneys and helpful social workers, and for assistance in navigating issues like obtaining custody or AFDC and Medicaid for the kids.

A group can also be a kind of way station, a place where basic needs can be gratified through, for example, a clothing exchange, a ride to a doctor's appointment, a new friend who might watch the kids for an hour. One support group in Las Vegas organized themselves to pay for medical exams and eyeglasses for disadvantaged grandparents. "We're not doing for the child," said its executive director. "We are doing for the grandparents so they can do for the child."[1]

FINDING A GROUP IN YOUR AREA

At last count there were over 400 grandparent groups already running in the United States.[2] Some of them are chapters or offshoots of larger organizations like Grandparents As Parents (GAP), Grandparents Raising Grandchildren, and Grandparents United for Children's Rights. Others are local, organized by individual grandparents, social workers, therapists, nurses, and even teachers. A number of support groups offer additional services, including dispensing of newsletters, resource directories, and how-to manuals; hotlines; and emergency assistance with basic needs like food, housing, and financial assistance. And many are active in political and legislative advocacy.

Appendix A is a small directory of resources; some may be able to point you to a group in your area. You should also call your local child guidance clinic or family service agency to see if the staff knows of any grandparent groups that are just starting up. If not, you may be able to convince them of the need to start one or to help you organize one.

STARTING YOUR OWN GAP GROUP

Before Your First Meeting

There are many kinds of grandparent groups across the country. Some focus on emotional support, some on basic needs and political action, and some on a combination of the three. Some of these groups are run by grandparents, others by social workers and therapists. Each, however, has had to resolve some of the same issues to get up and running.

Getting the Word Out

The first step is identifying your target population and letting them know about your group. Although GAP stands for "Grandparents As Parents," our membership extends beyond grandparents who are actually raising their grandchildren. We take grandparents who are fighting for visitation as well as grandparents whose grandchildren were returned to their parents by the system. We have even had a great aunt and a big sister show up at a meeting. I don't believe in turning away anyone who can benefit from the information and support GAP offers.

Once you get the ball rolling to start a GAP group, talk it up. Word of mouth does wonders. You never know who might know another grandparent raising a grandchild, and people strike up conversations all the time in the market, the bank, a doctor's office. In fact, most of our grandparents have GAP business cards. If they see a grandparent with a grandchild in a store, at a school meeting, or even on the street, they pass them out. There are also formal ways to spread the word:

▪ *Use your community.* You may not know other grandparents in your situation, but there are people who do. Contact local pediatricians, hospitals, social workers, attorneys, schools, churches, and synagogues. Tell them your plans and ask them to give your name and number to any grandparents they know. They cannot give you a grandparent's name—that's confidential—but they can give out your name or even send out a prepared letter. Their offices are also good places to post flyers, if you get permission first.

▪ *Use the media.* Not only are your local newspaper and radio and television stations a source of local news, they are your link to other isolated grandparents. There are two ways to get the word out through the media: meeting announcements and articles.

Most newspapers and radio stations have calendar listings of upcoming events. This is a simple way to spread the word. One group sent news releases to as many papers as possible, then followed up with a phone call to confirm. If you do this, be sure to include your name and contact number on your release.

A more challenging, but more effective, approach is the human interest story. Reporters are always on the lookout for personal stories that tie into a social trend. Contact a local newspaper and ask if they would like to do a story on your family. Make sure the article states that you are interested in starting a group for grandparents and includes a contact number. Do the same thing with local radio and television stations. When Peggy Plante wanted to start a GAP group in Quincy, Massachussetts, she called the *Patriot Ledger*. The paper ran a feature story on Plante and her GAP partner, Judy Kingston, and included the date and time of their first meeting.[3] Twenty grandparents showed up, and the group grew from there.

Encourage Grandfathers to Come

Many grandparent groups seem to be comprised mostly of women. This is because men are traditionally less inclined to seek out self-help and support, particularly men of an older generation. Many feel they don't need to talk about their problems or believe they should be able to cope without outside help. But grandfathers do need support. Like grandmothers, they can benefit from meeting others who have similar feelings and experiences. And your group will benefit from the perspective that grandfathers offer.

When you talk to grandfathers, assure them that they are welcome and that their input is important. And then be patient. A grandmother might come alone every week for months before the grandfather comes; then one meeting might hook him. We have several men who attend meetings religiously, and their presence is always valuable. Some grandfathers even find it helps their marriage to come and learn coping skills as a couple.

Where Will You Meet?

You will need a location for your meetings. Contact churches, libraries, senior citizens' centers, schools, hospitals, and any other community buildings that have space. If you get a newspaper or radio station interested, mention that you're looking for a donated meeting room. You'll be surprised how many people in the community come through for this type of program.

Word of mouth works, too. Talk it up. Don't be afraid to tell people what you need and to ask for it! One group approached their county council of churches and found a church where they could use a kitchen and a nursery. Another grandmother attended a parenting class at her grandchild's school and received permission to use a classroom for weekly meetings. The teacher even had her class leave valentines for the grandparents who use their desks at night.

A word about chairs: Look for a room that already has chairs and/or couches. Also try to find a variety of chairs: Some grandparents are overweight and need comfortable chairs whereas others have back problems and need sturdy support.

When Will You Meet?

Scheduling is tricky for grandparents, particularly scheduling something for themselves. Many work in the day and may not be able to find or afford a baby-sitter in the evening. Ask grandparents about times when you first contact them, and do the best you can for this first meeting. You won't please everyone, but try for a majority.

Will You Have Child Care?

From the beginning, GAP has offered child care at meetings. Many grandparents cannot afford baby-sitters and have no one to watch their grandchildren. Unless they can solve this problem, they will find it impossible to attend meetings, no matter when you schedule them. You will reach your widest population of grandparents and will

248 • III. STRENGTH IN NUMBERS

be able to help the most people if you make it as easy as possible for them to attend. That means child care.

When you talk to grandparents, ask if they will need child care to attend a group meeting and, if so, how many children they will be bringing. Perhaps you or the other grandparents know someone who would be willing to baby-sit during meetings. Sometimes you can find a volunteer from a church or temple or even a college student from a local child development program who might be able to get class credit for this. One of my groups is considering rotating the responsibility among the grandparents who regularly bring grandchildren to the group meeting. (You might consider having name tags for the children so the baby-sitter can call them by name. Make sure sitters know not to release children to anyone but their grandparents.)

Will You Charge for Meetings?

I think it is critical that support groups be free of charge. Otherwise, they just become one more place where grandparents have to give. Group should be a place where they can receive. Many grandparents are on a fixed income. They don't think about their own mental health needs, they think about the needs of their grandchild. If they have an extra $60 a month, they'll buy shoes and a haircut for their grandchildren before doing anything for themselves. Charging for meetings only creates one more barrier to people receiving the help they need.

The First Meeting

Here you are. You've found a meeting place and selected the time, the kids are coloring down the hall, and you are looking at a sea of faces in front of you. You have a few more things to consider . . .

Your Panic

If you're not used to speaking in front of people, you may be nervous at this first meeting. The thoughts may tumble past, one after the other: "How do I start? What do I say? Will all the grandparents get along?" Relax. These are normal thoughts and feelings. Regardless of the group composition—age, race, income, and so on—you are all there for the same reason: You are all dealing with grandchildren in one way or another. That is the focus. This is about emotional and moral support. You are not facing strangers, you are facing future friends.

The Welcome

Introduce yourself. Welcome everyone. Restate the reason for getting together. Stress the importance of confidentiality. Share briefly about yourself: how many grandchildren you are raising, why you have them, how long you have had them, your marital status. Let others do the same. Once grandparents start talking, the group takes off.

For many grandparents, this will be their first opportunity to meet others in the same predicament and to discuss feelings and issues. There is a tremendous sense of relief the first time you walk into a room filled with people who will understand and accept you. Some, however, may not choose to talk until they feel more comfortable in the group setting. They may be perfectly happy just listening. Let them know that they are welcome even if they keep silent. And don't worry—each grandparent will wade in at his or her own pace.

Consider using name tags for this first meeting. It helps to connect names and faces in case more than a few people show up. On the other hand, don't be disappointed if you only get one or two the first night. Those two people still need help. Be patient and persistent. Some groups grow slowly, but they do grow.

Group Decisions

During this first meeting you will want to make several decisions:

▪ *Time:* Will the group keep this scheduled time? How often will it meet? I find that once a week for two to three hours works best. It depends on the number of grandparents at a given meeting—5 people can address their crises in less time than 12 people can—and on what your schedules allow. Consistency of meetings is probably more important than frequency. If the group can't meet weekly, schedule a meeting for twice a month or once a month, but make it something reliable to look forward to.

▪ *Format:* What format will you use? Will you start with all members recapping their week, or will you start with whomever is in crisis? Let the group decide what format is most comfortable, and recognize that it may change from time to time. One thing I do recommend is setting aside a few minutes for business items and announcements midway through the meeting; this way you catch people who come late and the ones who must leave early.

▪ *Time-limited or open-ended?* The majority of therapy groups are limited to a set number of weeks and don't allow new members after the first or second session. That was my plan when I started GAP. However, I soon realized that the issues grandparents encounter are much too complex and ongoing to be handled in a limited time frame. All of my groups are open-ended, with new members joining at any time. I have a policy that everyone is welcome, and I never turn anyone away. When new grandparents come into the group, they get great support and guidance from the ones who have been there longer. The grandparents are wonderful about helping each other, and that is one of the joys of the group.

▪ *Refreshments:* Will you have them? How will you handle them? If you plan to take turns, a sign-up sheet is helpful. If you prefer to pitch into a kitty with one person responsible for buying the refreshments, consider rotating the responsibility every few months.

▪ *Cleanup:* Will you have a volunteer cleanup committee to leave the room in shape? Rotate that, too.

Don't forget to have a sign-in sheet for a directory, exchange names and addresses, and keep a box of tissues handy!

Once You're Under Way

Attendance

Attendance is a changeable thing with grandparents. You will find that a core group will come to each meeting without fail. They will become your educators, helping each other out. They may even become politically active, pursuing changes that might not help their grandchildren but could save someone else's. Other grandparents will come only occasionally. Perhaps they work and can't take time off. Maybe they have medical appointments, sick grandchildren, unreliable transportation, or poor health. Encourage other members to call them and see how they're doing. Let them know they're missed.

Inevitably, a few people may drop out if this is not what they are looking for. Groups are not for everyone.

Participation

It is important that everyone at a meeting has time to share. Some grandparents may not be as verbal as others. Encourage quiet, shy grandparents to participate; as time goes by, they may become more comfortable sharing their feelings. At times, you may have to gently and politely interrupt one grandparent to give others a chance to talk.

A wonderful part of a group is that members benefit from each other's experiences, as well as from the support given and received. It's important to share positive experiences as well as negative experiences, because you learn from both.

Be Patient with Evolution

It is tempting, when you give support and advice, to push for quick changes. It is easy to become impatient with people who seem to be stuck in a situation and yet continue to suffer because of it. But change rarely comes quickly or easily, particularly where the heart is involved. Ultimately, grandparents will make the changes that they can in the time frame they can handle—and no sooner. I have heard grandparents talk for two years before they could take any action, such as getting an adult child out of the house. As a group, you can only support and encourage them. Be there when they need to cry and when they want to laugh. When they're ready to make a change, they will do it. But remember, it will be in their time frame.

There are also situations that have no answers, no clear course of action. Sometimes the only thing to do is talk, cry, and feel the understanding of people who have been there. To air your feelings, to see them as natural, and to know you're not alone and not crazy is the beginning of the healing process.

Topics

There is no standard format for subject matter in an ongoing group. Sometimes grandparents will talk about the system; sometimes they will talk about parenting issues, their own childhood, community resources, even their jobs. There is rarely an absence of topics.

(However, Appendix B offers a list of common grandparenting issues for those moments when the discussion runs dry.)

Outreach

I do a lot of outreach work. I will spend months on the phone with a grandparent in crisis; sometimes I give one grandparent the phone number of another in a similar situation. Some will eventually come out for a meeting; others will just call to hear a supportive voice.

It can be difficult to get certain grandparents to attend a group, particularly in communities that have a strong emphasis on privacy and keeping problems in the family. If you have trouble with group attendance, plan a picnic for the kids. Grandparents may not make time to come out for themselves, but they will try harder for the children.

Kicking into High Gear

Once you have a cohesive group, there are a few other things you might want to try:

Outside Experts

I have found it beneficial to occasionally invite outside experts to address my groups. Attorneys, health care specialists, and representatives from the welfare department are among those who have been kind enough to attend our meetings and share their expertise. You might also ask a local mental health professional to conduct a series of parenting classes—a lot has changed since you raised your first set of kids. But do not invite experts until your group has become a cohesive whole.

Family Activities

About once or twice a month, I plan a weekend activity that involves both grandparents and grandchildren. It is important for the children to realize that they are not alone; that many other kids are raised by grandparents; that "they're not the only ones with a Momma with gray hair," as one Grandma puts it. Group activities raise everyone's morale. We frequently have potluck picnics at a local park, reserving in advance a shelter area to guarantee some shade. Events like these give kids space to run and allow grandparents time to relax and socialize with other adults.

Donated Tickets

Many families I work with are on fixed incomes, making it difficult to do the extras they would like to do for their grandchildren. I have, on occasion, been able to obtain donated group tickets to Disneyland, Barnum and Bailey Circus, Ice Capades, Disney on Ice, local children's theaters, and various sporting events. It takes lots of phone calls and letters (often just to find out who can make the decision to donate to a group). Don't get discouraged if you ask for something and get turned down. Persistence generally does pay off.

Shared Skills

Your group is composed of grandparents who have diverse talents and abilities. You may decide to exchange these skills to help each other. For instance, in my groups I have grandparents who are willing to cut hair, repair appliances, fill out forms, and provide occasional respite care for other grandparents. Some grandparents have even volunteered to accompany each other to court. It can make you feel so much better to have someone there who cares, even when the outcome isn't positive. Exchange of these favors and services encourages mutual support.

Shared Goods

When good people come together, wonderful things happen, from clothing exchanges to acts of great generosity. Hand-me-downs were often easy pickings when you were young parents with friends who were also starting families. But when this second shift arrives late in life, you face childrearing alone—until you join a group.

One of the things my groups have organized is a clothing exchange. Grandparents bring in their grandchildren's outgrown clothing to share, and there are always families with younger grandchildren who are delighted to receive them. The same goes for toys, furniture, and other child accessories. If you do start something like this—and why not?—make sure that all donations are in good condition.

And then there is the magic . . .

When a grandfather in my group bought a new car, he and his wife donated their old one to a grandmother who didn't have one. When another grandmother could not afford to visit her dying brother, the group pooled its resources and came up with a round trip ticket to send her to see him. One grandmother was mugged immediately after cashing the check to cover her rent and food; the grandparents came to her rescue with food and donations. And a few grandparents regularly help out several families with groceries. You can't plan or schedule magic like this, it just happens. But by keeping a group together, you do set the stage for great things.

Will Your Group Need a Mental Health Professional?

One of the things you need to consider when you set up your group is if you will need a mental health professional (i.e., a social worker, psychologist, or counselor) and, if so, what his or her involvement will be.

A GAP group can work without a leader or therapist. You can become a big family, calling and supporting each other in times of stress. But there are some situations grandparents cannot cope with on their own. At some point you may have a grandparent who is in a crisis that is beyond your capacity to handle. You could, for example, have a grandparent who is suicidal and needs to be hospitalized. As a fellow grandparent, you might not know where to start. Sometimes a grandparent or grandchild needs an outside referral or needs individual therapy in addition to a self-help group. Georgia Hill is a 49-year-old grandmother who has raised her grandson since her daughter died in a car accident four years ago. A recent car accident of her own jolted her back into the grieving process, opening up all kinds of old wounds. Georgia needs more intense therapy than a group alone can provide. I referred her to someone who specializes in bereavement counseling.

I would hate for any grandparent to give improper information to another grandparent about their grandchildren, adult children, or themselves. People don't intend to hurt each other, but they can—through lack of knowledge. For example, the line between discipline and child abuse is much thinner these days than when you were raising your own children, and a lot of grandparents are capable of unwittingly giving poor advice. Washing a child's mouth out with soap, for instance, used to be a perfectly acceptable way of punishing a foul mouth; by today's standards, it is considered abusive.

It can also destroy a group if someone gives the wrong information at a meeting and it backfires. It is always better to admit you don't know something and offer to try to find out. Write down such questions and find an outside resource. Meanwhile, you might consider connecting with a mental health professional.

There are several ways a mental health professional can be involved in a GAP group:

- As a group leader
- As a regular consultant
- As an on-call consultant
- As a visiting expert

For most groups it's good to have someone on the sidelines who might not show up every week but is available to consult on complicated issues. Perhaps he or she could attend the first few meetings, while your group is becoming cohesive. At the very least, I recommend having someone do a series of classes on parenting issues. You could even arrange a group for grandchildren, who also need to know they're not alone.

How to Find a Mental Health Professional

If you are in therapy or know another grandparent in therapy, talk to the therapist. He or she may be able to recommend someone. Perhaps a local counselor or social worker is already working with three or four grandparents. Check with your local child guidance or mental health clinic for referrals. Also, any place that does outpatient therapy is a good resource.

A Word to the Mental Health Professional

Several years ago I went on vacation and left another professional to fill in for me. She couldn't wait for me to return. "All I did was answer phone calls and deal with problems," she told me. "I didn't have time to do anything else." All she saw was a group of complaining, demanding old people. She was expecting it to be easy and got a real education. If you are a professional who is considering working with a GAP group, there are two questions you need to ask yourself: Do you have a special place in your heart for this population? Do you understand how these groups differ from traditional therapy groups?

When you work with a family in outpatient therapy, you work with their mental health needs, not with the washer breaking down and the car breaking down. You may see the children in outpatient therapy for an hour a week. Grandparent groups can be much more time consuming. We are dealing with whole families and many kinds of problems, and their needs are great. GAP groups deal with more than just emotional support. From the start, my philosophy has been that if you do not deal with basic needs, you cannot begin to deal with mental health needs.

When you work with traditional therapy groups, you have rules and commitments about time, frequency, and attendance. Grandparents may show up for a group meeting once a week or once in six months; they may pop in for half an hour between doctors' appointments or before a second-shift job. They are under incredible stress, and their own care is not their first priority. They may only come when they have a crisis, or they may call regularly for advice, feedback, suggestions, and resources. I have regular contact with a lot of grandparents I never see face to face but who call when they are in need.

You do end up giving more of yourself in a GAP group than in a traditional client–therapist relationship. But if you have a feeling for grandparents, grandchildren, and their concerns, working with grandparent groups can be rewarding work.

CHAPTER 15

The Call to Action

> The seventies were a time when people became
> sensitive to single-parent families. Now we need
> awareness of a new family type—grandparents
> raising their grandchildren.
>
> *—Jessie Taylor*[1]

Here are some snapshots from the GAP political album:

Two grandmothers testify on grandparent issues before a Senate committee in Washington.[2]

Three sets of grandparents talk to Phil Donahue on national television.[3] Thousands of Americans hear what it's like to be a second-time parent.

Six grandmothers meet in chambers with a Los Angeles judge to discuss the possibility of running an information table at the county juvenile dependency courthouse. She agrees to present the idea to her colleagues.

Grandparent leaders from approximately 30 states gather at a Washington, DC, church. They are joined by representatives from the American Association of Retired Persons (AARP), the University of Pennsylvania, and the Children's Rights Council, among others. Their purpose: to explore the possibility of working as a united front. The result: the National Coalition of Grandparents (NCOG). By the end of the weekend they have drafted a mission statement and a set of goals and have elected officers.

Several hundred California grandparents and grandchildren rally on the Capitol steps in Sacramento to put faces on their issues.

And you thought you were alone . . .

The struggle to raise your grandchildren and protect their interests starts on a very personal level: in your home and in your community. This is where you juggle your schedule and your finances; where you battle social workers, judges, and sometimes your own family; where you seek out help and support. But your struggle is not taking place in a vacuum; it is part of an enormous grassroots effort fighting for grandparent and children's rights. Call it a movement. Call it a crusade. Some people call it "Granny's March on Washington." But make no mistake about it: This is not just personal, it is political.

Across the country, grandparent activists are fighting tooth and nail to protect the interests of the next generation and to make sure that future grandparents don't have to struggle so bitterly to play a part in their grandchildren's lives. Margie Davis, founder of Grandparents Offering Love and Direction (GOLD) calls it a "quiet revolution," adding, "It is one of the more important revolutions because it is changing how we care for our nation's children as well as who cares for them."[4] And it is a revolution that is getting louder.

"People think you've got to know someone or have money to get laws changed," activist grandmother Jean Churder told a reporter. "It takes complaints, and it takes people like me letting it be known. . . . A person can do a lot. Look at what one person [Candy Lightner] did with MADD [Mothers Against Drunk Driving]."[5] Jean is a grandmother of 13 and founder of Grandparents and Grandchildren, a political action group in Riverside, California. An assembly speaker accidentally referred to her as "Mrs. Rock" after she described grandparents as the Rock of Gibraltar in their grandchildren's lives. That nickname would also be appropriate for the grandparent activists I work with. They are committed to seeing change. They work at all levels of activism, from facilitating support groups to traveling to Washington, DC, for Senate hearings. They meet with supervisors, judges, and social service agencies; serve on the executive committees of state and national coalitions; and have been a resource to grandparents all across the United States. Each one is like my right arm; I know I can rely on them.

HISTORY OF GRANDPARENTS' RIGHTS MOVEMENT

The idea of grandparents' rights is not a new concept. As far back as 1894 a Louisiana grandmother petitioned the courts for the right to visit her grandchildren.[6] What is new is how widespread the fight has become. The first generation of grandparent activists started in the mid-1960s. They were mostly third parties in custody battles and mostly unrecognized by the courts, and they generated attention and debate on one central issue: grandparent visitation.[7] These grandparents fought social workers, lawyers, and local lawmakers across the country, spurring the first grandparent statutes in a number of states. By the middle of the '80s all 50 states (but not the District of Columbia) had a grandparent visitation statute on their books.

The first wave of grandparent activism also caught the attention of Congress. Although Congress has no legislative authority over family law, it can pass "sense of Congress" resolutions, a kind of formal recommendation to the states. In 1985 former Congressman Mario Biaggi (D–NY) introduced a resolution (H. Con. Res. 67) recommending that all states adopt uniform grandparent visitation laws—in the case of death, divorce, or dissolution of marriage of the parents. The resolution passed unanimously, although state action is slow in coming.[8]

Then, in the late '80s a new generation of grandparents hit the streets. They don't just want to *see* their grandchildren, they are raising them. And they are lighting political fires to protect their interests. They have formed support groups—with names like Grandparents United for Children's Rights, Grandparents Raising Grandchildren, Grandparents Reaching Out, and my own Grandparents As Parents (GAP)—and are pursuing not only visitation issues but issues of custody, government aid, and even the very definition of *family* in today's society. "Network!" is their rallying cry. They network in their own communities with sympathetic judges, lawyers, lawmakers, and social services personnel; with other grandparent groups through state and national coalitions; and with congresspeople and senators by participating in state and federal hearings.

This generation of grandparents is educating themselves about the system so they can work through the system. "Until 15 years ago, people were in awe of legislation," says Ethel Dunn, executive director of Grandparents United for Children's Rights. "Now they see that it's just a law, and we can change it." They are also educating the system about themselves and their issues. "The granny in the sensible shoes and blue hair—you don't see her anymore," says Dunn.[9]

Much of this book has been about loss and stark realities. There is no question that you have been dealt a mean hand in this game, and the stakes are high against you. But this book is also about hope and the difference one person can make. One person, a grandparent, makes an enormous difference in the life of a neglected child. One person who starts a group helps each person who joins it. And one person joining forces with another person, and another, and another can changes laws and move mountains. "The only way to make any changes in children's rights is for us to find each other and help each other," says Barbara Kirkland, founder of Grandparents Raising Grandchildren.[10]

You do have power. I know it is hard to believe, especially when a nameless, faceless welfare worker cuts your benefits or a harsh judge gives unsupervised visitation to your abusive son-in-law. But as a group you have clout. "Supervisors are afraid of people like you," says attorney Michael Salazar. "You're the ones who vote. You've got the country on the run, under tremendous political pressure."[11] Former Congressman Thomas Downey (D–NY) would agree. "It's a well known fact that seniors are the most active lobby in the country," he said in a 1991 congressional hearing. "And when it comes to grandparents, there is no one group more united in their purpose."[12]

Strength in numbers. Unity. That is your power. It is surprising how few letters or phone calls it takes to make legislators look at something. They get no feedback on most of what they work on, so it doesn't take much mail to make something an issue. And people in government do listen. Already we are making headway, and every victory is a milestone! Here are some of our achievements:

▪ *States are beginning to understand that grandparents do have a role to play in the family.* Visitation statutes are being tested, state by state and even at the U.S. Supreme Court level. Some states even have "intact family" bills, which allow grandparents to petition for visitation even though the parents are still married.[13] Arizona allows grandparents to petition even if the parents were never married.[14] Nevada passed a law in 1991 giving grandparents and other relatives preference for child placement even when they live outside the state.[15] Texas grandparents who have guardianship of their grand-children may include them on their group health insurance.[16] Maine passed a bill in 1994 that gives grandparents the right to petition for standing in child protection proceedings.[17]

▪ *Communications are improving between grandparents, social workers, and the courts.* GOLD has worked with the San Diego County Department of Social Services to establish an information table at the San Diego courthouse. It is staffed by trained grandparent volunteers and offers court-approved information from GOLD and other groups. According to Margie Davis, founder of GOLD, the judges, attorneys, and social workers all love it.[18]

▪ *We have the ear of legislators.* Ethel Dunn and I get calls from various local and state senators asking for feedback on legislation. I have even had three-way conference calls with local senate aides and the American Bar Association in Washington, DC, to change the language of a proposed bill.

▪ *We have the attention of congresspeople and senators.* From 1990 to 1992 grandparents testified before three congressional hearings on the issues of grandparents and children, including the first Senate hearing on the subject.[19]

▪ *The National Coalition of Grandparents (NCOG) was formed.* I don't think there is a better signal to grandparents that your voice will be heard, and with groups constantly cropping up in different states, our ranks keep growing.

▪ *Local coalitions are on the rise.* Support groups in several areas have begun to network and organize themselves to create a stronger voice on local issues. California has a statewide coalition of grandparent and relative caregivers; Washington, Oregon, and Idaho have created a tristate coalition; and similar efforts are taking place in other regions of the country.[20]

▪ *We have a national resource center.* In 1993 the American Association of Retired Persons created the AARP Grandparent Information Center in Washington, DC. The center is a clearinghouse for national and local resources. It includes a database of hundreds of grandparent support groups across the country and received 2,100 calls for information in its first four months of operation alone.[21]

These are all signs of progress. Still, NCOG copresident Ethel Dunn cautions patience. "Individually, when you talk to grandparents,

262 III. STRENGTH IN NUMBERS

they'll be very frustrated. They're not winning their case now, and they see the clock ticking; they recognize that their grandchildren are losing time with them, and they are losing time with their grandkids. But in the overall sense, grandparents are making headway. We're gaining respectability."[22] It is that very frustration itself that drives people into the grandparent movement. Political action gives them a place to channel their anger and their energy. "You feel as though you're doing something," she explains. "You're not sitting and wallowing in your pain."

"This has become a passion with me," says GAP member Barbara Wasson. "When I got involved I thought that the state protected children. I found out the state does not protect them. I want to be a part of helping these children have a voice, with education, changing laws, whatever it takes."[23]

Rosalie Cauley no longer has her grandson with her; he was returned to his mother by a dependency judge. Still, Rosalie is a staunch advocate for grandparents' and children's rights. "When Jeremy was first taken, we were absolutely devastated," she explains. "We didn't know what to do with our time or our energy, where to put all this anger. We wanted to work towards improving the system and protecting children. We have told Jeremy that we may not be able to help him, but maybe some other little kid won't have to go through what he's gone through."[24]

LIGHTING THE POLITICAL TORCH

Don't let the word *political* scare you. There are many ways to make a difference without actually rallying on the Capitol steps—although some of our grandparents found that to be an exciting experience. You can work behind the scenes with legislators by sponsoring a bill, shaping a bill, or just supporting it with calls and letters. You can work with judges, attorneys, and social workers, offering them resources and educating them about your concerns. You can work with the media and the community, creating public awareness and public education about children's rights and grandparents' rights. But if you do want to impact policy, you need to be armed with knowledge about the issues, the process of government, and the players. You need to make yourself heard.

Know the Issues

To be taken seriously, you have to know your subject: the history of the issue, the stories, the statistics, anything that will make your concerns real to the people who can help you. If you can do this and be specific, detailed, and well organized with your information, you will have a valuable perspective to offer those you are working with.

You must also know the bills. Is there something already under consideration? It may need your support—perhaps a letter to your legislator or your testimony at a hearing. Is this a new area that needs to be introduced to your legislators? You may want to provide model bills from other states or join forces with a politically savvy attorney who can work with legislative offices to draft a new bill. Many attorneys feel strongly about issues like children's rights and kinship care; perhaps you can work with one who is willing to volunteer the time.

Trust what you know. Many grandparents assume that they are only "bumbling little grannies" and that other people know more than they do. As they move forward, they discover they have a wealth of information and insight to offer.

Know the Process

Before you can fight the system, or even work within it, you must know how it works—not just the courts and the agencies but the workings of your local, state, and federal governments as well. You know what the problems are, but who causes them? Where do they start? Who can change them? Is the problem one of process or one of law? It makes a difference. "Trial judges and jurors must interpret the laws as written by legislators," a California court judge told us. In other words, don't picket the court, picket the capitol. Is it a federal issue or a local one? Most issues that are important to grandparents originate at the state and local levels. It's not worth sending thousands of letters to a federal representative when it is a local law in question.

Know the Players

Political advocacy is a big field with many issues and just as many players. Some people can help you, others cannot. You need to know the difference. Who is on your side—and can you work together? Who is against you—and can you sway them? Who is undecided? To answer these questions you need to know the following groups:

▪ *Your representatives:* Do you know who your council member is? Your delegate in Congress? Your state senator or assembly member? These are the people most likely to listen to you. You are one of the people they were elected to serve, and you are one of those who will keep them in office. Your concerns should be their concerns. But before you contact them, here are some things you might want to know about them: their concerns and interests, their voting record on family issues, the stands they are taking now, and the committees they serve on. The more you know in advance about your representatives, the better you can focus your appeal. After all, you will approach a sympathetic listener differently than someone who is antagonistic or on the fence.

▪ *Your allies:* Few issues exist in a vacuum. For every issue that you promote or oppose, there is probably another group working with the same agenda. For instance, Grandparents United for Children's Rights joined forces with the National Foster Parents Association to support a national kinship mandate;[25] both groups would like to see a uniform law requiring all child welfare agencies to look to family members before placing a child in unrelated foster care. Whatever your goal, network with other groups in your area. Find out who shares your position and whether you can work together. At least make sure you don't double someone else's efforts. Remember, numbers count. A coalition has more clout than one grandparent or even one group alone.

There are many groups that keep an eye on family and child legislation; the Foster Parent Association, Children Now, Child Welfare League, and the National Association of Social Workers are just a few. Many of these groups have state chapters. Your group could join forces with one of them, and their newsletters are a good way to follow current developments.

▪ *Your opposition:* It's great to sit and agree with your friends, but at some point you have to turn and face your enemies. Every issue you support may have someone who opposes it; the more you know about them, the better chance you have of answering their arguments, perhaps even of swaying them to your side. Be willing to negotiate.

Make Yourself Heard!

None of your passion or knowledge will help your cause if no one hears about it. Don't just tell your friends and neighbors, tell your government officials. If they are to represent you, they must know how issues and actions affect you. They have the clout to make the changes.

Letter Writing

Letters do count. Legislators don't get tired of hearing from their constituents. Legislators read their mail, and what they read can affect their position on a bill or issue. Remember, most bills don't get any letters at all, so a little mail goes a long way.

One California grandmother wrote a letter that was so eloquent it was copied into every senator's folder as part of the legislative analysis of the bill it was supporting. "That's history here in the Senate," says legislative assistant Leza Davis. "Five years from now, if someone wants to get the bill folder from the archives, they will see Rosalie's letter."[26] Incidentally, the bill passed. So don't think your letter is unimportant. This is a case of the squeaky wheel getting the grease—if it is handled properly.

Who Should Get Your Letter?

Knowing where to send a letter sounds simple, but you'd be surprised at how many people write letters to officials who can't help them. A well-targeted letter does more good than randomly papering your capitol with mail. Here are some suggestions to help you target your letters:

▪ *Write to your own representatives.* You have more influence with senators from your state and representatives from your district than with anyone else. Give them your support if they agree with you. If they don't, explain why a different position makes sense right now. Show your familiarity with the issue, and cite your firsthand experience.

▪ *Write to the relevant committee members.* If you have facts you think should influence their thinking, send them to the chairperson

How to Write Effective Political Letters*

1. Begin with the appropriate heading and address. Elected officials are addressed as "The Honorable," followed by their name. In the letter use the proper title: "Dear Senator Jones," "Dear Assembly Member Thomas," "Dear Congressman Smith," "Dear Governor Jackson."

2. Be specific. State the actual bill number, if you can, or at least provide the bill's title.

3. State your opinion in the first sentence.

4. Identify yourself and explain why you are concerned about this issue. Give factual information to support your view. If you are writing on behalf of a group, include the group's name and the size of its membership—there is strength in numbers.

5. State how this bill will address the problem and how it will affect your district.

6. Close by urging your representative to take appropriate, specific action.

7. Sign your name legibly and include your address on the letter itself; sometimes envelopes get lost or pitched.

8. Include any pertinent materials, for example, editorials from local papers.

Remember to . . .

- Write about one subject only.
- Be brief and to the point; one page should do it.
- Write legibly, or type if you can. But don't put off writing just because you don't type; every letter counts.
- Use your own words instead of a form letter. Use your own stationary, unless you are writing on behalf of a group or organization (then use the organization letterhead).
- Keep letters individual. If you write several legislators, don't send identical letters. And don't send photocopied letters, form letters, or printed post cards.
- Be courteous and reasonable.

A Few Don'ts

- Don't be self-righteous. Your legislators know you are a citizen and a taxpayer; you don't have to flaunt it.

(continued)

(continued from previous page)

- Don't apologize for taking your legislator's time. Just be concise and specific.
- Don't make comments like "I hope this gets by your secretary." This only irritates and alienates office staff.
- Don't be rude or threatening.
- Don't be vague.

---

*Adapted from "A Walk through Policyland" by Grandparents United for Children's Rights.

or the members of a committee that will hear a bill. If you do this, send a copy to your own legislator with a short personal note.

- *Don't complain to legislators from other districts.* Just because you disagree politically with your own legislators does not mean that it is a good idea to write to a member of another district. Write to your legislator directly.
- *Write to the fence-sitters.* Before a bill goes to vote, find out who is on your side and who is not. You have a better chance of swaying the ones who are undecided than in reversing the position of someone who is dead-set against you.
- *Write to the governor.* Even if a state bill passes both houses, the governor will still have to sign it. But don't wait for a bill to reach the governor's desk before starting your letter-writing campaign.

When to Write

Timing is critical when you are writing political action letters. Whether you are writing to propose, support, or oppose a bill, you want to make sure your letter arrives at the right stage of the process to be effective. Here are some general guidelines on timing:

- To propose a bill or submit ideas for legislation, write during your state's legislative recess. This gives the staff time to research your issue.
- To affect the writing and language of a bill, write when it is being considered in committee.
- To advocate for or against a bill, write at the beginning of committee hearings if your representative is on the committee; if not, write just before the bill comes to the floor.

▪ If the bill has passed both houses, write to your governor. Make sure your letter goes out early enough to be considered; this is your last chance for input.

When time is of the essence, you can send a telegram or Mailgram or even make a phone call or send a fax to your official's office. If enough calls come in, he or she will get the message. Your public officials also need positive feedback. Write to let them know when they've done a good job for you, not just to complain or to oppose their actions.

Working with Legislators

If you want to influence the writing of new laws, you will want to establish a relationship with your public officials. Once you do that, you can educate them about your concerns and position yourself as a reliable sounding board for grandparent issues. Lawmakers can't possibly know every implication of the laws they write; they must rely on outside experts. You can get to know your legislators by inviting them to one of your meetings or by scheduling private appointments with them. Don't be discouraged if you start out meeting with their aides. Aides and consultants are good people to know. They are advisers and often gather information for their senator, representative, or council member.

The Visit

When you visit a legislator in his or her office, try to be as organized and professional as possible. Remember that legislators must make time in a busy schedule to see you, and let them know that you know their time is valuable by arriving early and keeping your meeting brief. Be honest and courteous; remember, you are trying to create a relationship with this person, not just win one vote. Some other techniques for an effective visit include the following:

▪ *Be prepared and be concise.* Have your information ready ahead of time and get to the point quickly; keep your presentation simple and specific.
▪ *Bring a written position paper.* Writing it will focus your thoughts, and it gives you something to leave with your legislator.

▪ *Keep your group small.* Too many people with too many voices can overwhelm a person and dilute your message.

▪ *Offer solutions.* "[Lawmakers] don't have time to solve your problems for you," says GOLD founder Margie Davis.[27] "Never take a problem without a solution."

▪ *Avoid arguments.* You want your legislator to see the issues from your perspective, you don't want to create an adversary. Be composed, not confrontational.

▪ *Avoid war stories.* You want your legislator to see this issue as one that affects more than one grandparent. You can do this by showing the broad picture, not your personal story. "You watch sometime," says one grandparent activist. "If you're with an official and a grandmother starts talking about 'My granddaughter . . . ,' you can see the curtain close, and they're not listening."[28] If you want to be heard, stay impersonal.

▪ *Always end your visit with a question.* For example: "Will you support this issue?" "What can you do to help us?" Grandparent issues need legislative support; don't be afraid to come out and ask for it.

▪ *Don't forget to thank your legislator for his or her time.*

▪ *Remeber to follow up your visit with a letter.* Remind your public official of any commitment he or she made and express your gratitude yet again for his or her time and support.

Step by Step

Remember, each piece of legislation is a step, not a cure. This is a slow process, and not every effort will succeed. But even small changes make a big difference. You don't always need to write a new law; you can help change (or enforce) existing laws. For instance, a Virginia grandmother and foster parent wanted to help change foster care laws in her state. She took one issue—the amount of time children remain in the foster care system—and worked with her state legislature. She was persistent, organized, and diplomatic. Today, a child can be in the Virginia foster care system no more than two years, instead of five, before a permanent plan is established.[29]

Expect changes in your original amendments. Your public officials are trying to balance the concerns of many people, departments, and interest groups at the same time. Be willing to work with your opponents and stay open to discussion. You might end up with a better product. And don't forget: Each grandparent situation is different. Many issues will continue to be decided court by court and case by case. Legislators write laws, but judges still interpret them.

Public Awareness and Political Education

Political action goes beyond writing and rewriting legislation. Laws must be passed, they must be interpreted, and they must be carried out. While it is important to work with legislators, for real change to come about you must also educate the people who vote on, interpret, and execute new legislation. The trick is to know your audience and how to approach them.

Judges and Attorneys

Like legislators, judges and attorneys are not able to keep track of all issues that affect their work. They need outside sources of information—but these need to be impersonal sources. It doesn't do to approach these professionals with your own story and needs; they can't address individual cases, and they will, unfortunately, stop listening to you. You can set up an office visit with a judge, but, as with a lawmaker, be sure to come in representing the larger issues and don't bring a problem without a proposed solution. The basic question you are posing is "How can we work together?"

You can also try tapping into continuing education. Judges and attorneys must earn a certain number of educational credits a year to keep up with new trends. Grandparent issues definitely present a new trend in law. A well-organized grandparent group could offer to create a panel of grandparents and legal experts for one of these educational programs. This may take some salesmanship and advance planning, but it offers you a chance to educate decision makers in a nonthreatening environment. Remember, however, that your goal is to educate, not complain.

Social Services and Social Workers

The more thoroughly social workers can understand the plight of grandparents in general—outside their individual caseload—the better chance they have of being sensitized to grandparent issues. Working with local legislators, attorneys, and activists in children's rights and foster parent organizations will bring you into networking contact with social service administrators; you can also contact them directly. Again, position yourself as a positive resource.

The Media

The media is on a constant hunt for human interest stories. As grandparents raising grandchildren, your stories are lightning rods for many social ills. This is one place where individual details and strong emotions are appropriate. Remember, the media shapes public opinion, and public opinion shapes government.

DOWN THE ROAD: REDEFINING THE FAMILY

Family renification and parental rights are the key stumbling blocks you encounter as a grandparent with a grandchild in crisis. The courts are pledged to support family reunification, and parental rights are closely guarded. These are important ideals. The problems don't lie with the importance our society attaches to family and parents, the problems lie with the definition of *family* and *parent*.

For centuries the family was a wide net that included grandparents, uncles, aunts, cousins, even great-grandparents. Today, however, law and society define family in the narrowest of terms: mother, father, and child. When the law breaks the relationship between a parent and child, all of the child's other blood ties cease to exist. This kind of thinking is absurd. To quote psychiatrist Arthur Kornhaber, M.D., "Nature doesn't limit the family to two generations; why should the law?"[30]

The concept of parent is even more complicated. Traditionally, parents gave birth to a child and then raised him. Today, increasing numbers of children are raised by stepparents, foster parents, adoptive parents, grandparents, and other relatives—people who have no direct biological connection to the child but have cared for and bonded with him on a day-to-day basis. Still, we repeatedly see the courts take a child away from one parent, place him with relatives, and then go looking for the "real" father or mother—whether that person knows the child or not. Some grandparents angrily refer to these absent parents as "sperm donors" and "egg carriers," but the law remains on their side.

We need to redefine the word *parent*, and we need to consider more than biology in our definition. Until we do, we can expect more and more painful battles between parents and grandparents, between biological and foster parents, and between adoptive parents and birth mothers. The advent of artificial insemination, *in vitro* fertilization, surrogate motherhood, and test-tube babies raises whole new questions about parenthood. As one scientist told GOLD founder Margie Davis, "If those in the social service end of the world do not redefine the word *parent*, we in the scientific community will do it for you."[31] The grandparent movement, by its very existence, is helping to broaden the definitions of parent and family. With every lawsuit, with every hearing, with every magazine article, grandparents and other child advocates are informing the public about parenthood and family issues. Only through education, discussion, and public acceptance will true change occur.

Remember, anyone can make a baby. It takes a parent to raise a child.

CHAPTER 16

Conclusion

> You know they say blood is thicker than water?
> Well, for us, love is thicker than blood.
> —*Jonathan Williams, 37, raised by*
> *step-grandmother and grandfather*[1]

In an issue of "The Intergenerational Hookup," the newsletter of Grandparents United for Children's Rights, executive director Ethel Dunn wrote a moving article about Las Madres de la Plaza de Mayo (the mothers of the Plaza de Mayo). These were the middle- and upper-class mothers and grandmothers of Argentina who gathered each Thursday in the square outside Argentina's White House to protest the disappearance of thousands of children and grandchildren during the military government's campaign against "subversives" in the mid-1970s and early 1980s. As many as 4,000 of these children were believed to have been kidnapped and turned over to military families for adoption. These grieving mothers and grandmothers translated their fear into anger and their anger into advocacy; they walked in a large silent circle, week after week, carrying pictures of missing children. It is a story of courage, love, and determination.

In our own country there is no military government spiriting away children. But since the 1980s the threat of drugs and alcohol, violent crime, child abuse, AIDS, and a bureaucratic court system have endangered far more than 4,000 children. Here, too, there are thousands of grandparents who are turning grief and fear into advocacy. "Sometimes we, too, march, picket, carry signs, and demand," writes Dunn. "We never stop trying to educate. We sometimes become angry, often frustrated. Once in a while we smell the passionate fragrance of success and allow ourselves a short period of time to rejoice. Always, however, we persevere."[2]

Persevere. It means to continue in spite of difficulty and opposition. It doesn't matter if you are on a picket line or in a grocery line; every grandparent trying to raise a grandchild perseveres. Each morning your grandchildren wake up safe and each night they go to bed well loved and well cared for, you have succeeded. Each grandparent who has lost a grandchild perseveres, and each day that grandparent survives the sorrow, he or she has succeeded.

Grandparents in Los Angeles, California, and Paducah, Kentucky, have as much to tell about courage, love, and determination as Las Madres de la Plaza de Mayo. If you ever wonder where the rewards come from, consider the following letter, which was written by my nephew Kevin, now in college.[3] It is addressed to my mother, the grandmother who raised him:

Nona,

On July 31st, 1983, you unexpectedly became a mother again. You took an 8-year-old boy into your home and treated him like he was your son, as if it was normal.

Your life was turned upside down. You lost the most precious thing in the world to you—your daughter. In the middle of your pain and suffering you found the time to take care of a scared, confused, and uncertain little boy who had just lost his mother.

As the little boy got older, he learned how to push your buttons. He had a knack for making your day miserable. Making life hard for you was his way of saying he didn't want another mom. He did everything he could to push you away, but you wouldn't leave him alone. The more problems he caused, the more you were there for him—getting him out of trouble and pushing him to do something with his life. You never thought twice about helping him when he needed it. When he was sick, you nursed him back to health. When he wanted a ride to a friend's house, you took him there. You always tried your hardest to make him happy.

Now he has grown up and understands the sacrifices you made for him.

Nona, this little boy is a very grateful young man now, and I want you to know how much I appreciate all you've done for me.

I want you to know that I'm proud to be your grandson. But most of all, I want you to know I love you.

Kevin

The great American poet Carl Sandburg once said, "A baby is God's opinion that the world should go on." When you take in a grandchild, you do more than help one family; you preserve our future.

Appendices

Resources for Grandparents and Relative Caregivers

FOR FINDING GROUPS IN YOUR AREA

AARP Grandparent Information Center
AARP Headquarters
601 E St., N.W.
Washington, DC 20049
(202) 434-2296 Weekdays, 9:00 A.M. to 5:00 P.M. EST

You can write to them or call. If you call, you will hear a recorded message asking for your name and phone number. Center staff will return your call, keeping your expense to a minimum.

Grandparents As Parents (GAP)
P.O. Box 964
Lakewood, CA 90714
(310) 924-3996
(310) 839-2548
Fax: (714) 828-1375

Grandparents United for Children's Rights
137 Larkin St.
Madison, WI 53705
(608) 238-8751

SOURCES OF ADDITIONAL SUPPORT

Al-Anon (also Alateen and Alatot)
Al-Anon Family Group Headquarters
P.O Box 862
Midtown Station, NY 10018-0862
(212) 302-7240

You can also look up Al-Anon in your telephone book for information on local groups.

Compassionate Friends
P.O. Box 3696
Oakbrook, IL 60522-3696
(708) 990-0010

This is a group for bereaved parents who have lost children of any age, for any reason.

PARENTING RESOURCES

American Council for Drug Education
204 Monroe St., Suite 110
Rockville, MD 20850
(800) 488-DRUG

Boy Scouts of America
1325 W. Walnut Hill Lane
Irving, TX 75015-2079
(214) 580-2000

This organization can work with learning disabled children. It also runs a major antidrug program, which includes the publication of a booklet for children.

Children and Adults with Attention Deficit Disorder (CHADD)
499 N.W. 70th Ave., Suite 109
Plantation, FL 33317
(800) 233-4050
Fax: (305) 587-4599

Educational Resources Information Center (ERIC) System
1600 Research Blvd.
Rockville, MD 20850-3172
(800) 538-3742

ERIC is a promotional and outreach arm of the U.S. Department of Education's Office of Educational Research and Improvement. It offers free materials on topics like "How Can I Be Involved in My Child's Education?" It publishes a free education journal, *The ERIC Review*, three times a year. Call for a subscription or to order free brochures.

Learning Disabilities Association (LDA)
4156 Library Rd.
Pittsburgh, PA 15234
(412) 341-1525

This association is for children and adults with learning disabilities.

Mothers Against Drunk Driving (MADD)
511 E. John Carpenter Freeway, Suite 700
Irving, TX 75062
(214) 744-6233

In addition to legislative action, MADD offers programs to help young children develop positive self-esteem and refusal skills.

National Association for Perinatal Addiction Research and Education (NAPARE)
200 N. Michigan Ave., Suite 300
Chicago, IL 60601
(800) 638-2229

In addition to its national help line, NAPARE offers free information on caring for drug-exposed children. Ask for their *Foster Parent* and *Adoptive Parent* packets.

National Clearinghouse for Alcohol and Drug Information
11426-28 Rockville Pike
Rockville, MD 20852
(800) 729-6686

This is a federal clearinghouse that provides pamphlets, booklets, posters, fact sheets, and directories on alcohol and drugs.

National Information Center for Children and Youth with Disabilities (NICHCY)
P.O. Box 1492
Washington, DC 20013
(800) 695-0285

NICHCY is a clearinghouse for free information on disabilities and disability-related issues involving children and youth. NICHCY publications include explanations of special education laws and school services for children with disabilities, state resource sheets, and information on individual disabilities. Some materials are printed in Spanish. Call or write NICHCY for a free copy of their publications list.

National Institute on Drug Abuse (NIDA)
5600 Fishers Lane
Rockville, MD 20857
(800) 729-6686

NIDA provides drug information and a counseling hotline.

National PTA Drug and Alcohol Abuse Prevention Project
330 N. Wabash Ave., Suite 2100
Chicago, IL 60611-3690
(312) 670-6782

Open Arms Family Support Network
P.O. Box 50982
Pasadena, CA 91115-0982
(818) 383-6800

Publishes the *Open Arms Baby Book: Special Care Techniques for Infants Prenatally Exposed to Drugs or Alcohol.* Available by mail for a $2.00 donation.

CHILD-FOCUSED BOOKS

Ages Four to Eight

Do I Have a Daddy? (Jeanne Warren Lindsay). Buena Park, CA: Morning Glory, 1991. Age level: five to eight years old. This story provides a model for how to respond to children's questions about a parent they have never seen.

Nonna (Jennifer Bartoli). New York, NY: Harvey House, 1975. Age level: four to seven years old. A boy tells the story of the death of his grandmother, portraying how young children respond to the death of a loved one.

The Saddest Time (Norma Simon). Morton Grove, IL: Whitman, Albert & Co., 1986. Age level: four to eight years old. Death is the subject of these three gentle stories.

When Grandpa Died (Margaret Stevens). Chicago, IL: Children's Press, 1979. Age level: four to eight years old. A little girl learns to accept the death of her grandfather.

Ages Eight to 13

Aarvy Aardvark Finds Hope (Donna O'Toole). Burnsville, NC: Celo Press, 1988. Age level: all ages. An aardvark's delayed grief over the loss of family begins to heal through the support of a caring friend.

Blew and the Death of the Mag (Wendy Lichtman). Albion, CA: Freestone, 1975. Age level: 10 and up. After her mother dies, a young girl explores her feelings of love, fear, anger, and, finally, understanding.

How It Feels When a Parent Dies (Jill Krementz). New York, NY: Alfred A. Knopf, 1981. Eighteen children, ages seven through 16, tell how it feels to lose a parent through death.

Older Children

Unlocking Potential: College and Other Choices for Learning Disabled People— A Step-By-Step Guide (Barbara Scheiber and Jeane Talpers). Chevy Chase, MD: Adler & Adler, 1987. Available only through Woodbine House, 6510 Bells Mill, Bethesda, MD 20817. (800) 843-7323. $12.95 plus $4.00 shipping/handling.

LEGAL ORGANIZATIONS AND ASSOCIATIONS

American Bar Association
750 N. Lake Shore
Chicago, IL 60611
(312) 988-5000

Legal Services for Prisoners with Children
474 Valencia St., Suite 230
San Francisco, CA 94103
(415) 255-7036

This organization publishes several state manuals for grandparent/relative caregivers and their advocates.

National Association of Protection and Advocacy Systems
900 Second St., N.E., Suite 211
Washington, DC 20002
(202) 408-9514

Protection and advocacy agencies pursue legal, administrative, and other solutions to protect the rights of people who are developmentaly disabled or mentally ill.

LEGAL BOOKS AND PUBLICATIONS

Family Law Dictionary (Robin D. Leonard and Stephen Elias). Berkeley, CA: Nolo Press, 1990.

The Guardianship Book: How to Become a Child's Guardian in California (David Brown). Berkeley, CA: Nolo Press, 1989.

POLITICAL ACTION RESOURCES

American Association of Retired Persons (AARP)
AARP Headquarters
601 E St., N.W.
Washington, DC 20049
(202) 434-2296 Weekdays, 9:00 A.M. to 5:00 P.M. EST

National Coalition of Grandparents (NCOG)
137 Larkin St.
Madison, WI 53705
(608) 238-8751

Western Union
(800) 325-6000

Western Union has a reduced rate for messages to public officials. Personal Opinion Messages (POMs) carry a flat rate for 20 words and will reach your legislator in one day. The voice response system will prompt you through the various choices.

Conversation Topics for Grandparent Support Groups

THE STORIES

- How many grandchildren you have and how you came to have them.

LIFE CHANGES

- The decrease in your social life now that you're a parent again
- How your life is different from that of your friends
- How your grandchildren have changed your work life
- Your feelings about work
- The financial strain of raising a second family
- The dreams and plans that have been put on hold
- The toll on your health

INTENSE FEELINGS

- Grief over the loss of your child
- Anger at your child, the situation, the system, everything
- Guilt
- Depression
- Feeling you don't want to raise your grandchildren, but not wanting them split up or placed with strangers
- Feeling you don't belong anywhere, neither with young parents nor with adults your age

- Fears
- Hopes for your grandchildren
- The small rewards

PARENTING ISSUES

- Changes in childrearing techniques since you brought up your own kids
- The effects of the parent's visits on the child's behavior and emotions
- Dealing with school problems children might have
- Setting limits with grandchildren and adult children; what behaviors you will or will not tolerate
- Setting age-appropriate consequences
- How to raise your grandchild's self-esteem
- How to help children who were born drug exposed
- Learning to accept that some grandchildren might need more help than you can provide

YOUR ADULT CHILDREN

- Learning to accept the fact that your son or daughter is choosing to be an irresponsible parent
- When to decide that you have done enough for your adult child and that it's time to let go
- Protecting yourself and your grandchildren from your adult child

THE REST OF YOUR FAMILY

- The reaction of other children and family members to your becoming a parent again
- Handling sibling rivalry
- The effects of second parenthood on your marriage

THE BUREAUCRACY

- How to negotiate the bureaucracy of government agencies and "the system"

- The frustration with a system that was set up to protect your grand-children but often doesn't
- What groups can do to help change the system

A Guide to the Grandparents Mentioned in This Book

Liz Andersson, in her 70s, raising five grandsons, ages 18 months to 12 years, in Seattle, Washington

Rose and Gerald Avery, in their 50s, raising two grandsons in Boston, Massachusetts

Janet Baker, in her 50s, raising three granddaughters in Los Angeles, California

Jewell Baxter, in her 60s, raising two grandsons, ages three and four, in Anaheim, California

Alice Brody, in her 60s, raising three grandchildren in Wilmington, Delaware

Marjorie Brown, in her 40s, raising three-year-old Jessica and two-year-old Billy in Chicago, Illinois

Charlotte Buckley, in her 40s, raising four-year-old Joey in Los Angeles, California

Maggie Butler, in her 50s, raising two granddaughters in Columbus, Ohio

Henrietta Casper, in her 70s, raising 15-year-old Adam in Long Beach, California

Ruth Castle, in her 60s, raising two grandsons in Los Angeles, California

Rosalie Cauley, in her 50s, lives in Lakewood, California, and is no longer raising 14-year-old Jeremy

Sandra Cobb, in her 60s, raising seven grandchildren in Washington, D.C.

Katherine Connor, in her 60s, raising five grandchildren in Long Beach, California

Leah Croft, in her 60s, raising nine-year-old twins and three-year-old Josh in Woodland Hills, California

Lucy Davis, in her 50s, raising seven-year-old Lindsey in Studio City, California

Wanda Davis, in her 50s, raising eight-year-old Monica in Tuscon, Arizona

Andre and Ginette de Toledo, in their 60s, raised 19-year-old Kevin in Culver City, California

Barbara Douglas, in her 80s, raising eight-year-old Max in Warwick, Rhode Island

Beth and Alan Grafton, in their 60s, raising three grandchildren in Boston, Massachusetts

Joyce Griffin, in her 60s, raising five grandchildren in Houston, Texas

Nancy Harper, in her 50s, raising eight-year-old Marissa in Los Angeles, California

Georgia Hill, in her 40s, raising seven-year-old Stephen in Long Beach, California

Marlena Hunt, in her 40s, raising two-year-old Tiffany in Anaheim, California

Ivy Johnson, in her 50s, raising five grandchildren in Baltimore, Maryland

Dorcas King, in her 70s, raising two grandchildren in Los Angeles, California

Victor Lane, in his 60s, raising three grandchildren in Long Beach, California

Pam and Robert Marshall, in their 60s, raising five-year-old Megan in Long Beach, California

Frances Morgan, in her 70s, raising two grandchildren in Tarzana, California

Ethel Murray, in her 70s, raising nine-year-old Scott in Springfield, Illinois

Carolyn Parker, in her 50s, raising six-year-old Eric in Los Angeles, California

Emily and Carter Petersen, in their 60s, raising four-year-old Amanda and three-year-old Jared in Buffalo, New York

Claire and Evan Powers, in their 60s, in Santa Monica, California, no longer raising 12-year-old Sarah, but see her one weekend a month

Sue Ellen Rice, in her 50s, raising four-year-old Martin and two-year-old Alice in San Diego, California

Jay and Brenda Saunders, in their 70s, raising six-year-old Anthony in Hartford, Connecticut

Jack and Betty Segal, in their 60s, raising eight-year-old Beth in Portland, Oregon

Frank and Gloria Simon, in their 60s, raising eight-year-old Stephanie and six-year-old Jill in Los Angeles, California

Donna and Hal Smith, in their 50s, raising ten-year-old David and six-year-old John in Sacramento, California

Esther Smith, in her 80s, in Scottsdale, Arizona, no longer has her grandsons living with her

Diane Snyder, in her 50s, raising seven-year-old Andrea in Azuza, California

Marta Sobol, in her 50s, raising eight-year-old Christopher in Woodland Hills, California

Julia Stone, in her 60s, raising four grandchildren in Los Angeles, California

Fay and Jim Strassburger, in their 60s, raising two grandsons in Los Angeles, California

Jane and Doug Sullivan, in their 60s, raising nine-year-old Elisa, five-year-old Shannon, and four-year-old Mark in Sherman Oaks, California

Alice Sutherland, in her 50s, raising 13-year-old Suzanne, 12-year-old Faith, and nine-year-old Tommy in Van Nuys, California

Anne Sutter, in her 60s, raising six-year-old Gregory in Long Beach, California

Arlene Townsend, in her 60s, raising seven-year-old Stuart in San Francisco, California

Rebecca Tybor, in her 70s, raising 16-year-old twins in Los Angeles, California

Grace and Marcus Tyler, in their 50s, raising five-year-old Jason in Pittsburgh, Pennsylvania

Dave and Milly Walsh, in their 70s, raising four grandchildren in Redondo Beach, California

John and Carol Waters, in their 60s, raising eight-year-old Brian in Long Beach, California

Notes

INTRODUCTION

1. Linda L. Creighton. "Silent Saviors," *U.S. News & World Report*, December 16, 1991, p. 83.
2. Mary Lou Wilson. "Recycled Parents," *The Reporter* (Vacaville, CA), March 19, 1990.
3. Andrew H. Malcolm. "Helping Grandparents Who Are Parents Again," *The New York Times*, November 19, 1991.
4. Lenora Madison Poe. *Black Grandparents as Parents*. Berkeley, CA: Lenora Madison Poe, 1992; Meredith Minkler and Kathleen M. Roe. *Grandmothers as Caregivers: Raising Children of the Crack Cocaine Epidemic*. Newbury Park, CA: Sage Publications, 1993; Irene M. Endicott. *Grandparenting Redefined: Guidance for Today's Changing Family*. Lynwood, WA: Aglow Publications, 1992.

CHAPTER 1

1. Jill Smolowe. "To Grandma's House We Go," *Time*, November 5, 1990, p. 90.
2. Ibid., p. 86; Meredith Minkler and Kathleen M. Roe. *Grandmothers as Caregivers: Raising Children of the Crack Cocaine Epidemic*. Newbury Park, CA: Sage Publications, 1993, pp. x, 4–5.
3. U.S. House of Representatives Select Committee on Aging. *Grandparents Rights: A Resource Manual*. Washington, DC: U.S. Government Printing Office, 1992, p. 15.
4. *Grandparent Information Center* (Handout). Washington, DC: AARP Grandparent Information Center.
5. *Grandparents Rights: A Resource Manual*, op. cit., p. 15.
6. Susan R. Pollack. "The Grandparent Trap," *The Detroit News*, July 17, 1991.

7. Mike Yorkey. "Picking Up the Pieces," *Focus on the Family*, September 1993, p. 13.
8. Patricia Edmonds. "Those Caught in Middle Are 'Missing a Lot,'" *USA Today*, July 23, 1991.
9. Laurie Becklund. "I Wanted Somebody to Love," *Los Angeles Times*, March 14, 1993; Center for the Study of Social Policy. *Kids Count Data Book: State Profiles of Child Well-Being.* Washington, DC: Annie E. Casey Foundation, 1993, p. 14.
10. Kristin A. Moore. *To Individuals and Organizations Concerned about Teen Pregnancy and Childbearing* (Memo). Washington, DC: Child Trends, February 1995.
11. U.S. Senate Committee on Labor and Human Resources. *Falling through the Crack: The Impact of Drug-Exposed Children on the Child Welfare System* (March 8, 1990). Washington, DC: U.S. Government Printing Office, 1990, p. 109.
12. Ellen Barry et al. *Manual for Grandparents and Caregivers* (3rd ed.). San Francisco: Legal Services for Prisoners with Children, 1993, p. 5.
13. *Falling through the Crack*, op. cit., pp. 18–21.
14. Ibid., p. 108.
15. Felicia R. Lee. "AIDS Toll on Elderly: Dying Grandchildren," *The New York Times*, November 21, 1994.
16. *Falling through the Crack*, op. cit., pp. 6, 9.
17. Interview with Mary Hayes (Division Chief, Foster Care Division, Department of Children and Family Services) by authors. Los Angeles, December 27, 1994.
18. There is no denying that the African American community is harder hit by the grandparenting phenomenon. According to the 1990 census, 12 percent of black children live with their grandparents, compared with four percent of white children. However, the actual *numbers* of black and white children are nearly equal: 1.2 million black children and 1.8 million white children. The discrepancy is due to the fact that there are five times more white children in the United States than black children. Hispanic children represent the smallest numbers, but they still number nearly half a million. See *Grandparents Rights: A Resource Manual*, p. 15.
19. Ibid., p. 15.
20. *Falling through the Crack*, op. cit., pp. 34, 161.
21. Ibid., p. 159.
22. Ibid., p. 94.
23. Karen Greene. "The Great American Grandparent: Reinventing Families," *Children's Advocate*, March/April 1992.
24. *Falling through the Crack*, op. cit., p. 36.
25. Interview with Michael Jones by authors (via telephone). June 22, 1994.

26. Linda L. Creighton. "Silent Saviors," *U.S. News & World Report*, December 16, 1991, p. 87.

CHAPTER 3

1. Andrew H. Malcolm. "Helping Grandparents Who Are Parents Again," *The New York Times*, November 19, 1991.
2. *Donahue*. April 11, 1991.
3. Susan R. Pollack. "The Grandparent Trap," *The Detroit News*, July 17, 1991.
4. Miriam Durkin. "When Grandparents Start Over," *Charlotte Observer*, November 3, 1991.
5. Tony Link. "When Kids Come to Grandma's House to Stay," *Daily News* (Los Angeles), December 19, 1989.
6. Laura Accinelli. "Starting Over," *Daily Breeze* (Torrance, California), September 11, 1988.
7. Madeleine Wild. "Grandmas Forced to Become Moms," *Woman's World*, July 16, 1991, p. 21.

CHAPTER 4

1. Eileen Beal. "Grandparents Raising Grandchildren," *Cleveland Jewish News*, November 23, 1990, p. 15.

CHAPTER 5

1. *Seniors Speak Out*, KPBS TV, San Diego, November 26, 1992.
2. Muriel Dobbin. "Grandmothers Fill In for Drug-Abusing Parents," *Senior Highlights*, March 1990, p. 5.
3. Harriet Goldhor Lerner. *The Dance of Intimacy*. New York: Harper & Row, 1989, p. 27.

CHAPTER 6

1. Robin Worthington. "The Second Time Around," *San Jose Mercury News*, March 22, 1992.
2. Sherry Angel. "Starting Over: Grandparents Who Step In and Raise Their Grandchildren," *Los Angeles Times/Orange County*, April 15, 1991.

3. Ingrid Watson. "Rocking the Cradle," *Fort Worth Star-Telegram*, November 13, 1988.
4. For a full definition of ADHD see: American Psychiatric Association. *Diagnostic and Statistical Manual of Mental Disorders* (4th ed.). Washington, DC: American Psyciatric Association, 1994, pp. 78–85.
5. Claudia Wallis. "Live in Overdrive," *Time*, July 28, 1994, p. 43.
6. Ibid., p. 43.
7. *Diagnostic and Statistical Manual of Mental Disorders*, op. cit.
8. Interview with Michael Jones by authors (via telephone). June 22, 1994.
9. Jane Glenn Haas. "It Can Be Grand to Be Raised by Grandparents," *The Orange County Register*, March 25, 1992.

CHAPTER 7

1. "General Information about Learning Disabilities." *National Information Center for Children and Youth with Disabilities. Fact Sheet Number 7* (FS7). Washington, DC: National Information Center for Children and Youth with Disabilities (NICHCY), 1993.
2. "Eight Famous Persons with Learning Disabilities," *Their World*, January 1981.

CHAPTER 8

1. Muriel Dobbins. "Grandmothers Fill In for Drug-Abusing Parents," *Senior Highlights*, March 1990, p. 5.
2. JoBeth McDaniel. "The Second Shift," *Life*, June 1, 1992, p. 65.
3. Thomas C. Holt, Eric Foner, and John A. Garraty, eds. *Reader's Companion to American History*. Boston: Houghton Mifflin Company, 1991, p. 297.
4. Ibid., p. 298.
5. Laura Feig. *Drug Exposed Infants and Children: Service Needs and Policy Questions*. Washington, DC: U.S. Department of Health and Human Services, 1990, p. 1; Interview with Jacqueline Battle, Infants of Substance Abusing Mothers Clinic, Los Angeles County–University of Southern California Medical Center, by authors. Los Angeles, October 1, 1993.
6. Information on the rise and effects of crack cocaine from : U.S. Senate Committee on Labor and Human Resources. *Children of Substance Abusers* (February 5, 1989). Washington, DC: U.S. Government Print-

ing Office, 1990; U.S. Senate Committee on Labor and Human Resources. *Falling through the Crack: The Impact of Drug-Exposed Children on the Child Welfare System* (March 8, 1990). Washington, DC: U.S. Government Printing Office, 1990; "Drugs and Narcotics," *Guide to American Law Supplement 1990*. St. Paul, MN: West Publishing Company, 1990, pp. 94–96.

7. *Falling through the Crack*, op. cit., pp. 18–19.
8. Anastasia Toufexis. "Innocent Victims," *Time*, May 13, 1991, p. 58.
9. *Falling through the Crack*, op. cit., p. 7.
10. Ibid., p. 65.
11. Ibid., p. 65.
12. Ibid., p. 96.
13. Ibid., p. 125.
14. Information on addiction has been adapted from several interviews and printed sources, including: *The Disease of Chemical Dependency*. Carson City, NV: Serenity Support Services, 1991; *What Everyone Should Know about Drug Abuse*. South Deerfield, MA: Channing L. Bete, 1990; *About Addiction*. South Deerfield, MA: Channing L. Bete, 1991.
15. "The Second Shift," op. cit., p. 66.
16. *Falling through the Crack*, op. cit., p. 58.
17. Ibid., p. 164.
18. *Donahue*, April 11, 1991.
19. "Drugs and Narcotics," op. cit., p. 95.
20. Interview with Jacqueline Battle, Infants of Substance Abusing Mothers, Los Angeles County–University of Southern California Medical Center, by authors. Los Angeles, October 1, 1993.
21. Interview with Dorsey Nunn, Legal Services for Prisoners with Children, by authors. Los Angeles, November 4, 1993.
22. *Falling through the Crack*, op. cit., p. 108.
23. *Children of Substance Abusers*, op. cit., p. 3.
24. *Falling through the Crack*, op. cit., p. 34.
25. Ibid., p. 95.
26. "Minimal Protocols for Response to Births Involving Indications of Prenatal Substance Abuse" (Memo from California Superior Court), January 31, 1994 (factsheet). Pasadena, CA: Open Arms Family Support Network, 1993; *Falling through the Crack*, op. cit., pp. 209–211; "Fetal Alcohol Syndrome," *Public Health Education Information Sheet*. White Plains, NY: March of Dimes Birth Defects Foundation, 1989.
27. Interview with Jacqueline Battle, op. cit.
28. Ibid.
29. Cathy Trost. "Born to Lose: Babies of Crack Users Crowd Hospitals, Break Everybody's Heart," *The Wall Street Journal*, July 18, 1989.
30. "Innocent Victims," op. cit., p. 59.

31. Interview with Fay Strassburger, California grandmother, by authors. Los Angeles, May 18, 1994.
32. Melissa Balmain Welner. "A Testament to Survival," *Orange County Register*, June 14, 1992.
33. Marie Kanne Poulsen. *Perinatal Substance Abuse: What's Best for the Children?* Garden Grove, CA: Orangewood Children's Foundation, 1992, p. 3.

CHAPTER 10

1. "Family 'Kin Care' Trend Increasing," *NASW News* (National Association of Social Workers), May 1992.
2. Trish Johnson. "'Older' Parents Need Support," *Katy Times*, February 25, 1990.
3. Interview with Ted Youmans, California attorney, by authors. Long Beach, California. October 22, 1993.
4. Ingrid Watson. "Rocking the Cradle," *Fort Worth Star-Telegram*, November 13, 1988.
5. Robin D. Leonard and Stephen Elias. *Family Law Dictionary*. Berkeley, CA: Nolo Press, 1990, p. 20.
6. Ibid., p. 44.
7. "Rocking the Cradle," op. cit.
8. Susan Swartz. "When Grandparents Are Parents Again," *Press-Democrat* (Santa Rosa, California). July 14, 1991.
9. Interview with Harold LaFlamme, California attorney, by authors. Buena Park, California, February 20, 1993.
10. Ibid.
11. Legal guardianship ends at age 18 in California; your state may differ.
12. Interview with Ted Youmans, California attorney, by authors. Santa Ana, California, March 6, 1993.
13. River Ginchild and Ellen Barry. *Manual for Grandparent–Relative Caregivers and Their Advocates.* San Francisco: Legal Services for Prisoners with Children, 1994, p. 10.
14. Ellen M. Barry et al. *Legal Manual for Children's Caregivers in Illinois.* San Francisco: Legal Services for Prisoners with Children and Chicago Legal Aid to Incarcerated Mothers, 1993, p. 1.
15. Ibid., p. 5.
16. See Lisa Goldoftaz and David Brown. *The Guardianship Book: How to Become a Child's Guardian in California* (revised). Berkeley, CA: Nolo Press, 1993.
17. Interview with Pamela Mohr, Executive Director, Alliance for Children's Rights, by authors. Los Angeles, May 10, 1994.

18. Judicial Council of California. *Guardianship Pamphlet*, p. 4.
19. Interview with Robert Walmsley, California attorney, by authors. Buena Park, California, February 20, 1993.
20. Ellen C. Segal and Naomi Karp. *Grandparent Visitation Disputes: A Legal Resource Manual*. Washington, DC: American Bar Association, 1989, p. 5. Additional information on grandparent visitation state by state is available in: U.S. House of Representatives Select Committee on Aging. *Grandparents Rights: A Resource Manual* (December 1992). Washington, DC: U.S. Government Printing Office, 1992, pp. 65–107. (This is a reprint of a 1991 report put out by the Congressional Resource Services, *CRS Report for Congress: Legal Overview of Grandparent Visitation Rights*, by Gina Marie Stevens and Gloria Sugars.
21. *Grandparents Rights: A Resource Manual*, op. cit., pp. 80–81.
22. Joan Schrager Cohen. *Helping Your Grandchildren through Their Parents' Divorce*. New York: Walker and Company, 1994, p. 132.
23. Interview with Michael Salazar, California attorney, by authors. Los Angeles, September 12, 1994.
24. Fran H. Zupan. "Love is Grand," *State Newspaper* (Columbia, South Carolina), April 9, 1992.
25. Interview with Michael Salazar, op. cit.
26. *Manual for Grandparent–Relative Caregivers and their Advocates*, op. cit., p. 24.
27. Interview with Charles Ollinger, Arizona attorney, by authors (via telephone). September 9, 1994.

CHAPTER 11

1. Interview with Ted Youmans, California attorney, by authors. Santa Ana, California, March 6, 1993.
2. Ibid.
3. Ibid.
4. Joan Schrager Cohen. *Helping Your Grandchildren through Their Parents' Divorce*. New York: Walker and Company, 1994, p. 139.
5. The petition of dependency must be filed within 48 hours in California. River Ginchild and Ellen Barry. *Manual for Grandparent–Relative Caregivers and Their Advocates*. San Francisco: Legal Services for Prisoners with Children, 1994, p. 29.
6. Social Security Act, Title IV-E, 42 USC 670 et seq., § 475. Note: The Federal Code uses the term *disposition hearing* for the establishment of a permanent plan; many states refer to this stage as the *permanent planning hearing*.

7. Interview with Pamela Mohr, Executive Director, Alliance for Children's Rights, by authors. Los Angeles, February 24, 1993.
8. 42 USC 670, op. cit.
9. Interview with Pamela Mohr, op. cit.
10. *Manual for Grandparent–Relative Caregivers and Their Advocates*, op. cit., p. 24.
11. Interview with Pamela Mohr, op. cit., March 29, 1994.
12. Interview with Charles Ollinger, Arizona attorney, by authors (via telephone). September 9, 1994.
13. Ibid.
14. Interview with Michael Salazar, California attorney, by authors. Los Angeles, September 12, 1994.
15. Interview with Pamela Mohr, op. cit.
16. Interview with Ted Youmans, op. cit.
17. Interview with Michael Salazar, California attorney, by authors. Buena Park, California, February 20, 1993.
18. Ellen Palmer. "Grandparents Raising Grandchildren—The Golden Years: Cancelled," *Valley Magazine* (Orange County Beach Cities, California). December 1990.
19. Ingrid Watson. "Rocking the Cradle," *Fort Worth Star-Telegram*, November 13, 1988.
20. Interview with Michael Salazar, op. cit., February 20, 1993.
21. U.S. Senate Committee on Labor and Human Resources. *Falling through the Crack: The Impact of Drug-Exposed Children on the Child Welfare System* (March 8, 1990). Washington, DC: U.S. Government Printing Office, 1990, p. 8.
22. Ibid., p. 58.
23. Interview with Ethel Dunn, Executive Director, Grandparents United for Children's Rights, by authors (via telephone). September 19, 1993.
24. Interview with Charles Ollinger, Arizona attorney, by authors. Long Beach, California. October 22, 1993.
25. Ibid.
26. Interview with John C. Wooley, California judge, by authors. Buena Park, California, February 20, 1993.
27. Interview with Charles Ollinger, Arizona attorney, by authors (via telephone). September 9, 1994.

CHAPTER 12

1. Miriam Durkin. "When Grandparents Start Over," *Charlotte Observer*, November 3, 1991.

2. Linda L. Creighton. "Silent Saviors," *U.S. News & World Report*, December 16, 1991, p. 80.
3. Michele L. Norris. "Grandmothers Who Fill Void Carved by Drugs," *Washington Post*, August 30, 1991.
4. These figures are based on 1989 maintenance benefits for children under the age of two in Missouri, multiplied by five. This is the minimum a family of five might have received in Missouri in 1989. U.S. House of Representatives Committee on Ways and Means. *Overview of Entitlement Programs: 1990 Green Book.* Washington, DC: U.S. Government Printing Office, 1990, p. 767.
5. *Overview of Entitlement Programs*, op. cit., pp. 556–557.
6. Interview with Pamela Mohr, Executive Director, Alliance for Children's Rights, by authors. Los Angeles, March 28, 1995.
7. River Ginchild and Ellen Barry. *Manual for Grandparent–Relative Caregivers and Their Advocates.* San Francisco: Legal Services for Prisoners with Children, 1994, p. 52.
8. Interview with Yolanda Vera, staff attorney for the National Health Law Program, by authors. Los Angeles, November 4, 1993.
9. *Aid to Families with Dependent Children (AFDC) Action Transmittal (No. ACF-AT-94-5).* Washington, DC: U.S. Department of Health and Human Services, February 28, 1994.
10. Interview with Pamela Mohr, op. cit.
11. Foster care benefits are defined in Title IV-E of the Social Security Act, 42 USC 670 et seq., and are known as IV-E Foster Care. They may also be known as AFDC-FC (AFDC-Foster Care).
12. Legal Aid Foundation of Los Angeles Government Benefits Unit. *Foster Care Manual.* Los Angeles: Legal Aid Foundation of Los Angeles, 1993, p. 17; *Miller v. Youakim Fact Sheet*, photocopied.
13. *Foster Care Manual*, op. cit., pp. 15–16.
14. Jeffrey Miller. "Woman Fights Social Service Agencies," *Los Angeles Times*, January 3, 1988.
15. *Foster Care Manual*, op. cit., p. 29.
16. Social Security Administration. *Social Security and SSI Benefits for Children with Disabilities.* Baltimore: U.S. Department of Health and Human Services, Social Security Administration, 1993, p. 7.
17. Michele Melden. *An Introduction for Advocates to SSI for Children.* Los Angeles: The Alliance for Children's Rights, 1992, p. 13.
18. Ibid., p. 13.
19. *Social Security and SSI Benefits for Children with Disabilities*, op. cit., p. 9.
20. Interview with Pamela Mohr, op. cit.
21. Social Security Administration. *Survivors* (SSA Publication No. 05-10084). Baltimore: U.S. Department of Health and Human Services, Social Security Administration, 1993, p. 3.

22. Interview with Pamela Mohr, op. cit.
23. 42 U.S.C. § 1396d(r)(5) of the Medicaid Act. Cited in Jane Perkins. *Advocate's Medicaid EPSDT Reference Manual.* Chapel Hill, NC: National Health Law Program, 1993, p. 21.
24. Bonnie Armstrong. *An Agenda for Children's Health Care in Los Angeles County.* Los Angeles: Los Angeles Roundtable for Children, 1993.
25. Interview with Anne Rutherford, fiscal and program service coordinator, WIC, Portland, by authors (via telephone). August 30, 1993.

CHAPTER 13

1. Attributed to Walter Barbee. Source unknown.
2. "Legal Rights because of Learning Disabilities," *L/D Law,* 1990, p. 13.
3. Ibid., p. 13.
4. Rehabilitation Act of 1973. 29 USC 794 et seq., § 504, as explained in *L/D Law,* op. cit.
5. Individuals with Disabilities Education Act (Public Law 101-476) is an amendment of the Education for All Handicapped Act (Public Law 94-142). 20 USC 1401 et seq. in *NICHCY Briefing Paper: Individualized Education Programs (IEPs): Federal Regulations and Appendix C to Part 300.* Washington DC: National Information Center for Children and Youth with Disabilities (NICHCY), update March 1994.
6. Interview with Larry Hanna, California attorney, by authors. Los Angeles, May 13, 1993.
7. Pamela Darr Wright. *Your Child's IEP: Practical and Legal Guidance for Parents.* Richmond, VA: Pamela Darr Wright, Licensed Clinical Social Worker, 1994.
8. Interview with Peter Wright, Virginia attorney, by authors (via telephone). April 3, 1995.
9. Interview with Larry Hanna, California attorney, by authors. Sherman Oaks, California, August 11, 1993.
10. Interview with Peter Wright, Virginia attorney, by authors (via telephone). August, 1994.
11. Interview with Larry Hanna, op. cit., May 13, 1993.
12. *How to Participate in our Child's IEP Meeting.* Chicago, IL: Coordinating Council for Handicapped Children.
13. National Information Center for Children and Youth with Disabilities (NICHCY) *A Parent's Guide to Accessing Programs for Infants, Toddlers, and Preschoolers with Disabilities.* Washington, DC: NICHCY, 1992.
14. Interview with Larry Hanna, op. cit.

CHAPTER 14

1. Warren Harris. "Raising Second Family," *Las Vegas Sun*, June 19, 1989.
2. AARP Grandparent Information Center statistics, as of April 1994.
3. Catha McSweeney. "Filling the GAP," *Patriot Ledger*, October 27, 1989.

CHAPTER 15

1. "'Washington Summit' on Grandparent Caregiving," *Brookdale Grandparent Caregiver Information Project Newsletter*, February 1992, p. 2.
2. Senate Hearing: Joan McMillin (California) and Mary Ruth Shaheen (Maine) appeared before the U.S. Senate Special Committee on Aging on July 29, 1992. U.S. Senate Special Committee on Aging. *Grandparents as Parents: Raising a Second Generation* (July 29, 1992). Washington, DC: U.S. Government Printing Office, 1992, pp. 34, 37.
3. *Donahue*, April 11, 1991.
4. Sandy Pasqua. "Grandparents Mobilize to Demand Their Rights," *Senior World of Los Angeles*, September 1992.
5. Donna Kennedy. "When Grandparents Raise the Grandkids: 'Mrs. Rock' Battles to Change the Law," *Press-Enterprise* (Riverside, California), August 2, 1989.
6. In 1894 a Louisiana grandmother petitioned for visitation with her grandchildren, and lost, in the landmark case *Succession of Reiss*. The ruling supported the argument that grandparents' rights would interfere with parental rights and would undermine the parent's authority. Marie Purnell and Beatrice H. Bagby, "Grandparents Rights: Implications for Family Specialists," *Family Relations*, April 1993; Interview with Ethel Dunn, Executive Director, Grandparents United for Children's Rights, by authors (via telephone). September 19, 1993.
7. Interview with Ethel Dunn, op. cit.
8. U.S. House of Representatives Select Committee on Aging. *Grandparents Rights: A Resource Manual*. Washington, DC: U.S. Government Printing Office, 1992, pp. 1–2.
9. Interview with Ethel Dunn, op. cit., October 21, 1993.
10. Patty Housen. "Retiring to the Nursery: Grandparents Raising Kids' Kids," *Senior Beacon: In Focus for People Over 50*, May 1990, p. 1.
11. Interview with Michael Salazar, California attorney, by authors. Culver City, California, November 12, 1992.
12. U.S. House of Representatives Select Committee on Aging. *Grandparents Rights: Preserving Generational Bonds* (October 2, 1991). Washington, DC: U.S. Government Printing Office, 1991, p. 2.

13. Stephanie Edelstein. "Do Grandparents Have Rights?" *Modern Maturity,* December 1990–January 1991, p. 41–42.

14. Carolyn Pantier. "Many Grandparents Parenting Again," *Senior World of Los Angeles,* September 1993, p. 7.

15. Patrick Burke. "Grandfolks Win a Round," *Senior Spectrum,* August 1991, p. 1.

16. Patty Housen. "Retiring to the Nursery: Grandparents Raising Kids' Kids," *Senior Beacon: In Focus for People Over 50,* May 1990, p. 1; Interview with Barbara Kirkland, founder of Grandparents Raising Grandchildren, by authors (via telephone). April 11, 1994.

17. Act Regarding the Rights of Grandparents in Child Protection Proceedings, 22 MRSA 4005-B, § 1. (State of Maine)

18. Interview with Margie Davis, GOLD founder, by authors. Los Angeles, July 7, 1993.

19. Three hearings took place in the United States House and Senate between 1990 and 1992: "Grandparents Rights: Preserving Generational Bonds," House Select Committee on Aging, October 2, 1991; "Grandparents: New Roles and Responsibilities," House Select Committee on Aging, June 8, 1992; "Grandparents as Parents: Raising a Second Generation," Senate Special Committee on Aging, July 29, 1992.

20. "Coalitions Forming in Support of Grandparent Caregivers," *Brookdale Grandparent Caregiver Information Project Newsletter,* June 1992, p. 1.

21. "New Beginnings . . . The Grandparent Information Center Opens." *AARP Grandparent Information Center Newsletter,* Winter 1994, p. 1.

22. Interview with Ethel Dunn, op. cit.

23. Interview with Barbara Wasson, grandparent activist, by authors. Long Beach, California, March 2, 1994.

24. Interview with Rosalie Cauley, grandparent activist, by authors. Long Beach, California, October 21, 1993.

25. Margaret Collins. "Foster Parents a Safety Net," *Capital Times,* March 30, 1993.

26. Interview with Leza Davis, California legislative assistant, by authors (via telephone). October 30, 1994.

27. Interview with Margie Davis, op. cit., May 17, 1993.

28. Interview with Barbara Castro, grandparent activist, Long Beach, California, March 4, 1994.

29. *Grandparents Rights: A Resource Manual,* op. cit., p. 6.

30. Interview with Dr. Arthur Kornhaber, president and founder of the Foundation for Grandparenting, by authors (via telephone). March 23, 1995.

31. Interview with Margie Davis, op. cit., July 7, 1993.

CHAPTER 16

1. Alice Hornbaker. "Parents Second Time Around," *Cincinnati Enquirer*, September 10, 1991, p. 2.
2. Ethel Dunn. "Those Wonderful Abuelas," *Intergenerational Hookup*, Winter/Spring 1993, p. 1.
3. Reprinted with permission of Kevin de Toledo.
4. Donald O. Bolander, Dolores D. Varner, Gary B. Wright, and Stephanie H. Greene (compilers). *Instant Quotation Dictionary*. Little Falls, NJ: Career Publishing, 1981, p. 30.

Bibliography

BOOKS/MANUALS/HEARINGS

American Psychiatric Association. *Diagnostic and Statistical Manual of Mental Disorders* (4th ed.). Washington, DC: American Psychiatric Association, 1994.

Armstrong, Bonnie. *An Agenda for Children's Health Care in Los Angeles County*. Los Angeles: Los Angeles Roundtable for Children, 1993.

Barry, Ellen, David20 Fortier, Gail Smith, and Joanne Archibald. *Legal Manual for Children's Caregivers in Illinois*. San Francisco: Legal Services for Prisoners with Children and Chicago Legal Aid to Incarcerated Mothers, 1993.

Barry, Ellen, Dorsey Nunn, Carrie Kojimoto, Nancy Jacot-Bell, and Gabriela Lujan. *Manual for Grandparents and Caregivers* (3rd ed.). San Francisco: Legal Services for Prisoners with Children, 1993.

Center for the Study of Social Policy. *Kids Count Data Book: State Profiles of Child Well-Being*. Washington, DC: Annie E. Casey Foundation, 1993.

Cohen, Joan Schrager. *Helping Your Grandchildren through Their Parents' Divorce*. New York: Walker and Company, 1994.

Endicott, Irene M. *Grandparenting Redefined: Guidance for Today's Changing Family*. Lynwood, WA: Aglow Publications, 1992.

Ginchild, River, and Ellen Barry. *Manual for Grandparent–Relative Caregivers and Their Advocates*. San Francisco: Legal Services for Prisoners with Children, 1994.

The Guide to American Law Supplement 1990. St. Paul, MN: West Publishing Company, 1990.

Holt, Thomas C., Eric Foner, and John A. Garraty, eds. *Reader's Companion to American History*. Boston: Houghton Mifflin Company, 1991.

Keller, Helen. *We Bereaved*. New York: Leslie Fulenwider, 1929.

Leonard, Robin D., and Stephen Elias. *Family Law Dictionary*. Berkeley, CA: Nolo Press, 1990.

Lerner, Harriet Goldhor. *The Dance of Intimacy*. New York: Harper & Row, 1989.

Minkler, Meredith, and Kathleen M. Roe. *Grandmothers as Caregivers: Raising Children of the Crack Cocaine Epidemic.* Newbury Park, CA: Sage Publications, 1993.

Poe, Lenora Madison. *Black Grandparents as Parents.* Berkeley, CA: Lenora Madison Poe, 1992.

Segal, Ellen C., and Naomi Karp, eds. *Grandparent Visitation Disputes: A Legal Resource Manual.* Washington, DC: American Bar Association, 1989.

Tamborello, Frank, ed. *How to Get Food and Money in Los Angeles County.* Los Angeles, CA: Southern California Ecumenical Council Interface Hunger Coalition, 1993.

U.S. House of Representatives Committee on Ways and Means. *Overview of Entitlement Programs: 1990 Green Book.* Washington, DC: U.S. Government Printing Office, 1990.

U.S. House of Representatives Select Committee on Aging. *Grandparents: New Roles and Responsibilities* (June 8, 1992; Comm. Pub. No. 102-876). Washington, DC: U.S. Government Printing Office, 1992.

———. *Grandparents Rights: A Resource Manual* (December 1992; Comm. Pub. No. 102-898). Washington, DC: U.S. Government Printing Office, 1992.

———. *Grandparents Rights: Preserving Generational Bonds* (October 2, 1991; Comm. Pub. No. 102-833). Washington, DC: U.S. Government Printing Office, 1991.

U.S. Senate Committee on Labor and Human Resources. *Children of Substance Abusers* (February 5, 1989). Washington, DC: U.S. Government Printing Office, 1990.

———. *Falling Through the Crack: The Impact of Drug-Exposed Children on the Child Welfare System* (March 8, 1990). Washington, DC: U.S. Government Printing Office, 1990.

U.S. Senate Special Committee on Aging. *Grandparents as Parents: Raising a Second Generation* (July 29, 1992; Serial No. 102-24). Washington, DC: U.S. Government Printing Office, 1992.

BROCHURES/PAMPHLETS/PAPERS

About Addiction [Pamphlet].South Deerfield, MA: Channing L. Bete, 1991.

Advocacy . . . Why Bother? Sacramento, CA: On the Capitol Doorstep, 1989.

Aid to Families with Dependent Children (AFDC) Action Transmittal (No. ACF-AT-94-5). Washington, DC: U.S. Department of Health and Human Services, February 28, 1994.

Aid to Families with Dependent Children (AFDC) Fact Sheet. Sacramento, CA: Western Center on Law and Poverty, September 1991.

Alliance for Children's Rights. *A Manual on the Adoption Assistance Program*. Los Angeles: Alliance for Children's Rights, 1992. (Adapted from article by Alice Bussiere and Ellen C. Segal, "Adoption Assistance for Children with Special Needs" and a manual prepared by Pamela Mohr for the Children's Rights Project of Public Counsel).

————. *1992 Dependency Laws* (California). Los Angeles: Alliance for Children's Rights, October 1992. (Based on a manual by Pamela Mohr for the Children's Rights Project)

Anderson, Terry K., Susie Kaylor, and Joan Flaherty. *The Legislative Process: You Really Do Matter*. Sacramento, CA: Senate Select Committee on Citizen Participation in Government, 1989.

Barnes, Ellen. *IEP Checklist* (On-line). Syracuse, NY: Developmental Disabilities Rights Project and Direction Service Center on Human Policy, 1993. (Compuserve, ADD+ Forum, iepdoc.txt)

Battle, Jacqueline, Kathryn Payne, and Maureen S. Wilson. *Open Arms Baby Book: Special Care Techniques for Infants Prenatally Exposed to Drugs or Alcohol*. Pasadena, CA: Open Arms Family Support Network, 1995.

California Superior Court. *Minimal Protocols for Response to Births Involving Indications of Prenatal Substance Abuse* (Memo). January 31, 1994.

Coordinating Council for Handicapped Children. *How to Participate in our Child's IEP Meeting* (On-line). Chicago, IL: Coordinating Council for Handicapped Children, n.d. (Compuserve, ADD+ Forum, iep.txt)

Council for Exceptional Children and ERIC Clearinghouse on Handicapped and Gifted Children. *Providing an Appropriate Education to Children with Attention Deficit Disorder* (ERIC Digest No. E512) (On-line). Reston, VA: ERIC, Education Resources Information Center, 1992. (Compuserve, ADD+ Forum, appro.txt)

County of San Diego Department of Social Services. *Juvenile Dependency Court Information* (Brochure). San Diego: County of San Diego Department of Social Services, 1992.

————. *A Parent's Guide to Child Welfare Services* (Brochure). San Diego: County of San Diego Department of Social Services, October 1992.

Desk Guide: Rights and Responsibilities of Legal Guardians/Adoptive Parents (Handout). Los Angeles: County of Los Angeles Department of Children's Services, 1991.

Feig, Laura. *Drug Exposed Infants and Children: Service Needs and Policy Questions*. Washington, DC: U.S. Department of Health and Human Services, 1990.

"Fetal Alcohol Syndrome," *Public Health Education Information Sheet*. White Plains, NY: March of Dimes Birth Defects Foundation, 1989.

Finnegan, L. P., and B. A. Macnew, *American Journal of Nursing*, Vol 74., No. 4, April 1974. (As adapted in the handout "Comforting Techniques for an Infant Exposed to Drugs Prenatally," courtesy of Infants of Substance Abusing Mothers at Los Angeles County–University of Southern California Medical Center)

Fowler, Mary. *NICHCY Briefing Paper: Attention Deficit Disorder* (On-line). Washington, DC: National Information Center for Children and Youth with Disabilities (NICHCY), 1991. (Compuserve, ADD+ Forum, nbpadd.txt)

Frost, Diane, ed. *Children Who Learn Differently*. Sacramento, CA: California Association for Neurologically Handicapped Children (CANHC), Contra Costa West Chapter, 1975.

(Grandparent Information Center handout). Washington, DC: AARP Grandparent Information Center.

Grandparents Offering Love and Direction. *GOLD Court Assistance Program (CAP) for Relatives*. San Diego: Grandparents Offering Love and Direction, March 1992.

Grandparents Offering Love and Direction and San Diego County Department of Social Services. *Handbook for Relatives*. San Diego, CA: 1993.

Grandparents Rights: An Overview of the Law (Handout). Santa Ana, CA: Law Office of Van Deusen, Youmans and Walmsley, 1992.

Grandparents United for Children's Rights. *A Walk through Policyland: A How-To Manual on Dealing with Your Legislators*. Madison, WI: Grandparents United For Children's Rights, 1991.

Janov, Brooke. *AFDC, AFDC-FC, and Youakim Benefits: A Comparative Overview for Advocates and Clients*. Los Angeles: Alliance For Children's Rights, 1993.

Legal Aid Foundation of Los Angeles Government Benefits Unit. *The Foster Care Manual*. Los Angeles: Legal Aid Foundation of Los Angeles, 1993.

Lokerson, Jean. *Learning Disabilities* (ERIC Digest No. 516) (On-line). Reston, VA: Council for Exceptional Children, 1992. (Compuserve, ADD+ Forum, ericdi.ld)

Melden, Michele. *An Introduction for Advocates to SSI for Children*. Los Angeles: Alliance For Children's Rights, 1992.

Mental Health Law Project. *SSI: New Opportunities for Children with Disabilities, Checklists and Topic Sheets for Advocacy Training*. Washington, DC: Mental Health Law Project, 1991–1992.

Mohr, Pamela A., and Greg Bordo. *Legal Guardianship of the Person* (Draft). Los Angeles: Children's Rights Project, n.d.

Moore, Kristin A. *To Individuals and Organizations Concerned about Teen Pregnancy and Childbearing* (Memo). Washington, DC: Child Trends, February 1995.

Morgan, Daniel P. *Parents' Rights and Responsibilities* (On-line). Reston, VA: Educational Resource Information Center, 1984. (Compuserve, ADD+ Forum, right.txt)

National Information Center for Children and Youth with Disabilities. *Definition of Learning Disabilities* (Fact Sheet No. 7) (On-line). Washington, DC: National Information Center for Children and Youth with Disabilities (NICHCY), 1993. (Compuserve, ADD+ Forum, lddef.txt)

——. *General Information about Public Agencies* (On-line). Washington, DC: National Information Center for Children and Youth with Disabilities (NICHCY), 1993. (Compuserve, ADD+ Forum, public.txt)

——. *NICHCY Briefing Paper: Individualized Education Programs (IEPs): Federal Regulations and Appendix C to Part 300.* Washington, DC: National Information Center for Children and Youth with Disabilities (NICHCY), update March 1994.

——. *NICHCY New Digest* (Vol. 1, No. 1). Washington, DC: National Information Center for Children and Youth with Disabilities (NICHCY), 1991.

——. *NICHCY News Digest* (Vol. 3, No. 2). Washington, DC: National Information Center for Children and Youth with Disabilities (NICHCY), September 1993.

——. *A Parent's Guide to Accessing Programs for Infants, Toddlers, and Preschoolers with Disabilities* (On-line). Washington, DC: National Information Center for Children and Youth with Disabilities (NICHCY), 1992. (Compuserve, ADD+ Forum, access.txt)

——. *Questions Often Asked about Special Education Services* (Fact sheet). Washington, DC: National Information Center for Children and Youth with Disabilities (NICHCY), update 1993.

Perkins, Jane. *Advocate's Medicaid EPSDT Reference Manual.* Chapel Hill, NC: National Health Law Program, 1993.

Poulsen, Marie Kanne. *Perinatal Substance Abuse: What's Best for the Children?* Garden Grove, CA: Orangewood Children's Foundation, 1992.

Repetto, Jeanne, and Donna Wandry. *Transition Services in the IEP* (On-line). Washington, DC: National Information Center for Children and Youth with Disabilities (NICHCY), 1993. (Compuserve, ADD+ Forum, iep-1.txt)

Serenity Support Services. *The Disease of Chemical Dependency.* Carson City, NV: Serenity Support Services, 1991.

Social Security Administration. *Social Security and SSI Benefits for Children with Disabilities* (SSA Pub. No. 05-10026) (Brochure). Baltimore: U.S. Department of Health and Human Services, Social Security Administration, 1993.

——. *SSI: Supplemental Security Income* (SSA Pub. No. 05-11000) (Brochure). Baltimore: U.S. Department of Health and Human Services, Social Security Administration, 1993.

——. *Survivors* (SSA Pub. No. 05-10084) (Brochure). Baltimore: U.S. Department of Health and Human Services, Social Security Administration, 1993.

Stevens, Gina Marie, and Gloria Sugars. *CRS Report for Congress: Legal Overview of Grandparent Visitation Rights.* Washington, DC: Congressional Resource Services, 1991. (In U.S. House of Representatives Select Committee on Aging. *Grandparents Rights: A Resource Manual* [Comm. Pub. No. 102-898]. Washington, DC: U.S. Government Printing Office, 1992.

Vera, Yolanda. *Most Frequently Asked Questions Regarding Foster Care Children.* Los Angeles: Legal Aid Foundation of Los Angeles.

What Everyone Should Know about Drug Abuse (Pamphlet). South Deerfield, MA: Channing L. Bete Co., 1990.

Wright, Pamela Darr. *Your Child's IEP: Practical and Legal Guidance for Parents* (On-line). Richmond, VA: Pamela Darr Wright, 1994. (Compuserve, ADD+ Forum, ieps&c.txt)

MAGAZINES/NEWSPAPERS/JOURNALS

Accinelli, Laura. "Starting Over," *Daily Breeze* (Torrance, California), September 11, 1988.

Angel, Sherry. "Starting Over: Grandparents Who Step In and Raise Their Grandchildren, *Los Angeles Times/Orange County*, April 15, 1991.

Beal, Eileen. "Grandparents Raising Grandchildren," *Cleveland Jewish News*, November 23, 1990.

Becklund, Laurie. "I Wanted Somebody to Love," *Los Angeles Times*, March 14, 1993.

Burke, Patrick. "Grandfolks Win a Round," *Senior Spectrum*, August 1991.

"Coalitions Forming in Support of Grandpaent Caregivers," *Brookdale Grandparent Caregiver Information Project Newsletter*, June 1992.

Collins, Margaret. "Foster Parents a Safety Net," *Capital Times*, March 30, 1993.

Creighton, Linda L. "Silent Saviors," *U.S. News & World Report*, December 16, 1991.

Dobbin, Muriel. "Grandmothers Fill In for Drug-Abusing Parents," *Senior Highlights*, March 1990.

Dunn, Ethel. "Those Wonderful Abuelas," *Intergenerational Hookup*, Winter/Spring 1993.

Durkin, Miriam. "When Grandparents Start Over," *Charlotte Observer*, November 3, 1991.

Edelstein, Stephanie. "Do Grandparents Have Rights?" *Modern Maturity*, December 1990–January 1991.

Edmonds, Patricia. "Those Caught in Middle Are 'Missing a Lot,'" *USA Today*, July 23, 1991.

"Eight Famous Persons with Learning Disabilities," *Their World*, January 1981.

"Family 'Kin Care' Trend Increasing," *NASW News* (National Association of Social Workers), May 1992.

Greene, Karen. "The Great American Grandparent: Reinventing Families," *Children's Advocate*, March/April 1992.

Haas, Jane Glenn. "It Can Be Grand to Be Raised by Grandparents," *The Orange County Register*, March 25, 1992.

Harris, Warren. "Raising Second Family," *Las Vegas Sun*, June 19, 1989.

Hornbaker, Alice. "Parents Second Time Around," *Cincinnati Enquirer*, September 10, 1991.

Housen, Patty. "Retiring to the Nursery: Grandparents Raising Kids' Kids," *Senior Beacon: In Focus for People over 50*, May 1990.

Johnson, Trish. "'Older' Parents Need Support," *Katy Times*, February 25, 1990.

Kennedy, Donna. "When Grandparents Raise the Grandkids: 'Mrs. Rock' Battles to Change the Law," *Press-Enterprise* (Riverside, California), August 2, 1989.

Lee, Felicia R. "AIDS Toll on Elderly: Dying Grandchildren," *The New York Times*, November 21, 1994.

"Legal Rights because of Learning Disabilities," *L/D Law*, 1990.

Link, Tony. "When Kids Come to Grandma's House to Stay," *Daily News*, December 19, 1989.

Malcolm, Andrew H. "Helping Grandparents Who Are Parents Again," *The New York Times*, November 19, 1991.

McDaniel, JoBeth. "The Second Shift," *Life*, June 1, 1992.

McSweeny, Catha. "Filling the GAP," *Patriot Ledger*, October 27, 1989.

Miller, Jeffrey. "Woman Fights Social Service Agencies," *Los Angeles Times*, January 3, 1988.

"New Beginnings . . . The Grandparent Information Center Opens." *AARP Grandparent Information Center Newsletter*, Winter 1994.

Norris, Michele L. "Grandmothers Who Fill Void Carved by Drugs," *The Washington Post*, August 30, 1991.

Palmer, Ellen. "Grandparents Raising Grandchildren—The Golden Years: Cancelled," *Valley Magazine* (Orange County Beach Cities, California), December 1990.

Pantier, Carolyn. "Many Grandparents Parenting Again," *Senior World of Los Angeles*, September 1993.

Pasqua, Sandy. "Grandparents Mobilize to Demand Their Rights," *Senior World of Los Angeles*, September 1992.

Pollack, Susan R. "The Grandparent Trap," *The Detroit News*, July 17, 1991.

Purnell, Marie, and Beatrice H. Bagby, "Grandparents Rights: Implications for Family Specialists," *Family Relations*, April 1993.

Smolowe, Jill. "To Grandma's House We Go," *Time*, November 5, 1990.

Swartz, Susan. "When Grandparents Are Parents Again," *Press-Democrat*, (Santa Rosa, California), July 14, 1991.

Toufexis, Anastasia. "Innocent Victims," *Time*, May 13, 1991.
Trost, Cathy. "Born To Lose: Babies of Crack Users Crowd Hospitals, Break Everybody's Heart," *The Wall Street Journal*, July 18, 1989.
Wallis, Claudia. "Live in Overdrive," *Time*, July 28, 1994.
"'Washington Summit' on Grandparent Caregiving," *Brookdale Grandparent Caregiver Information Project Newsletter*, February 1992.
Watson, Ingrid. "Rocking the Cradle," *Fort Worth Star-Telegram*, November 13, 1988.
Welner, Melissa Balmain. "A Testament to Survival," *Orange County Register*, June 14, 1992.
Wilson, Mary Lou. "Recycled Parents," *The Reporter* (Vacaville, California), March 19, 1990.
Wild, Madeleine. "Grandmas Forced to Become Moms," *Woman's World*, July 16, 1991.
Worthington, Robin. "The Second Time Around," *San Jose Mercury News*, March 22, 1992.
Yorkey, Mike. "Picking Up the Pieces," *Focus on the Family*, September 1993.
Zupan, Fran H. "Love Is Grand," *State Newspaper* (Columbia, South Carolina), April 9, 1992.

MISCELLANEA

Social Security Act, Title IV-E, 42 USC 670 et seq., § 475.
Federal Register, Vol. 48, No. 100. May 23, 1983.
Rehabilitation Act of 1973. 29 USC 794 et seq., § 504.
Individuals with Disabilities Education Act (Public Law 101-476) (An amendment of Education for All Handicapped Act [Public Law 94-142]) 20 USC 1401 et seq.
Act Regarding the Rights of Grandparents in Child Protection Proceedings, 22 MRSA 4005-B, § 1. (State of Maine)
Donahue. April 11, 1991.
Seniors Speak Out, KPBS TV, San Diego, November 26 1992.

Index

MODERN TIMES

Modern Times is the third volume of the series, *The Canadian Novel*. Volume I, *Here and Now*, is a study of contemporary Canadian novels and their authors; Volume II, *Beginnings*, considers the major early works in the Canadian tradition. A fourth volume, a study of recent and avant garde Canadian fiction to be called ''Present Tense,'' is in preparation and another volume, on the novel in French Canada, is being planned.

The Canada Council
Conseil des Arts du Canada
1957-1982

THE CANADIAN NOVEL
VOLUME III

MODERN TIMES

A Critical Anthology
Edited with an Introductory Essay by

JOHN MOSS

NC Press Limited
Toronto

Cover illustration: Charles Comfort, *Young Canadians*, 1932 By permission of Hart House, University of Toronto

Canadian Cataloguing in Publication Data
   Main entry under title:
   The Canadian Novel

   Contents: v.3 Modern Times
   ISBN 0-919601-88-X (bound v.3)   ISBN 0-919601090-1 (pbk v.3)

   1. Canadian fiction (English) – 20th century – History and
      criticism – Addresses, essays, lectures. I. Moss, John, 1940 –

PS8187.C36   C813'.5'09   C78-1385-9
PR9192.5.C36

We would like to thank the Ontario Arts Council and the Canada Council for their assistance in the production of this book.

New Canada Publications, a division of NC Press Limited, Box
4010, Station A, Toronto, Ontario, M5W 1H8, (416) 593-6284

CONTENTS

INTRODUCTION

Modern Times is the third book in a series on the Canadian novel. The second contains essays on fiction that is important to our literary heritage. From a Canadian perspective, the works discussed are classics. Their lasting value is as much for their contribution to our cultural history, however, as for their intrinsic literary worth. Some of them, such as *The History of Emily Montague* (1769), *Wacousta* (1832) and *The Imperialist* (1904), are remarkably readable today, depending on taste, but clearly they are beginnings, they belong to the past. The first book in this series offers essays on the contemporary achievement of the Canadian tradition, its culmination here and now. The novels considered, by such writers as Alice Munro, Margaret Laurence and Mordecai Richler, are fine works in their own right, without deference to a particular context. They may have special meaning for Canadians, but this has little bearing on their merit as art. Between these two phases, when the literature's significance is primarily because it was Canadian and when its Canadian origin is incidental to its achievement (though we may take pride in its quality, and assurance from its source in the community we share), there is a transitional phase which vigourously resists coherent definition. This phase is the concern of the present volume.

The transition between the past that is clearly past and the unequivocally contemporary does not correspond to an exact historical period. The National Gallery of Canada recently mounted an exhibition on "Modernism in Quebec Art, 1916-1946". No such ready perimeters can be applied to the Canadian novel. It is generally easy to distinguish "early" Canadian writing, and the contemporary virtually identifies itself. Leacock belongs to the past; Laurence to the present. Of contemporary writers, only Robertson Davies is apparently out of step with his times, and that may be because he is ahead of them, rather than behind.

But what of those writers, some of them still writing, who provide a link between past and present, whose works are modern but not contemporary, whose works are immediate, dynamic, relevant, but redolent of times that have slipped away? To what period in our literary development do we assign the novels of

Morley Callaghan, whose canon extends through seven decades? What of Hugh MacLennan, whose most recent novel, *Voices in Time* (1981), expresses the world view of another era, in form and content very much of the present? What of W. O. Mitchell, whose work, the older he gets, seems ever more irrepressibly young?

Such writers are modern, by any definition of the term. Yet their fiction has more in common with the self-conscious modernism of Frederick Philip Grove and Martha Ostenso than with the aggressive contemporaneity of Robert Kroetsch or the casual authority of Mavis Gallant. They are writers upon whose work the Canadian tradition is built, and while they have continued to publish new fiction in the 1980s, their importance has been established for a generation and more.

And what of *The Double Hook* (1959) by Sheila Watson, and Elizabeth Smart's *By Grand Central Station I Sat Down and Wept* (1945)? Both novels are more avant-garde, even now, than anything by Margaret Atwood or Rudy Wiebe. In their lyricism, their narrative unconventionality, their rhetorical inventiveness, they are on the leading edge of modernism. Yet they are part of our heritage, and speak to us from the past. They have more in common with *As For Me and My House* (1941), *The Mountain and the Valley* (1952) and *Swamp Angel* (1954) than with *Surfacing* (1972) or *The Temptations of Big Bear* (1973). They speak with voices that are immediate but not contemporary, and they see from perspectives that are impossible in the present, except in fiction.

This book is an attempt to provide a common field for the consideration of work that falls between and yet overlaps two clearly defined phases in our cultural development. The challenge has been to bring together novels written as much as half a century apart, by people of widely dissimilar temperament and experience, in styles ranging from stolid to evanescent, forms from lumbering to ethereal, without intruding on their integrity as separate works of art, and without relying on inevitably misleading generalizations about their cultural and historical relevance. The concept implied by the title *Modern Times* seems appropriate in this regard. In terms of Canadian history, modern times probably originate in the trenches of World War I and extend into the present era of constitutional sovereignty. Culturally, the burgeoning West, the Depression, the Canadian Broadcasting Corporation, Mackenzie King, World War II, the National Film Board, are at the very centre of modern times in Canada, a centre from which we are inexorably drifting away. The word "times" represents an era, but also a sequence of separate events, all in the past, or passing.

"Modern" is a more elusive term, and conveniently more elastic. Modern thought may be said to originate with the Renaissance, and the modern sensibility with the Enlightenment; or modern thought with Darwin, Marx and Freud, and the modern sensibility with the holocausts of world war and genocide, very much within the living memory of many among us. Modern architecture, poetry and painting are determinedly of the present century, yet seem curiously dated now; arbitrary, solipsistic, ironically encumbered with preoccupations of the nineteenth century. The modern novel is equally a thing of the past; to describe a new work as modern is to indicate its limitations, its inappropriateness to our present experience of the world. The modern novel in English may be said to begin with Defoe, or a century later with Austen, or a century after that with Joyce, depending on perspective, and modern novels are still being written and will always be read, but we are no longer speaking of a tradition that culminates in the present. It was possible to say of Faulkner's *The Sound and the Fury* (1929), "this is what the novel has been building to." But with the best fiction of the 1970s and 1980s one would more likely say, "this is where the novel is now," and leave it at that. Its achievement is no less than in the past, but it is going in new directions not yet understood. The novel today speaks for the postmodernity of our experience, in a world of rampant television, the ubiquitous computer, and imminent universal annihilation, whether it participates in literary postmodernism or not.

Modernism in literature is characterized by a particular set of illusions which many of us came to accept as truths: these are the precepts of objectivity, impersonality, realism, rationalism and linguistic neutrality. The writer does not exist in his fiction; the reader certainly does not exist, except as a consumer. What is described is what is; the created world is more real, more coherent, lucid and meaningful than our own. Events and personalities within the fiction are logically formulated and subject to reasonable inquiry. The world and consciousness of the world are interdependent, yet consciousness has no control over the world, though the world does over consciousness (this unbalanced equation, in my opinion, provides the best possible definition of literary naturalism, a deterministic variant of realism). Words and syntax, style, remain under the writer's control, even when he no longer exists, and have no significant meaning but what the context intends; in other words, writing does not make literature, the writer does.

Modernism in the novel has become virtually synonymous with realism. But realism, ironically, has come to mean romance — in which the moral, social or psychological predispositions of the author are exercised, but the illusions of objectivity, autonomy and rationalism are sustained. In Canadian fiction, romantic-realism begins with the novels of Frederick Philip Grove and remains the dominant mode to the present day. There have been a few outstanding exceptions, but not until the super-realism of Munro, the psycho-romance of Davies, the expository confessionals of Laurence, the documentary visions of Wiebe, the confessional satire of Richler, did the modernist conventions in Canada begin to crumble.

Certainly the conventions of modernism are devoutly upheld by the fictions of Callaghan, MacLennan and Wilson, and in the major works of Buckler and Ross. Grove's *Settlers of the Marsh* and Ostenso's *Wild Geese*, both published in the mid twenties, blend romance with realism as early examples of Canadian modernist fiction; and Mitchell's novels, the most recent of which was published only last year, conforms in content and style if not always in form to the tenets of modernism. Perhaps the masterworks of Watson and Smart defy such conventions, but both are thoroughly modern, philosophically (and possibly postmodern as well). These writers and their works dominate the modernist movement in Canadian fiction. It is their writing we regard from a self-consciously Canadian perspective, in coming to terms with our developing tradition, during the transition from outpost of Empire to nation-state, as, by degrees, we lay claim to a sovereign Canadian imagination. These writers and their novels occupy the interval, not historical but aesthetic and ontological, between Leacock and Laurence. They and their work are the subject of this volume, which is intended to provide an appropriate context for their consideration.

Altogether, the work of ten Canadian novelists is represented on the following pages in essays by fifteen different critics. Most of the essays were written especially for this book. Several have been previously published and are reprinted here because it seemed important to make or keep them accessible. A number of writers or works are the subject of two essays. This is less a measure of their special merit than of the need I felt as editor to redress their neglect. Five of the writers are known for a number of works. Grove published nine novels, and Callaghan, MacLennan, Wilson and Mitchell are similarly celebrated for the variety of their achievement. The reputation of the other five rests primarily on the critical acclaim given a single work by each. In addition to *The Double Hook*, Sheila Watson has published only a few short stories, but Martha Ostenso, Sinclair Ross, Elizabeth Smart and Ernest Buckler have written other novels, some of which were very well received. Nevertheless, their contribution to the Canadian tradition centres on the singular works of outstanding merit which are discussed. The critics represent fifteen different perspectives on literature, fifteen different critical approaches. The fact that such diversity can be coherently gathered into a single volume is a tribute to the rich heritage of modern literature in Canada.

Grove's *Settlers of the Marsh*, originally published in 1925, marks a great leap forward for Canadian fiction into a morally and psychologically complex modern world, a turning away from the idyllic and gothic distortions of the past. Grove was not alone: others, like Ostenso, Douglas Durkin and Robert Stead, all writing from the West, participated in the modernist revolution. For Grove, however, this was just the beginning and what followed is a remarkably varied body of work extending over three decades. Grove may now seem to hover above the modern era like a great mechanical bird; but the intriguing thing is, he is still there. In this book, two critics consider the machinery that keeps him aloft.

Both Lee Thompson and Henry Makow write about *Settlers of the Marsh*, which many regard as Grove's most accomplished novel. Thompson illuminates the deliberate design of a work determined to be art — Grove's aspirations were never to anything less. Makow goes back to the drawing board, as it were, to compare the author's intent for his novel with his misleading responses to its less-than-enthusiastic reception. For Makow the text is important primarily as document; for Thompson, as structure. They work in ways utterly distinct from one another that are, nonetheless, complementary. Together they reveal much of what makes this Grove's best work, and something of its limitations.

Ostenso's *Wild Geese* appeared in the same year as *Settlers* and met with Grove's contempt, possibly for its financial and critical success. There is really no accounting for the subsequent neglect of Ostenso by critics. Stanley Atherton's essay in this volume is a fresh and eclectic attempt to offset the slight. Atherton, in effect, starts from the beginning; he relates *Wild Geese*, Ostenso's best known work, to her personal experience and to actual places and events, but he also offers revealing insights into the novel itself.

No one novel by Callaghan offers a similar focal centre for an assessment or appreciation of his work. Callaghan's principal metier has been the short story. His novels, when taken together, however, are of major significance. Even if one does not stand out, as a group they embody an austere moral and aesthetic determination unparalleled in our literature. A Callaghan novel does not suffer analysis gladly: any attempt to see what makes it work either reduces it to parable or inflates it into myth. Wilf Cude's unusual perspective fortunately reveals the author's achievement without dismantling or distorting it for critical convenience.

Sinclair Ross is also celebrated for his short stories. It is the novel *As For Me and My House*, however, that assures his paramount place in the Canadian tradition. Much has been written about this novel, including a number of fine essays by critics represented in this book. Nothing I have read, though, seemed to get inside the enigma of the novel, rather than explain it away. Since I had a definite idea of what was needed, rather than subject someone else to editorial imposition, I undertook the job myself. An essay with emphasis on the text of *As For Me and My House* and its impact on the reader is the result.

MacLennan offers an unusual problem for the critical anthologist. Since a number of his novels are arguably of comparable stature, which, if any, is to be taken as representative? *Each Man's Son* (1951) contains some of MacLennan's most sensitive writing and the powerful themes of *Two Solitudes* (1945) seem ever more relevant. *The Watch that Ends the Night* (1959), however, holds within it the greatest depths of experience, and *Barometer Rising* (1941) remains the most popularly appealing. Elspeth Cameron's approach to *The Watch* provides fascinating insight into both the novel and the author as she draws extensively on researched materials to explicate MacLennan's method and intent. David Arnason adeptly relates the form of *Barometer Rising* to its historical context, illuminating a primary source of the novel's power and lasting appeal.

The most satisfying thing about criticism of good writing is that it can take such varied forms with equal effectiveness. Arnason and Cameron display entirely different relationships to author and text, yet each shows splendid originality. Lorraine McMullen in her fine treatment of Elizabeth Smart's unusual poetic novel, *By Grand Central Station I Sat Down and Wept*, proves equally imaginative, and necessarily so. She responds to the generic ambiguity of the author's art and to its neglect by critics with an agile analysis that combines a broad overview with specific inquiry, much as if it were a lyric poem. A very different but complementary approach to Smart is John Goddard's personal essay on her life and work, reprinted for its disconcerting insight into both from a popular periodical. Together the journalist and the scholar go a great way towards penetrating the shroud of obscurity that has surrounded Smart's Canadian reputation until now.

In her discussion of Ethel Wilson's *Swamp Angel*, Donna Smyth concentrates on its feminist aspects, bringing into focus the subtle power of the novel and the sources of its profound and lasting impact. In contrast to Smyth's singular approach, George Woodcock takes in the whole of Wilson's remarkable canon with a critical sweep of great perception and wit. As usual Woodcock is the equal of his subject and the reader is treated to what amounts to a critical dialogue between peers — Wilson through her fiction and he, through the art of his essay.

With an obvious affection for the combination of research and speculative thought (which he shares with Henry Makow), Alan R. Young leads the reader through an exhaustive and exhilarating quest for the creative origins of Buckler's *The Mountain and the Valley*. George Bowering, in an idiosyncratic essay that reveals a great deal about the postmodern aesthetic of Bowering's own work, draws everything that has been written about *The Double Hook* into summation and offers a fresh new beginning for our appreciation of Watson's genius.

The two final essays in this book are devoted to works by W. O. Mitchell. Mitchell is underrated or ignored by many critics because of his populist style and apparently simplistic themes, yet as Ken Mitchell and Catherine McLay show, there is depth, breadth and subtlety to his work, if you know where to look, and how. Both *Who Has Seen the Wind* (1947), long rather solemnly regarded as a classic without being taken seriously as art, and *The Vanishing Point*, the most recent novel (1973) considered in this book, receive comprehensive introductory analyses by Mitchell and McLay, the kind of thorough and thoughtful treatment that lesser works could not sustain.

W. O. Mitchell is popular, although MacLennan remains our most celebrated novelist and Callaghan our most enduring. Perhaps the least known of our major writers is Elizabeth Smart. Yet for those who open to her complex and allusive poetic prose, hers is a moving achievement. Smart is just coming into her own, although her novel was published nearly forty years ago. Oddly enough, our most analyzed novel is also highly poetic. However, Sheila Watson draws image, form and style not from her own private anguish and ecstasy, as Smart does, but from mythology and literature. *The Double Hook* remains so haunting in the reader's mind because it is a violent fusion of the familiar; *By Grand Central Station*, because it renders the familiar alien and bizarre.

Perhaps the most accessible of all our novelists is Ethel Wilson. Her prose is pellucid; her narratives immediate, direct, subtle and without ambiguity. She writes humane stories; treats her characters with compassion, even those she despises; treats the world warily but with affection. Her greatest gift, though, is in the scope she allows for the reader's imagination, the finesse she demands of it. She does not lay everything before the reader the way, for instance, Mitchell does; she draws on the reader's own experience of the world and himself. One reacts to Mitchell's writing; one becomes, reading Wilson.

There are many other writers and other works which might have been included under the rubric "modern times". Adele Wiseman's powerful novel, *The Sacrifice* (1956), is a major Canadian work, as disturbing to read now as when it appeared over a quarter of a century ago. Critically, A. M. Klein's brilliant and eccentric novel, *The Second Scroll* (1951), belongs with those included, as does *Tay John* (1939), by Howard O'Hagan. Some would argue that Gwethalyn Graham's *Earth and High Heaven* (1944) should have been considered, though I would strongly disagree — personally, I would have included Patricia Blondal's fine flawed novel, *A Candle to Light the Sun* (1960), and Charles Bruce's evocative regional novel, *The Channel Shore* (1954), and Thomas Raddall's *The Nymph and the Lamp* (1950), a mature and moving story of love in a lonely place. However, personal preference gave way to editorial discretion. As editor, I had to make decisions based on my perception of the Canadian literary tradition. Those novels represented, those novelists discussed, seemed to me the most central to an understanding of the novel in modern times in a Canadian context. There are other works which might have been considered, and were not; but none I hope which were, and should not have been.

John Moss
Bellrock, 1982

FREDERICK PHILIP GROVE

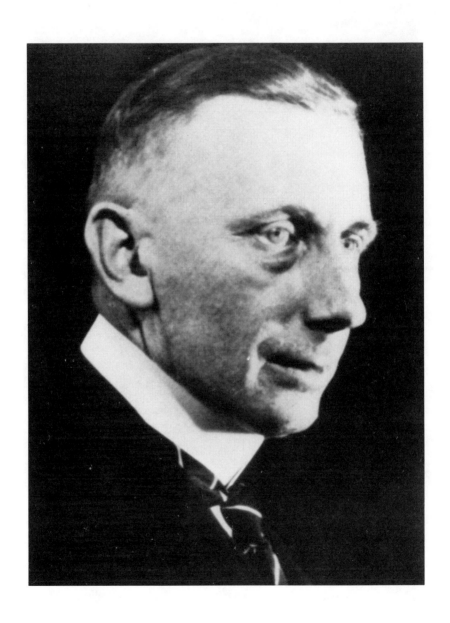

IN SEARCH OF ORDER: THE STRUCTURE OF GROVE'S *SETTLERS OF THE MARSH*

Lee Briscoe Thompson

In his pseudo-autobiographical *In Search of Myself* (1946), Frederick Philip Grove pilloried "that terrible, three volume novel which I called *Pioneers*" and was no less sparing of its abbreviated form, "a garbled extract" which was published "in 1925, under the title of one of its parts, *Settlers of the Marsh.*"[1] He decried the process of condensation as a "ruthless cutting-down" in which he claimed he was forced by the publishers to go "to work slashing the book [*Pioneers*] to *Settlers* as "some of my best work" and followed it with a straightfaced comparison of that novel with Flaubert's *Madame Bovary*, terming each "a serious work of art."[3]

Grove's vacillation is shared by many who subject *Settlers* to close scrutiny. His characterizations are not quite felt upon the pulse; dialogue is frequently stilted; plot developments occasionally seem incredible to readers unaccustomed to the extremes that prairie environment may encourage. Yet the novel as a whole works for the majority of readers, and indeed is often so engrossing as to mask the complexity and subtlety of its structure. Nor is it merely an exercise in craft; Grove is as concerned with idea as order. Interwoven upon a primary framework of themes considered by Grove to be of cosmic significance are intricate subordinate themes, symbols, and images, producing a tight fabric deserving of the name art.

There are four major themes; four structural pillars of the novel, to which the symbols, images and sub-themes direct themselves and lend support. These "themes" cannot easily be wedged into tidy pigeonholes, any more than human experience can be rigidly compartmentalized. But certain designations will conveniently indicate the various patterns revealed by close analysis. Speaking in simplified and sweeping terms, one may say that Grove has built his story of Niels upon:

    i.   Visions and dreams;
    ii.   Fatedness and freedom;
    iii. Passion and its frequent associate, sin;
    iv. Isolation.

Examination of the text will show how structurally dominant these "pillars" are.

I

The most arresting theme of the novel is "Visions", with Niels' recurring and subtly altering dream constantly modulated by the visions of others. The first mention of such imaginings comes early in the novel, when, in the midst of a prairie snowstorm, a modest "vision of some small room, hot with the glow and flicker of an open fire" seizes Niels.[5] Mrs. Lund more ambitiously hopes for "everything as it should be. A large, good house; a hot-bed for the garden; real, up-to-date stables; and ... everything .... We want Bobby to go to college ..." (p. 33). Left at this, the revelation of her dream would seem unrelated and meaningless, but the author continues:

> ... suddenly he understood far more than the mere words. He understood that this woman knew she was at the end of her life and that life had not kept faith with her. Her voice was only half that with which we tell of a marvelous dream; half of it was a passionate protest against the squalor surrounding her; it reared a triumphant vision above the ruins of reality. It was the cry of despair which says, It shall not be so! (p. 33)

We now have a dramatic indication of the futilities and set-backs that are inherent in any vision, Niels' no exception. It is also Grove's first suggestion of the Promethean nobility of the struggle in which, he avows, each person must engage.

Olga Lund, like Niels, is said at this point to nurture a "dream of the future ... capable of fulfillment, not fraught with pathos as her mother's ... " (p. 34). Then, in corroboration of the damage that unrealized dreams can deal to human dignity, the elder Lunds proceed to strip each other of harmless little illusions they have cherished, reduced by frustration to spite (p. 35).

Despite these ominous incidents, Niels' dream continues to blossom and flourish undaunted, and the author's articulation of it binds Niels' individual longings to those of the human race. "Suddenly, ... a vision took hold of Niels: of himself and a woman, sitting of a mid-winter night by the light of a lamp and in front of a fire, with the pitter-patter of children's feet sounding down from above: the eternal vision that has moved the world and that was to direct his fate" (p. 36). The mechanics of human dreaming increase in complexity when Grove reveals that the vision of land, house, and wife is rooted in a negative vision of the past: "that vision of himself as a child, as a poor child, [which] had haunted him when he grew up till fierce and impotent hatreds devastated his heart" and planted the seeds of his New World vision in the ash heap of aspirations impossible in Sweden (p. 39).

If we are not disturbed by the unpromising derivation of Niels' dream, we are certainly alarmed by his reaction to the very first suggestion of its attainability. Women, he muses, have thus far been only a symbol in his dreams; he sees no specific face in the visions. "Now that he was in the country of his dreams and gaining a foothold, it seemed as if individual women were bent on replacing the vague, schematic figures he had had in his mind. He found this *intrusion* strangely disquieting" (p. 40, italics supplied). Is there, then, something within him that will resist or impede the realization of the very goals he seeks?

The vision theme becomes all the more intricate when closely interwoven with a subordinate theme concerning mothers. Part of the reason that Niels' vision has had no clearly defined woman and that the possibility of a real wife disturbs him is that he has subconsciously filled the position: "Niels was hushed with a sense of longing for his own old home, for his mother..." (p. 42). That Ellen does not mother him is the source of "a trace of resentment" against her "unyielding aloofness" (p. 44). For both Niels and Ellen, part of the struggle of life is presented in the process of resolving distortions of the mother-child relationship.

The land and Ellen make their impressions on the young Swede, who finds himself more and more dominated by his vision. The woman in the image becomes Ellen, and Niels finds himself impatient to progress and succeed. Now, "in the first flush of reality; now, when all that was needed seemed to be a retracing in fact of what had already been traced in vision: now that vision became an obsession" (pp. 48-9). In these days of exalted agony, Clara Vogel re-enters the picture. Fleeing her company is, for Niels, like "waking up from a terrible dream" (p. 53). In spite of, perhaps because of, his innocence, he can sense the threat to his dream that she represents. The dream, in a life spent with Mrs. Vogel, will indeed be a nightmare.

Naturally, in retreating from Clara, he aches for security. Again he longs "to be with his mother, to feel her gnarled, calloused

fingers rumpling his hair, and to hear her crooning voice dron-
ing some old tune ..." (pp. 55-6). The vision taking shape before
his eyes undergoes a peculiar series of transformations. Niels is
at his mother's knee. We suddenly become aware that the maternal eyes gazing pityingly at him are the "sky-blue eyes" of Ellen.
But the transposition is not yet complete. The vision clarifies and
the young Swede is crouching in a childless home before the third
female competitor for his soul, Clara. In this single sequence,
Grove has granted a glimpse at the close and complex interrela-
tionships of the three women and has given a definite indication
of the imprecision of perception that will prove Niels' downfall:
the confusion of sexual allure with mother love.

Random encounters with Ellen reaffirm her place in Niels' vision. As the moment for Ellen's revelation of her abhorrence of
sex nears, Niels' sense of vision loses its former clarity. In the
presence of half-mad Sigurdsen he comes to participate in "wild
visions", "as if he could have got up and howled and whistled,
vying with the wind ..." (p. 84). Instinct warns him of
"Something dreadful ... coming, coming ..." (p. 85). A confrontation in the field after the summer storm is postponed by Ellen,
but Niels walks in the subsequent silence "as through a vacant
dream devoid of feeling." Then just before Ellen begins the story
of her mother, Niels finds that "His vision [is] a blank" (p. 104).

The profound effects that their mothers have had on the couple's formative years is revealed. The crisis comes and goes, a
mere moment in the interminable life cycle of men. Nature fills
part of the void created by Ellen's rejection with the passage of
time and incessant work. The change wrought in Niels by the
"gradual negation of his old dream" has become common talk:

> ... it gave him such an air of superiority over his en-
> vironment that the few words which he still had to
> speak were listened to almost with deference. They
> seemed to come out of vast hidden caverns of meaning.
> His face, scored and lined so that it sometimes seemed
> outright ugly, held all in awe, some in terror ....
> The truth was, lightning flashes of pain sometimes
> went through his look, giving him the appearance of
> one insane; or of one who communed with different
> worlds ....
> A new dream rose: a longing to leave and to go to

the very margin of civilisation, there to clear a new
place; and when it was cleared and people began to settle about it, to move on once more, again to the very
edge of pioneerdom, and to start it all over anew ....
That way his enormous strength would still have a
meaning. Woman would have no place in his life ....

He looked upon himself as belonging to a special race
— a race not comprised in any limited nation, but one
that cross-sectioned all nations: a race doomed to
everlasting extinction and yet recruited out of the
wastage of all other nations ....

But, of course, it was only the dream of the slave who
dreams of freedom .... (p. 119)

This final remark refers to Grove's reintroduction, on the very
next page, of the widow Vogel, "a dismal dream, almost forgotten." Niels' new vision is as imperilled as was his old. The subsequent marriage immediately confirms this impression. The house,
so much a part of Niels' initial dream, becomes "much changed" (p. 127). The sweetish scents and luxurious, even decadent,
atmosphere Clara injects are beyond the understanding of his fatal
innocence. Children, an important part of the initial dream, are
another victim of mismating, for he decides that they "would be
a perpetuation of the sin of a moment ..." (p. 138).

Clara too appears to have thwarted dreams. As the marriage
disintegrates, her eyes more and more frequently hold "a new
expression ... a dreamy quality," "as if she [wishes] to erase reality" (p. 141). Her husband is aware that she, "a city woman, with
the tastes and inclinations of such a one," is "banished to the
farm .... [He realizes] the dreariness, the utter emptiness of her
life" (p. 139). Finally, as Clara prepares to leave the farm permanently, "the remnant of a happy dream" that has lain in her
eyes dies completely (p. 151). She falls into the nightmare confrontation with Niels, and upon awaking from that, proceeds to
create a nightmare for a Niels totally unaware of the furies he
has unleashed.

Maternal influences resurface as Clara ruthlessly anatomizes
their marriage. She says, "I thought you were a man" (p. 155);
but Niels is, as discussed before, essentially passive, with a child's
lack of insight into the emotional demands of adulthood. He
wants a mother; she does not want a child. We are left with the

reality of this "mother fixation" until after the murder and Niels' eventual release from jail. Restored to his farm, he experiences a vision which provides the final resolution of that identity problem: superimposed very gradually upon "the homely face of his mother" are "the features of his old man, of Sigurdsen, his neighbour whom he had loved" (p. 210). Herein lies recognition at last of Niels' relationship with Sigurdsen; this knowledge frees him from the need for further dependent relationships. He has embarked upon the self-sufficiency of adulthood.

A third dream of the future develops when Niels and Ellen are reunited: "the dream of the restful perpetuation of this state of dusk, of mutual wordless comprehension, of dispassionate friendship, brotherly love ..." (p. 213). And it is perhaps artistically necessary that Niels come to this level of sincerely platonic thought before the old dream, the dream of "the summer [rather than the autumn] of life" (p. 213), may reassert itself in all its creative vitality. The cycle of vision completes itself as Niels finds himself once more beginning to develop a "strange, new hope." He felt as if he must hold still so as not to frighten away what was building within him: "a new health, a new strength, a new hope, a new life ..." (p. 214).

In a final, triumphant confrontation, Ellen too resolves the distorted mother-child relationship under which she has struggled. She shows herself both willing and needing to assume her own role as a mother. With the deliberate caution of those who have suffered, the couple permit their dreams to reassert themselves and a mutual vision comes into view. It is a dream whose success is not to be perfect, is not guaranteed, for sin and ignorance have precluded that, but it is the hope which always follows on tragic suffering.

II

Settlers of the Marsh has as a second structural pillar, Grove's paradoxical views on man's Fatedness and man's Freedom. Many of Grove's personal pronouncements tend toward a view of man beset by the blind whims of an indifferent universe, "defending himself on all fronts against a cosmic attack."[6] A more specific and poignant statement of the frustrating, impersonal nature of these attacks is presented in Grove's unpublished poem, "The Gods". We are not even flies for wanton gods to kill in sport.

They, as we, are blind

And cannot see where leads their unled dance.
Above them, dangling, hangs the spider Chance,
And spins No-meaning, balm to soul or mind.[7]

Yet Grove also harbours the belief that the human spirit has a
responsibility to pit its strength against "the gods", and he often
sees the forces of fate operating from within the individual. This
brings us into the realm of human responsibility, an issue important both here and in later discussion of the passion-sin theme.

The transplanted Swede has every reason to feel that he is
master of his own destiny in the exciting New World atmosphere
of opportunity and success. "In Sweden it had seemed to him
as if his and everybody's fate had been fixed for all eternity. He
could not win out because he had to overcome not only his own
poverty but that of all his ancestors to boot ..." (p. 39). In comparison, the prairie setting, unconfined by finite spaces, open and
honestly challenging, seemed to offer freedom and the control
of one's destiny (p. 27). But the land counters the atmosphere
of freedom with a strong sense of both the immense inevitability
of timeless natural forces and the tremendous impersonal
ruthlessness of the forces which would move against him. "To
Niels his doings seemed inconsequential and irrelevant; such was
the influence of the boundless landscape which stretched away
in the dim light of the moon ... life had him in its grip and played
with him; the vastness of the spaces looked calmly on" (p. 34).

A multitude of details throughout the novel contribute to the
aura of fate, of external controls, molding the patterns of a man's
life. The countless calamities besetting the Lunds give rise to the
thought, "Success and failure! It seemed to depend on who you
were, an Amundsen or a Lund ..." (p. 36). Frequently, the snares
set for the unwary are embodied in one's acquaintances as in
Niels' "terrible destiny" in the form of Clara (p. 51). Still, it is
evident that however predetermined events may appear, there
is room for rebellion. Olga was able to escape; could not Niels?
He fled physically, but the horrible new knowledge had taken
hold that "he was a leaf borne along by the wind, a prey to things
beyond his control, a fragment swept away by torrents" (p. 55).
Niels' immediate response to this insight is the one to which he
would turn again and again when confronted with the unen-
durable or the incomprehensible: he would "cling to the landscape as something abiding, something to steady him" (p. 55).

Often it seems to Niels that stern fate has less to say in matters than sheer blind chance. "If he had remained in Sweden ... he would have accepted what is as immutable and pre-arranged." Instead, the uprooting and emigration "had awakened powers of vision and sympathy in him which were far beyond his education and upbringing. If one single thing had been different, everything might have run a different course ...." "How chance played into life," he mused, "with considerable fearfulness" (p. 60).

Crucially, however, Niels realizes "that the torrent which swept him away, the wind that bore him whither it listed came from his inner-most self. If, for what had happened to him anybody was to blame at all, it was he ...." (p. 56). Without this participation of self in the process, the drama would not achieve tragic dimensions.

Grove tends to play fate, chance, and freedom against one another throughout his narrative. Niels notes that the townspeople are bound to ennui and dissatisfaction by their own lack of imagination (p. 86). But it is the whims of fortune which persist in throwing Niels and Mrs. Vogel together. And outright necessity, "a tragic necessity no longer to be evaded," appears to control his relationship with Ellen. "The moment was coming. It was rushing along the lane of time where neither he nor she could escape it. Yes, it was already here. It stood in front of them; and its face was not smiling; it was grimly tragical ...." (pp. 94-5).

"Make your own life, Ellen, and let nobody make it for you!" (p. 112). So speaks a woman with whom, as with Mrs. Lund, life had not kept faith. But with these words, Mrs. Amundsen both frees and binds her daughter who has had to distort and suppress her natural needs for home, love and children to obey. It is in acquiescence to her female destiny that she paradoxically finds final freedom.

The images of slavery begin to make a cumulative impression. Niels, "the slave who dreams of freedom" (p. 119), meets Mrs. Vogel by "a blind chance happening" (p. 119). Like a beast under a yoke, tightly reined, the wedded Niels finds "no way of turning" (p. 126). Ellen asks in anguish, "Niels, how could you! ...." (p. 126), but the more relevant question seems to be, "How could you not?" Niels is cornered and haunted by "the feeling of disaster, of a shameful bondage that was inescapable. His doom had overtaken him irrevocably, irremediably: he was bond-slave to a moment in his life, to a moment in the past, for all future times ...." (p. 138). Then there is Niels peonage to the land. Time and again we are reminded that "The farm was a law unto itself ...." (p. 149). Finally, there is the bondage of the ultimate force grinding his fate, Niels own nature. Repeatedly the solution to a situation lies in following the dictates of intuition or impulse.

> But it was a peculiarity of his nature that, having thought out and laid down a plan, he must go on along the demarcated line and carry out that plan even though circumstances might have arisen which made it absurd. Thus he had broken his land, thus built his house, thus made himself the servant of the soil .... It was his peasant nature going on by inertia .... (p. 152)

As the action moves towards the murder, the references to forms of slavery, a fitting preface to rebellion and self-assertion, pile up. The paradox of Clara's view of freedom is revealed in the impassioned kitchen scene. An artificial, possessive woman, she desires a similar love. To feel loved, she needs her freedom curtailed. Indeed, her three tests of Niels' love all centre on freedom, and he fails in declining to restrict her (p. 155). Once convinced that he does not love her, Clara changes her tune. "I cannot stay here, a prisoner, condemned to a life-sentence. I won't" (p. 158). The restriction she seeks in love has become vile imprisonment in hatred.

In probing the raw nerves of the marriage which his wife has exposed, Niels comes to understand the inevitability of his past course of action as well as the unaltered blame he bears for it. "He could not help himself; he was he; he could not act or speak except according to laws inherent in him. What must happen would happen. He had sinned. He saw no atonement. None, nowhere" (p. 161). These insights foster a new sympathy and understanding towards others fallen, now men of his own kind. But the composition of Niels' soul and mind fail to extend in the really crucial direction: toward his wife. "Had he made a single motion ... had he said a single word, even though it had been a word of forgiveness instead of desire, perhaps the worst might still have been averted; fate might have been stayed ..." (p. 165). This possibility of averting fate is, of course, illusory, for "fate" derives from the self and Niels' nature determines his "destiny".

In the process of investigating fully his own bondage, Niels unwittingly reduces his once-beloved Percheron team to slavery. "Horses know as well as dogs whether their masters feel friendly towards them or not. Unlike dogs, they do not cling to or fawn upon him who does not deserve their love. They cannot but do the work demanded of them; but they are henceforth mere slaves" (p. 165). The important point here is the qualitative difference in the types of slavery man and beast endure. Jock enslaved can assume at best only a dramatically stoic stature; Niels enslaved can utilize the human spirit and human reason to challenge his cosmic masters in Promethean, tragic terms. That these masters may issue primarily from within only accentuates the titanic scope of the inner struggle.

In dealing with Niels as he embarks upon the murder of his wife, Grove chooses a curious image, one of springs and clockwork. The impetus to murder appears totally mechanical: "There was not a spark of consciousness in Niels. He acted entirely under the compulsion of the spring" (p. 186). Does the author absolve Niels of responsibility through this device? It would seem more likely that Grove chose this technique simply to dramatize the power that forces, internal and external, working upon an individual, may exert. Niels becomes a sort of puppet, a tool, but controlled by what or whom? Surely a clue lies in the kitchen confrontation with Clara. At that time, "when his wife's revelations had hit him like so many hammer-blows, he had been stunned. Then, in life's first reaction against injury and death, he had been subject to fits of rage, sudden wellings-up in him of primeval impulses, of the desire to kill, to crush ..." (p. 159). The impetus is then a primeval instinct. Niels is both guilty and guiltless, in control and possessed, a murderer and victim of a nature he did not choose.

Grove is consistent regarding the fatedness of things. Chance no longer operates: Niels and Ellen, betrayed once by their own and others' natures, move together as inevitably and consciously as they once parted (p. 214). The now older couple are both free and destined. They deliberately reunite, but the forces which make their union acceptable and promising derive from sources more in the realm of the uncontrolled, the elemental — in a sense, fated. Niels has resolved the maternal dependency and blind morality which bound him and has expiated the sin those produced. Ellen has also freed herself from a legacy of fear and denial, and the indomitable procreative need of all living species has triumphed. In each instance, the integrity of the human spirit has been sustained throughout.

III

The themes of Passion and Sin, inextricable from a discussion of fate and freedom, are so thoroughly developed a structural support of *Settlers* as to warrant separate consideration.

Niels is a character completely "pure" in the ways of sex, "chaste to the very core of his being" (p. 40). For such a man, no mate could be more ill-chosen than "a being that was almost sexless," Ellen Amundsen (p. 38). Her rejection of natural processes, although based on traumatic experiences in childhood, was nevertheless a violation of nature for which she has paid in pain and loneliness. In the rarefied atmosphere of two such unnaturally virgin souls, sensations of passion and sensitivity to sin and guilt must play an accentuated role. Thus, early in the novel, Niels undergoes the stirrings of guilt-feelings without knowing why; "... whenever he had been dreaming of her [Mrs. Vogel] and his thoughts then reverted to Ellen, he felt guilty; he felt defiled, as if he had given in to sin" (p. 46).

Niels experiences "the ultimate, supreme, physical desire" (p. 49) for Ellen that he would have regarded with shame if directed toward the cloyingly intimate widow. Thus we find the word "glowing" used in his response to both women; but in the case of Ellen, the tone is ecstatic and reverent, while Mrs. Vogel's environment is one of fear (pp. 48, 51). "His chastity felt attacked" (p. 52). It does not seem accidental that "in order to save himself, he slipped out of the door and crossed the yard to where the children were playing ..." (p. 53). As, in times of trial, he longs for his mother, and seeks to be mothered by Clara, so, upon the instinct of flight and fear of sin, he tries to return to the state of innocence, to become one with childhood again.

The agony of Niels' situation and the mechanics of tragedy depend to a large degree on the Swede's unnatural innocence or ignorance. Gazing at Mrs. Vogel, he puts the nature of sin in the category of the ineffable. "She was incomprehensible." She "looked like sin" (p. 54). Therefore, sin is incomprehensible. The syllogism may be reversed, but the significance is the same: by neglecting this and other opportunities to increase his understanding of sin and passion, he exposes himself to inevitable disaster.

"His world, his workaday world of toil and worry, seemed suddenly so sane as compared with his own world of passion, desire, and longing" (p. 54). It is natural, then, that he would throw himself into work to release pent-up passions and soothe his spirit. In this novel Grove departs from his usual depiction of the land as a nearly personified force with which to fight for survival. The stark prairie, for all the hardships it represents, tends to ally itself with Niels in providing an external outlet for the true battle waged within.

Ellen's revelation of her mother's marital ordeals is a soliloquy on lust and its results. The sexual relationship is reduced to terms of power, and it is almost a foregone conclusion to hear Ellen say, "I vowed to myself: No man, whether I liked him or loathed him, was ever to have power over me!" (p. 112). In thus wanting on- ly the spiritual, she drives Niels to the purely physical.

As Niels proceeds toward his downfall, his feelings of guilt in- tensify. Playing against this is his stolid and incredible innocence, revealed in the conversation with Hahn. An incomplete sentence harboured the information that might have averted tragedy. "There's one like that Hefter woman in every district ....There's one in yours ..." (p. 118). Ironically, it is unselfish concern for Bobby's moral welfare that diverts Niels' attention at that critical moment from the gossip that might have prevented his marriage and preserved his own moral integrity.

Lindstedt's complex reactions to his first sexual experience en- compass all the fragmentary passion and guilt feelings he has previously undergone: the blood aflame, hatred of the seductress, desire for oblivion and death-in-life, fear and impulses to flight (p. 121). In literal and figurative darkness, he yields to sin. The wages of sin are soon apparent: "Already this marriage seemed to him almost an indecency" (p. 125). A new awareness of lust as "the defiling of an instinct of nature" arises (p. 138); but, amaz- ingly, Niels' innate innocence and, probably, aversion to such a truth, prevent his grasping the logical deduction of his wife's calling. And, his vitality drained away, he "could no longer res- pond with any great passion" (p. 125). Yet he has to meet the demand of "her strange, ardent, erratic desires" (p. 126).

The unnatural type of "love" the couple bear for each other in their earliest married days gradually turns to hate and Niels "felt as if he must purge himself of an infection, of things unimaginable, horrors unspeakable — the more horrible as they were vague, vague ..." (p. 149). It is convenient for Niels to speak of an infection, since the image shifts the blame for their situation from his shoulders to something external, mostly to Clara. But his wife does not permit him to maintain this fiction, charging Niels with having

> "...prostituted me if you know what that means ....
> After having made a convenience of me, when you
> married me, you committed a crime!" ...That woman
> was right! That was why he had married her! Not she,
> he stood indicted. (p. 154)

Wanderings in the labyrinths of guilt produce in Niels a sensitivity to similar failings in others. The pioneer Dahlbeck is now a "slave of passion" ruled by an evil genius of a woman (p. 161). Niels feels himself kin to that man, and realizes at last that he could never again judge others as he had in the innocent arrogance of his youth. Yet, refraining from judging, never does he go the step further to forgiveness that might have proved his salvation.

The extremity of Clara's new passion, hatred, made revenge her entire *raison d'être*. The marriage brings to her the death-in-life that Niels experiences through the shame of lust. It also brings on her madness. Nor is Niels untouched: "the decay in Niels consisted ... in a gradual disintegration of will and purpose" (p. 175). His "care for the farm was almost passionate. But it was the last flicker of a dying flame" (p. 172). Lust and its effects, however, are not yet finished with the Lindstedts. Clara, as part of her revenge, chooses to flaunt her lovers before Niels, prompting his eventual murderous anger. The Dahlbeck woman, whose lust, when thwarted, turns to vindictiveness and to cruel revelation, hisses at Niels, "You hypocrite .... You can't play the innocent with me! You married the district whore ..." (p. 177).

Two provocative facets of the nature of sin emerge after the murder. One is the tendency to involvement that a crime effects. Just as each man loses by another's death, so crime is not an exclusive thing, but spreads like ripples in a pond. Bobby, presumably uninvolved, becomes entangled in the guilt and the tragedy and the implications. "If it had not been for him, Bobby, there would have been no fire arms on the place .... He had been happy, constitutionally happy. He would never be quite so happy again; but he would be more thoughtful .... Bobby, young as he was, came to know the bitterness of regret and repentance" (pp. 188-9).

The other interesting aspect of the murder's aftermath is the pattern of ritual redemption and renewal. Niels falls into a profound and death-like sleep that initiates a dormant period for his soul. Although he wakes physically, his spirit comes "from another world" and his "voice, too, sounded as from an infinite distance" (p. 189). Niels then begins an elaborate cleansing ritual, "slowly, painstakingly, splashing and splashing for fully five minutes" (p. 189). By the time he leaves prison, he has achieved inward balance, "the peace of resignation" (p. 208).

One sin's weight lingers in his conscience. He "had done a great wrong; he had left alone a human being that had been in need of him" (p. 208). Niels' final peace of mind depends on Ellen's forgiveness. He still regards her through "mists of passion" (p. 209), but would suppress these entirely for the sake of brotherhood with her. The situation acquires delicacy and balance when Ellen meets Niels with, "I have been to blame towards you …. Can you forgive? …" (p. 213). They are reunited by the sorrows of the past, the needs of the present, and the hopes of the future. "Life has involved them in guilt; regret and repentance have led them together; they know that never again must they part. It is not passion that will unite them: what will unite them is love …" (p. 216).

IV

The fourth major structural pillar is "Isolation", a designation which serves to include both physical or natural separateness and the alienation of mind or soul. It is a theme which informs the novel from the first glimpse of the vast, depersonalized, bleak prairie setting. By nature a loner, Niels echoes the isolation of the prairie reaches and proves a vehicle as fit as the landscape for Grove's artistic response, tragic, and exulting, to geography unlocking cosmic significances.[8]

The general isolation Niels feels at Nelson's wedding becomes particularized as he realizes the effect marriage would have on their friendship. "Nelson had stepped aside; he was going to live in a world from which Niels was excluded. Niels was left alone" (p. 54). The desire to evade the world becomes "a desire to evade life's issues …," to return to the dependent, one-to-one relationship he has had with his mother (p. 55). One cannot really fault his wish to cut the world out, when one is aware of the almost sinister picture he has gained of human relationships. Mrs. Vogel confuses and frightens him; Ellen is cold and inscrutable; Olga marries to escape; the Lunds and the Amundsens present appalling views of married life.

The association between Niels and Ellen vacillates. For a while "an abyss seemed to yawn [between them] which nothing could bridge" (p. 68). Later there comes to be "no barrier between them: they looked at each other, as it were, stripped of all conventions, all disguises ..." (p. 95). But it is a candour which could be washed away by a summer storm: "... already something [had] stepped in between them: ... a great, infinite remoteness not to be bridged .... As he [sat] there and [looked], it [was] as if her face were receding and fading from view" (p. 99). The schism drives him again from society, "wishing it were winter and he were out, fighting the old, savage fight against the elements ..." (p. 100), a battle for which he is so much more suited.

It is significant that the same image of "the abyss" is used for the pain Ellen encounters in hearing her father force himself on her mother and for all the various moments of alienation that Niels experiences throughout the novel. This device neatly weaves individual incidents into the universal, tragic pattern of human alienation. The sense of isolation controls much of the force of Grove's tragic vision, for it is one thing to be engaged in heroic combat with actively interested and participating superhuman agents (e.g. gods, Nature), but quite another thing to swing blindly and frantically at random, yet inevitable, disinterested cosmic forces (e.g. fate, Nature).

The separation of Ellen and Niels finds its objective correlative in the actual road-chasm where the two inadvertently meet after Niels' marriage. It serves also to presage the social and personal isolation that his new wife has brought: "... not a congratulation, not an invitation for neighbourly intercourse: nothing. ... Niels could not but be aware of enveloping reticences; he felt as if he were surrounded by a huge vacuum in which the air was too thin for human relationships to flourish ..." (p. 129). More painful is Niels' grim picture of his life with Clara, existing side by side: "without common memories in the past, without common interests in the present, without common aims in the future. ... decades upon decades of exactly the same thing ahead, ... facing eternity alone! ..." (p. 137). The emotional separation of the couple becomes concrete in physical separation, with each move away from one another compounded by misunderstandings, absences and reticences into a "demoralization of all human relationships" (p. 141). Finally, faced with Clara's accusations, Niels finds himself "walking along an abyss, blindfolded" (p. 157). Their relationship has hit a depth from which there seems no return. The "blindfolded" Niels fails to interpret his wife's penetrating analysis in any other terms than that "She had given her body" (p. 157), and he misses the last opportunity for reconciliation in ignoring her proud displays of herself to him "as no woman could show herself to any man but her husband ..." (p. 164).

As the impact of Clara's mad revenge takes hold of Niels, he begins to show signs of instability himself. He clings to Bobby as "the last link that connected him with the world of living men: the last barrier between him and insanity ..." (p. 167). Yet he contradicts this in deliberately hiding from Bobby to avoid the judgement that he is mad (p. 166). In shaving and barbering Niels' wild unkemptness, Bobby finally serves as Niels' usher back to some bond with life and with people. It is significantly this shaved, "civilized" Niels who decides to destroy the active force in his life for isolation and nonliving, his wife.

The final sin which Niels and Ellen have to resolve involves, in both instances, violations of love which had produced alienation and loneliness. She has rejected Niels pledge of life, love, and secure intimacy, then lets him go away without a hint of change to sustain his hopes. He in turn does not return, but leaves Ellen alone to suffer. Through mutual contrition and forgiveness, they expiate their transgressions and bridge the crevasses which have too long held them captive and alien. "There is no barrier between them which would need to be bridged by words. They are not looking at each other; they are one" (p. 215). It is appropriate that the last word of the novel be "both", to stress that they have overcome isolation, achieved unity, and are united through love's power. The past is no barrier, but a bond.

V

Textual analysis reveals the domination of four themes — vision, fate, sinful passion, and isolation — in the structure of *Settlers of the Marsh*. These emerge as the strongest elements of the work, the elements about which all characters, incidents, and insights weave themselves. There are, in addition, a number of sub-themes which strengthen and enrich both the major themes and the work of art as a whole. It has been demonstrated, for example, how fully a major theme like "visions" may be informed by a secondary concern like the mother-child relationship. In the same way, motifs of life-death, success, and even the recurrence of the colour white substantially reward investigation. Nature, social issues, and the threads provided by individual characterizations, while comparatively minor structurally, also contribute to the organic quality of the fiction.

Probably the single feature of *Settlers* most troubling to critics' sense of a unified and tightly-knit novel has been the ending. Does it destroy or upset the cohesion and symmetry of the novel's structure? Is it not a shallow acquiescence to the popular demand for a "happy ending", the very phenomenon Grove repudiates in an essay by that name? Thomas Saunders feels that it "is not enough to blind us to the high quality of the narrative up to that point."[9] One might pose an even more loyal defense of Grove's artistic sensibilities by examining the original ending of *Settlers*, in which Niels and Ellen are portrayed in sugary domestic bliss, snug by the fire, with the howl of winter wind outside and "the pitter-patter of little feet" upstairs.[10] Realizing the artistic objections that would be raised to such a patently "happy" and convenient ending, Grove removed it from the novel. It was a decision totally in harmony with his view of tragedy.

What, then is tragic?

To have greatly tried and to have failed, to have greatly longed for purity and to be sullied; to have greatly craved for life and to receive death: all that is the common lot of greatness upon earth .... [In] acceptance or acquiescence lies true tragic greatness: it mirrors the indomitable spirit of mankind. All great endeavour, great ambition, great love, great pride, great thought disturb the placid order of the flow of events. That order is restored when failure is accepted and when it is seen and acknowledged that life proceeds by compromises only.[11]

The couple are now proceeding toward a vision as unguaranteed as their previous broken dreams. But they have tried and failed and have been exalted by the final acceptance of compromise. In Grovian terms, catharsis has been achieved. It becomes apparent how appropriate, consistent, and realistic the conclusion of *Settlers* actually is; indeed, how artificial, melodramatic, and clicheed the predictable "tragic" ending would have been.

Settlers of the Marsh, like all of Frederic Philip Grove's work, exhibits a constant awareness of the demands of the form-content relationship, a particular sensitivity to structure and motif. One might, with considerable support, claim that Grove meets these demands more fully in this novel than anywhere else. Each of the structural themes that the author employs has the status of a chain link: secondary and contributory but absolutely vital to the unity of the chain. The "parts" examined are naturally only parts, but they comprise an artistic totality greater than their sum. In coming to know the parts, then, we approach comprehension of the whole.

Grove's was an ordered mind in search of itself and its world, attempting to work out an ordered view of both. From first glance at the table of contents, wherein may be discerned complicated cycles and parallels of human destiny, one senses this artistic impulse to structure and unity. Time and again, in his "autobiographies" and through his characters, Grove went beyond the "givens" of a situation, attempting to establish patterns for a coherent reality. If the coherence went no further than the pattern itself, no matter. With tacit acceptance of the value of design in itself as a key to or manifestation of the cosmic mysteries, Grove assumes a legitimate place among form-content-reality theorists.

Notes

1   Frederick Philip Grove, *In Search of Myself* (Toronto: Macmillan of Canada, Ltd., 1946), p. 352.
2   *Ibid*, p. 379.
3   *Ibid*, pp. 370, 381.
4   Frederick Philip Grove, from "The Palinode, Part I" (University of Manitoba, the Grove Collection, Part III, no. 5, Box 15, Envelope No. 3).
5   Frederick Philip Grove, *Settlers of the Marsh* (New York: Doran, 1925; rpt. Toronto: McClelland and Stewart, 1966, introduction by Thomas Saunders), p. 17. Further references are to the 1966 edition.
6   *In Search of Myself*, p. 163.
7   Grove, from "The Gods" (University of Manitoba, the Grove Collection, Part III, no. 5, Box 15, Envelope No. 3).
8   For an account of the tremendous response of the author (imaginatively if not factually) to such stark, dramatic landscapes as the desert and Siberia, see *In Search of Myself*, pp. 149-50, 153-4, and 162. That the

author found Canada a parallel sort of experience is evidenced by remarks to that effect in his pseudo-autobiography and by a letter from Grove to Carleton Stanley, dated Simcoe, 14 May 1946: ''Yes, apart from the Canadian, Siberia was my deepest experience [sic].'' (Grove Collection, Box 5).

9 Thomas Saunders, introduction to Settlers of the Marsh, p. xiii.
10 Grove, The Grove Papers, Pt. II (Box No. 9, p. 196, dated 1917̇1924).
11 Frederick Philip Grove, It Needs to be Said (Toronto: Macmillan of Canada, Ltd., 1929), p. 87.

GROVE'S "GARBLED EXTRACT": THE BIBLIOGRAPHICAL ORIGINS OF *SETTLERS OF THE MARSH*

Henry Makow

Settlers of the Marsh is the most read of Grove's works and is widely regarded as one of his highest achievements.[1] Critics and students therefore are puzzled by Grove's repeated deprecation of the novel. In an oft-repeated passage from his autobiography, Grove writes that in 1920 he rewrote "that terrible, three-volume novel which I called 'Pioneers' ... of which a garbled extract was to appear in 1925, under the title of one of its parts, *Settlers of the Marsh*."[2] Elsewhere Grove fosters the impression that his publisher forced him to cut "Pioneers" ruthlessly, and that the dots which appear on almost every page of *Settlers of the Marsh* represent deletions. Grove writes to Desmond Pacey in 1943: "It was by the way, *Settlers* which was so ruthlessly cut down, from three long volumes to one short one. Hence the dots."[3] Grove's statements greatly influenced Pacey's assessment of the novel and subsequently that of many other critics.

On the basis of contemporary correspondence and a comparison of the "Pioneers" typescript with *Settlers of the Marsh*, Grove's statements can now be discounted. *Settlers of the Marsh* is not a "garbled extract"; the dots do not refer to deletions. The evidence indicates that Grove expected the novel to bring him international recognition. He was extremely disappointed with the uncomprehending reviews and miserable sales. The stories he invented were his way of "retracting" the novel, of rationalizing its failure. The published work accurately represents Grove's intentions. The manuscript was readily accepted by Ryerson Press in April, 1925, and published without significant changes. The previous year Grove had decided to condense the two completed volumes of the "Pioneers" trilogy into a shorter work. A comparison of "Pioneers" with the final version will show that nothing of importance was lost in the process. Finally, the evidence will suggest that Grove did not write a third volume of "Pioneers", although in his original conception of the trilogy he had intended to tell the story of Niels' and Ellen's marriage.

The first clue that *Settlers of the Marsh* faithfully represents Grove's intent is the affection the author felt for the work throughout his life. Despite his repeated disclaimers, he held the novel to be one of his most important achievements. In his autobiography, Grove writes of *Settlers of the Marsh*:

> ... I thought it a great book; ... I loved it as a beautiful thing; but .... To this day I am not quite sure that it conveys to others what it conveys to me. If it does, nobody had ever said so.[4]

In 1941, Grove wrote to Desmond Pacey that he considered *Settlers of the Marsh* "the most important of my prairie novels."[5] In his unpublished lectures, Grove refers nostalgically to the writing of *Settlers of the Marsh* as the novel in which most often the "miracle" took place, "that miracle by means of which words transcend themselves and shadow forth realities beyond the power of conscious intention."[6]

Grove had high expectations for *Settlers of the Marsh*, expectations encouraged by Arthur Phelps, an English professor at Wesley College in Winnipeg. Phelps read "Pioneers" in progress and communicated his enthusiasm in his letters to Grove. "I am sure it is a big thing, a very big thing. Somehow I know this. I have walked about in excitement over it."[7] Shortly after publication, Phelps predicted that *Settlers of the Marsh* would make Grove's name internationally known.[8]

Lorne Pierce, the editor of Ryerson Press, who published the novel, was equally sanguine about the prospects in store for the novel and its author. "Please take good care of yourself," he wrote Grove. "We are anxious to have more novels from you and you may yet find yourself sitting down enjoying an opulent old age."[9] Again, he wrote: "Should this prove a success — and we have no doubt that it will — we are hoping to create a Grove vogue before long."[10]

Any man would find these predictions tantalizing. A man such as Grove would find them particularly exciting. According to D. O. Spettigue's account, Felix Paul Grove was intent on making his mark on the world. He craved recognition and acclaim. "The trouble was, he was always on the margins and he wanted to be at the centre ...."[11]

After failing to gain recognition in the literary circles of Europe, Grove came to America in 1909. According to his autobiographical novel, *A Search for America*, he spent three years as an itinerant before becoming a high school teacher in Manitoba. There, under a new name, Grove unabashedly set about his aim which was to create literary works with the permanence of the pyramids.[12] With *Settlers of the Marsh* his first published "Canadian" novel, Grove no doubt hoped to achieve part of his ambition, and some of the recognition that had so far eluded him.

Grove was greatly disappointed. Despite a vigourous promotion campaign by Ryerson, the novel, published in October 1925, sold poorly. In the two years after publication, the novel sold only 1758 copies in Canada and the U.S.[13] Orders for the book had been so bad that in November Pierce suggested that Grove canvas his local drug store in Rapid City for an order.[14] In March, 1926, Pierce wrote Grove: "As we stand to lose a great deal on *Settlers of the Marsh*, I do not think you have any fault to find with the way it was handled in Canada. I think few novels have had more active promotion than this."[15]

The meagre royalties which Grove received were depleted by charges for corrections which he ordered at his own expense. (Despite his "exceeding care" in correcting proofs, he complained that the book "swarmed with misprints."[16] In Sept. 1926, Grove angrily returned to Ryerson a royalty cheque for ninety cents. The cheque had included a deduction of $27.81 charged for corrections by the New York printers.[17] In January, 1928, Grove learned to his surprise that a new, cheaper edition of the novel issued in New York had sold 1927 copies in the Christmas trade.[18] But these belated sales did not assuage Grove's initial humiliation and disappointment.

The public reaction to the novel contributed to Grove's disappointment. A controversy arose over Ellen's uninhibited account in *Settlers of the Marsh* of her mother's marital history. In his autobiography, Grove writes that the publication of *Settlers of the Marsh* became a "public scandal".

> Libraries barred it — London, Ontario, forming an honourable exception; reviewers called it "filthy" — W. T. Allison over the radio; Lorne Pierce nearly lost his job over it; people who had been ready to lionize me cut me dead in the street.
>
> As a trade proposition the book never had a chance; what sale it had was surreptitious. I resented this; it was the old story of Flaubert's *Madame Bovary* over again. A serious work of art was classed as porno-

graphy; but with this difference that the error in
Flaubert's case, increased the sales; he lived in France.
In my case, and in Canada, it killed them.[19]

M.R. Stobie quotes a letter by the Winnipeg librarian of the day
which indicates that no books were banned by the library.[20] The
false impression was created by a press report that some aldermen
had called for a cutback on purchases of "trashy" and "prurient"
novels. Nevertheless, by Stobie's own account, the controversy
was real enough. Many people believed the novel had been banned. Phelps wrote Grove: "The library has banned the *Settlers* and
Eatons sells it but quietly!" W.A. Deacon, the book editor of *The
Globe and Mail* waxed indignant, and *The Ottawa Journal* took up
the cudgel.

In 1962, Lorne Pierce recalled the controversy:

The publishing house was invaded by angry mail, and
by delegates of various sorts condemning us unsparing-
ly. Dr. Fallis, the head of the house was enraged by it
all and I believed my time also had come. Then one day
he walked into the office and laid a letter before me
having the Canadian coat of arms embossed on it. It
read roughly as follows: "I congratulate you on having
the literary insight to recognize a work of art when you
see it, and on having the courage to publish it. Yours
truly, Arthur Meighen, Prime Minister." The war was
over.[21]

Grove's novel shared the brunt of the criticism with Martha
Ostenso's *Wild Geese*, but this only contributed to Grove's frustration. Grove considered *Wild Geese* "deplorably, even unusually
immature." He was piqued that *Wild Geese*, also a first novel, had
won its 25-year-old author the $13,500 Dodd Mead prize as well
as critical accolades. A month after his own novel was published, Grove took time to upbraid a critic who had praised *Wild Geese*
at a meeting of the Canadian Authors' Association. Many
passages in *Wild Geese* "make a mature person smile," Grove
wrote to the critic. "In fact, how could a young girl know anything
of the fierce antagonisms that discharge themselves in sex?
Nobody will accuse me of prudishness. What I object to is the
incompetence, psychologic and artistic, in dealing with these
things ...." And he concluded: "It's an old story: only trash wins
a prize."[22]

Grove was also disappointed with the critical treatment of *Settlers of the Marsh*. The most obtuse reviews were from closest to home. In a *Winnipeg Free Press* review, November 2, 1925, the critic contended that the women of the settlement would not socialize with a well-known courtesan: "They will not condone immorality. That is simply not done, and in making his womenfolk do it, Mr. Grove, not for the first time in his story, forces the characters ruthlessly to follow his story instead of making the story flow naturally from them."

In a *Winnipeg Tribune* review, November 21, 1925, W. T. Allison, a professor at the University of Manitoba, says that Grove "should have had enough consideration for the majority of his readers to omit two nauseating passages. The introduction of the immoral widow into his novel is in itself enough to cause many people to refuse to allow his book on the family shelf."

However, the other reviews, while cursory, were generally positive. The influential *Montreal Star* reviewer, S. Morgan-Powell, wrote on October 31, 1925: "It is essentially a big thing to have done and I regard it as an important contribution to the contemporary fiction of the English speaking world." In general, however, Grove was not satisfied with the reviews. He wrote Ryerson advertising manager E. J. Moore on November 30, 1925:

> I wish to add that what I have seen of reviews, with the exception of Morgan-Powell's, is singularly unintelligent. And without any exception, they seem to me to miss the point.[23]

Grove felt that his novel was not understood by reviewers and the public. He tried to attribute blame for this to the dust jacket which boldly heralds the novel as a "North Country Romance." He wrote Moore on December 21, 1925:

> The jacket killed it. I know for a fact that the 3 leading reviews of what may be called "literature" ignored the book for the sake of the jacket (Danby, Sherman, Mencken). The buyer of North Country Romance, not getting what he wanted, returned the book to the booksellers. So it fell between two stools. I doubt whether even a few hundred copies were sold.[24]

In his reply, the Ryerson advertising manager defended Doran, the New York firm who published the novel and designed the jacket. He also deprived Grove of his rationalization: "Mencken and those other chaps you mention are rather too conversant with marketing methods to let the matter of a jacket influence them either pro or con if they were at all interested in the book itself."[25]

In late March, 1926, Pierce wrote to commiserate with Grove for the poor sales and reviews, the public outcry and other problems attending publication:

> I am sorry that Settlers of the Marsh has been such an unhappy undertaking for you throughout. From the time the Ms. was accepted until the present it seems to have brought you little pleasure.[26]

Even Grove's cordial relations with Pierce, however, were not to survive the debacle. In an attempt to relieve the gloom, Pierce made some flippant but insensitive remarks to Grove with reference to a review of Settlers of the Marsh by their mutual friend, Arthur Phelps.[27] Referring to Phelps' praise of Grove's "three dimensional characters," Pierce remarked that even a moron has three dimensions. He also assured Grove that by the time his next book is published, the "milieu created by the Settlers" will be "of only Paleozoic interest." Grove mistook both remarks and addressed the editor in recriminating tones. Pierce sought in vain to redress the injury. His reference to the milieu created by the novel was to the public outcry, not to the pioneer district depicted therein. He assured Grove that he had no intention of being "outright unkind," and that he was the staunchest supporter of the novel and its author. The slighted author, however, was not to be placated, and the relationship between the two men lapsed for more than a decade, and never regained its former warmth. Grove was not exaggerating very much when he wrote in his autobiography: "In the spring of 1926, the publication of Settlers of the Marsh had proved an unmitigated disaster...."[28]

Grove regarded his first Canadian novel as "a beautiful thing." It was the most important of his prairie works. Because the world did not share his opinion, he felt he had failed to communicate. Grove wrote Pierce explaining that when he feels he has failed to communicate, he becomes so nervous that he wishes he had not published.[29] Grove sought excuses, rationalizing his failure in terms of the obscenity controversy and the dust jacket. Later, he made Pierce his emotional scapegoat. Finally, the story of the "garbled extract" and the dots became Grove's lasting explanation for the novel's failure.

The correspondence shows that Grove recognized almost immediately that the reception of his novel would not meet his high expectations. The first suggestion that *Settlers of the Marsh* was not a bonafide expression of the author's intent is found in a review by Arthur Phelps in the *Winnipeg Free Press* of December 7, 1925. Phelps was replying to the negative review which the newspaper had run a month earlier:

> This last published book and first novel, *Settlers of the Marsh*, was originally planned as a work of 900,000 words in three volumes. As actually written it contained about 400,000 words. It was cut to 85,000 words to meet the publisher's demand in connection with a first novel. Hence the dots, which represent the loss to the reader of a rich quantity of supporting interpretive and descriptive material in the writing of which Mr. Grove's pen can be most satisfying. Hence the nervousness of the book and the seemingly rather sudden ending.

Most likely Phelps adopted the story of the publisher's demand and the dots after discussion with Grove. It was Grove who perpetuated the story. In lectures such as one he wrote in 1935, Grove said *Settlers of the Marsh* appeared in "a mutilated form."[30] He wrote Henry Miller of Graphic Publishers in November 1926: "Once before, in the case of the *Settlers*, I have spoiled a good book by cutting it to the bone."[30] Grove told Pacey in 1943 that "ruthless" cutting resulted in the dots and Pacey gave the story greater currency. In his book, *Frederick Philip Grove*, published in 1945, Pacey says *Settlers of the Marsh* has certain structural defects:

> Of these, perhaps the most obvious is a result of the ruthless process of abridgement to which the novel was subjected. Especially in the first half of the book, which was presumably reduced most severely, there is a plethora of scenes and sentences which trail off into a row of dots: [Pacey gives examples]. The dots, one assumes, indicate passages which were excised; but the critic must judge the work as it stands, and from this point of view these unfinished scenes and sentences are are a constant irritation .... They lend an air of the loose and episodic, the diffuse and scrappy, to the first half of

the novel. A few such passages, to indicate the passage of time, would have been acceptable; but there are too many of them.[32]

Watson Kirkconnell, a colleague of Phelps' at Wesley College and a friend of Grove's, expanded on Grove's rationalization in 1962:

> The novels also suffer because we do not get them in printed form as they were planned. *Settlers of the Marsh* for instance was just hewn out of a vast work on the pioneers that Art Phelps and I saw in Rapid City in the early 1920's. It was simply hacked out of his larger work in order to have something of such a limited length that a publisher would take at all. He is structually the best in novels like *Our Daily Bread* which were not formed by amputation from a larger work, but were planned entire.[33]

Grove's rationalization gets its widest currency in Thomas Saunders' *Introduction* to the New Canadian Library edition of *Settlers of the Marsh*, first issued in 1965. Saunders quotes Grove's statement that *Settlers* is no more than a "garbled extract" of the original version. Although he does not question Grove's statement, Saunders makes a germane point when he questions Pacey's contention that the dots are a defect. "One wonders, indeed, if he [Pacey] had had no knowledge of the abridgement, if he would have complained ...."[34]

Ronald Sutherland and D. O. Spettigue perpetuate Grove's rationalization in their 1969 books, both entitled *Frederick Philip Grove*.[35] Only Margaret Stobie in her book by the same title refers to the dots for what they are, "a fashion Grove took up for a while."[36] But critics continue to accept Grove's word about the editing, and are influenced by it. In an article originally published in the *Journal of Canadian Fiction*, J. Lee Thompson refers to Grove's contradictory claims for *Settlers* as both a "work of art", and a "garbled extract." She concludes: "Grove's vacillation is shared by many who subject the novel to close scrutiny."[37]

Contrary to the general assumption, Grove revised "Pioneers" of his own volition. He records in his autobiography that Volume One of "Pioneers" was submitted to Macmillan and rejected. "A letter accompanying the rejection stated that no book of the kind stood a chance in Canada .... Whereupon I went to work slashing the book to pieces and reducing it to its present one-volume form."[38] Macmillan's letter is in the Grove Collection. The letter is dated February 25, 1924, almost a full year before Grove submitted *Settlers of the Marsh* to Ryerson, who published it. Macmillan did not say that "no book of the kind stood a chance in Canada." They complimented Grove for his truthful portrayal of pioneer conditions. They said that the material might have been "much more effectively presented in a novel of two thirds the space."

> It seems to us that condensation is greatly to be desired and yet we feel that with your avowed purpose of a trilogy in mind, such a suggestion perhaps would not be particularly welcome to you.[39]

A month earlier, McClelland and Stewart also rejected the novel saying the Canadian market was not large enough for a commercial success. They recommended a New York literary agency and expressed interest in taking a Canadian edition.[40]

Volume One of "Pioneers", rejected by Macmillan, and McClelland and Stewart, consists of 203 pages of single-space type and covers Niels' story only until his marriage with Clara, and Ellen's exclamation: "Niels, how could you!" After hearing from the publishers, Grove decided to amalgamate this volume with the second one. Volume Two of "Pioneers", of similar length, continues Niels' story through the marriage, the murder, and ends with Niels' decision to turn himself in. For reasons that I will discuss later, I believe that the projected third volume of "Pioneers" was never written. Grove concluded his shortened novel with a new chapter entitled "Ellen Again" which describes Niel's trial and jail term, his return to the farm and his reconciliation with Ellen. A letter from Phelps to Grove dated January 20, 1925 indicates the novel was complete three weeks before it was submitted to Lorne Pierce in early February. Phelps refers to "the whole last part dealing with Ellen and Niels' ultimate coming together ...." Although prompted by publishers' rejections of Volume One, Grove decided of his own volition to recast his unfinished trilogy in one book.

Lorne Pierce was present February 9, 1925, when Grove gave a reading of his work to the Winnipeg branch of the Canadian Author's Association. In his autobiography Grove records that after the meeting, Pierce asked for the manuscript of *Settlers of the Marsh* and invited him to breakfast at his hotel the following morning.[41] At that time Grove gave an enthusiastic Pierce permission to take the manuscript back to Toronto with him. Here is Pierce's recollection of the breakfast meeting:

> I told Grove that I had been unable to lay down his manuscript and that I had read it on into the morning. I was so deeply impressed as a matter of fact that I assured him publication. He seemed pleased but not unduly elated especially when I told him that the great length of the manuscript would require drastic cutting. There was an episode in the story which did not seem essential, and I felt that those pages would cause more trouble than they were worth.[42]

Significantly, Pierce does not elaborate on the "drastic cutting" required but rather focuses on his objection to the episode dealing with Ellen's mother. He waived his objection when Grove, "white with anger," and "with surprising vehemence," staked his integrity on the inclusion of that episode. It is doubtful that any other cuts were requested. Pierce's account of the meeting, recorded in 1962, thirty-seven years after the event, was probably influenced by Grove's references to the novel as a "garbled extract."

There are compelling reasons for the conclusions that "drastic cutting" was not ordered. First, we have the evidence that Grove reduced "Pioneers" to its one-volume form after hearing from Macmillan the previous year. Second, Pierce likely would not have been kept awake reading a long manscript that required "drastic cutting." Third and most significantly, there was no time for major revisions. Grove's meeting with Pierce took place on February 10, 1925. On April 8, 1925, Pierce made an official offer to publish *Settlers of the Marsh*. Between early February and April there was no time for major revisions, let alone the transformation of an unfinished trilogy into one volume. Pierce's letter suggests that the editor took the finished manuscript to Toronto with him, as Grove says; and the intervening time was expended in consideration of the novel:

> My telegram expresses my great disappointment over the delay in getting word to you. It was impossible to move more rapidly. We are besieged with changes and committees of one sort or another which makes a meeting of the publication committee well nigh impossible.[43]

Pierce goes on to say he is "so impressed" with Grove's manuscript that he wants to arrange for simultaneous publication in New York and London. He says the novel will be set up during the summer and will be ready for late August. There is no mention of cuts in the letter or in any of the Grove-Pierce correspondence on the novel. Grove read the proofs in July and the novel was off the presses in the middle of October. The evidence suggests that the manscript which Grove submitted to Pierce in February 1925 was complete, and was published without significant changes.[44]

Extensive cutting and revision were a normal part of Grove's creative process. As *Settlers* was going to press, Grove wrote Pierce that *Our Daily Bread* must be cut to about 100,000 words: "The trouble with that book is the usual one with me — that it is far too long."[45] Grove tells us without complaint that he cut *A Search for America* by half from its original length of 600,000 words.[46] He claims to have cut *The Master of the Mill* from a first draft of 1300 pages to 400 pages.[47] He advised the young writer not to rest until he has cut his first draft to one quarter its length taking care that "nothing of what he omits actually disappears."[48]

A brief examination of how the "Pioneers" trilogy became *Settlers of the Marsh* is of value. "Latter Day Pioneers", the full title of the trilogy, was conceived in 1917 when Grove was teaching in the marsh country just west of the south tip of Lake Manitoba. In the conception of the trilogy, Grove appears to have had two distinct and ultimately incompatible aims. "Pioneers" was to be the story of Niels Lindstedt and his dream of Ellen as presented in *Settlers of the Marsh*. Grove wished imaginatively to express his vision of the tragic failure of man's highest aspirations. The abandoned white range line house which Grove passed on his journeys became the symbol of an unrealized ideal. The decrepit house became, in Grove's imagination, the magnificent mansion that Niels had built for Ellen but which she never occupied. The early drafts of "Pioneers" begin with a promise to tell the story of this house.

Grove's second aim in "Pioneers" was not related to the imagination. He wished to present a factual chronicle of life in a growing pioneer district. In a plan found at the beginning of the handwritten draft, Grove budgets for four national groups consisting of five characters, each of whom are typical of a pioneer district. The short epithets beside the names include: "middle aged, cattle in the bush the great idea: wife a slut, children lousy. But a dint of hard work makes success," "slow, incompetent as a farmer. Wife ambitious in a frivolous sense, sell to soldier, become store keepers. Lord car," "the man of hard luck, hail, fire," "the Poles, slovenly intelligent, but full of pride." These characters, some of whom never appear in "Pioneers" were probably based on real persons. Residents of the marsh country who were Grove's students say that the Lunds are based on a family Grove knew, the Brandons.[49] In his plan, the Lunds are described as "the typical failure." Fred Brandon was partially blind and borrowed money without repaying it. Bobby Brandon was an orphan who later looked after his mother. There was also a daughter named Olga. As well, there was a well-driller who answers Nelson's description and a giant who appears in the novel under his real name, "Hahn". In contrast to the "pioneer" figures, the three central characters of "Pioneers", Niels, Ellen and Clara were purely a product of Grove's imagination. There is no recollection of persons resembling them or of a young farmer who murdered his wife.

The reconciliation of his imaginative and chronicling impulses is one of Grove's perennial problems. In his book *Frederick Philip Grove*, Spettigue remarks: "To the end of his days Grove was to struggle to reconcile his interest in and awareness of the simple annals of the small town or farm family, with his desire for the fully charged stage, for tragedy wrought to its uttermost."[50]

In *Fruits of the Earth*, Grove opted for the chronicle over the imaginative aim. The first four drafts of the novel have a tragic ending. Rather than defer to authority, Spalding murders his daughter's seducer. Spalding says the man has flouted "every human and divine law," and his murder is intended as an example to future generations. Spalding is tracked down by a posse and spotter plane, and shot. However, Grove tells us in his autobiography that he intended the novel to serve a documentary function as the original title, "The Chronicle of Spalding District", suggests: "Abe Spalding's death, and what followed after, was necessary in order to round off his life before I could write it; but for the story of the district as I conceived it, it was irrelevant; and in the finished work it is never mentioned."[51]

With "Pioneers", a decade earlier, Grove made the opposite decision. He opted for the imaginative portrayal of the human tragedy over the chronicle account of the district. When he edited "Pioneers", Grove cut away an abundance of material which had been included for its documentary value only. *Settlers of the Marsh* therefore is not strictly speaking, a condensation of "Pioneers". The novel existed largely intact within the body of "Pioneers". Grove merely stripped away the documentary material, thereby throwing the story of Niels, Ellen and Clara into relief. With one minor exception, *every* scene in "Pioneers" in which Niels appears with Ellen or Clara has been reproduced in *Settlers of the Marsh* without significant change. This accounts for most of the novel and preserves the original pattern in which Niels' story unfolded.

The editing of "Pioneers" was nevertheless a painstaking process. Grove eliminated all details, characters and events which did not directly advance Niels' story. For example the stories, "The First Day of an Immigrant", "The Marsh Fire", "The Sale" and "Snow", which are found in *Tales from the Margin*, were all originally part of "Pioneers". Grove dropped discussions of subjects such as well-drilling and the virtues of barley as a crop. The progress of the neighbours — the topic of long sections in "Pioneers" — is suggested in a few paragraphs which also indicate the passage of time.

Superfluous anecdotes which only enforce our opinion of Amundson and Lund were dropped. Sigurdson's background, similar to that of the Sower in *The Turn of the Year* was left out. Long passages detailing Niels' introspection were carefully compressed. Details of Niels' progress — how he "proved up" or became a citizen — were dropped. Explicit statements of thematic importance were toned down or eliminated. Omissions were not indicated by dots or in any other manner. Grove placed dots in *Settlers of the Marsh* where no passages from "Pioneers" were omitted.[52]

On the other hand, all the "set pieces" in *Settlers of the Marsh* — among which Niels' moment of truth with Ellen and Clara are the most important — were reproduced without significant changes. It is not a great exaggeration to say that *Settlers of the Marsh* was lifted whole from its background in "Pioneers".

Finally, the question of whether Grove ever actually wrote the third volume of "Pioneers" is germane. As mentioned, the first two volumes takes Niels' story up to his decision to turn himself in for the murder of Clara. The third volume of "Pioneers", if it was ever written, is not extant. The final chapter of *Settlers of the Marsh* is not part of the "Pioneers" manuscript. The chapter, "Ellen Again", was found in 1964 in five examination booklets in Grove's handwriting almost as published. On the basis of a letter Phelps wrote to Grove on January 20, 1925, Stobie believes these booklets represent a condensation of the third volume.[53] Here is what Phelps said:

> My feeling at present ... is that (i) the jail description and (ii) the whole last part dealing with Ellen and Niels' ultimate coming together would bear some sort of compression; in the latter case it might not be compression I want. It may be something quite different; maybe I don't want anything. But on the first reading I wasn't "gathered up tight" by it as I was by some of the other "scenes" in the book.[54]

Stobie's view that the final chapter represents a condensation of the third volume of "Pioneers" is unlikely to be true for the following reasons. First, Phelps' advice was written on January 20, 1925, less than three weeks before Grove presented the finished manuscript to Lorne Pierce. It is unlikely that Grove, acting on Phelps' muddled advice, revised a whole volume in such short space. Second, we have Phelps' review in the *Winnipeg Free Press* of December 7, 1925, in which he says Grove completed only 400,000 of the contemplated 900,000 words of the trilogy. Third, according to Grove's plan, the third volume of "Pioneers" was tentatively entitled "Male and Female" and presumably would have dealt with the married life of Niels and Ellen, not just with their reunion. In the "Epilogue" which Grove deleted from the end of "Ellen Again", in the exam booklets, Niels' and Ellen's married life is "the subject of a different story." Finally, we have a seventeen-page fragment in Grove's handwriting which Spettigue calls "Ellen Lindstedt". The fragment appears to represent the beginning of the abortive third volume. "Ellen Lindstedt" begins with the marriage of Niels and Ellen, recapitulates their history and foreshadows possible areas of conflict before ending abruptly on an ominous note.

All the evidence suggests that Grove never completed the third volume of "Pioneers". Only two volumes were complete when, after hearing from Macmillan, Grove decided to shorten his novel. At that time he wrote the "Ellen Again" chapter to conclude the shortened work. "Ellen Lindstedt", which takes the marriage of Ellen and Niels as its starting point, was likely an attempt to write a sequel to *Settlers of the Marsh* based on Grove's earlier plans for a third volume entitled "Male and Female".

Critics may speculate on the nature of the projected sequel, but they need no longer guess about the authenticity of *Settlers of the Marsh* itself. Grove's repeated statements that *Settlers of the Marsh* is a "garbled extract" of the "Pioneers" trilogy, and that the frequent use of dots indicate omissions, may be discounted. Grove and his supporters had high expectations for his first Canadian novel which they all regarded as a great work. The novel's failure caused Grove to invent an elaborate rationalization which, valid for apologist and detractor alike, found widespread acceptance. Grove was reacting in part to the lack of perception displayed by the critics and public. Ironically his disavowal of the novel did his cause greater harm. It hampered future generations, who Grove said were his true public, from giving his novel the serious consideration which he desired. Grove's rationalizations now may be ignored and *Settlers of the Marsh* may be regarded as an accurate statement of Grove's artistic purpose.

Notes

1 As of June 30, 1975, *Settlers of the Marsh* had sold 29,832 copies in the NCL edition first published in 1965. *Fruits of the Earth*, published the same year, had sold 26,988. (McClelland and Stewart to Makow, July 14, 1975).
Ronald Sutherland and Wilfred Eggleston describe *Settlers of the Marsh* as Grove's finest achievement. W. E. Collins writes in 1946: "Le conflit tragique est souvent evoqué dans les livres de Grove mais nulle part avec autant de succès que dans *Settlers of the Marsh*, ou il atteint aux proportions d'une tragedie classique et represente une des plus grandes reussites artistiques de Grove."

2 F. P. Grove, *In Search of Myself*, introduction by D. O. Spettigue (Toronto: McClelland and Stewart, 1974), p. 352. (Hereafter referred to as *ISM*).

3 Grove to Pacey, June 1, 1943. Unless otherwise indicated, letters may be found in the Grove Collection at the University of Manitoba.

4 *ISM*, p. 379.

5 Grove to Pacey, April 2, 1941.

6 F. P. Grove, Unpublished Address: "Certain Phases of My Life", (1940), p. 11, Grove Collection. Grove also refers to this miracle in *ISM*, p. 409.

7 Phelps to Grove, July 12, 1923.

8 Phelps to Grove, November 15, 1925.

9 Pierce to Grove, June 15, 1925.

10 Pierce to Grove, June 24, 1925.
11 D. O. Spettigue, *FPG: The European Years* (Ottawa: Oberon, 1973), p. 68.
12 F. P. Grove, "Apologia pro vita et opere sua", *Canadian Forum*, XI (August, 1931), p. 420.
13 Grove to Kirkconnell, January 24, 1928.
14 Pierce to Grove, November 10, 1925.
15 Pierce to Grove, March 15, 1926.
16 Grove to Moore, November 17, 1925. (Lorne Pierce Collection, Queen's University).
17 Ryerson to Grove, October 4, 1926, January 29, 1927.
18 Grove to Kirkconnell, January 24, 1928.
19 *ISM*, p. 381.
20 Margaret Stobie, *Frederick Philip Grove* (New York: Twayne, 1973), pp. 111-114.
21 "The Search for Frederick Philip Grove" *CBC Wednesday Night* broadcast in December 1962. Tape transcript in Grove Collection. Part I, p. 17.
22 Grove to A. M. Bothwell, November 18, 1925.
23 Grove to Moore, November 30, 1925 (Queen's).
24 Grove to Moore, December 21, 1925.
25 Moore to Grove, December 30, 1925.
26 Pierce to Grove, March 24, 1926.
27 Pierce to Grove, April 21, 1926 and April 28, 1926.
28 *ISM*, p. 387.
29 Grove to Pierce, September 12, 1925 (Queen's).
30 F. P. Grove, Unpublished Address: "Some Aspects of a Writer's Life", (1935), p. 13.
31 Grove to Miller, November 14, 1926.
32 Desmond Pacey, *Frederick Philip Grove* (Toronto: Ryerson, 1945), p. 45.
33 "The Search for Frederick Philip Grove", CBC tape transcription, II, p. 37.
34 Thomas Saunders, "Introduction", *Settlers of the Marsh*, (Toronto: McClelland and Stewart, 1965), pp. vii, xii.
35 Professor Sutherland guesses correctly that the shorter version is "most likely a happy improvement over the original, ... for Grove had a tendency to overload his works with explanatory detail ...." But Sutherland goes on to state, incorrectly, that Grove indicates omissions "by the use of ellipses." *Frederick Philip Grove* (Toronto: McClelland and Stewart, 1969), p. 47. Professor Spettigue writes: "The number of dots in the printed *Settlers of the Marsh* testifies to the impatience of the editor with Grove's dogged perseverance." Spettigue goes on to cite a comment by Pierce that Grove had a slavish tendency to accumulate detail. *Frederick Philip Grove* (Toronto: Copp Clark, 1969), p. 90. Spettigue has told me that he would now retract the suggestions that Pierce edited Groves manuscript and inserted the dots.
36 Stobie, p. 83.
37 J. Lee Thompson, "In Search of Order: The Structure of Grove's *Settlers of the Marsh*", *Journal of Canadian Fiction*, III, 2, 1974, pp. 65-73. Reprinted in a somewhat altered form in the present volume.
38 *ISM*, p. 379.
39 Macmillan to Grove, February 25, 1924.
40 McClelland and Stewart to Grove, January 30, 1924.
41 *ISM*, p. 381. According to Pierce, he agreed to read the Ms. the

following day. If this is true, the breakfast meeting took place
February 11, 1925.

[42] "The Search for Frederick Philip Grove", CBC tape transcript, II, p. 16.

[43] Pierce to Grove, April 8, 1925 (Queen's).

[44] Although Stobie does not mention and refute Grove's statements, her brief account is consistent with these conclusions. *Frederick Philip Grove*, p. 78.

[45] Grove to Pierce, September 12, 1925.

[46] *ISM*, p. 351.

[47] Grove to Carleton Stanley, November 3, 1945.

[48] F. P. Grove, Unpublished Address: "The Novel", April 10, 1934, p. 16.

[49] Interview with Mr. and Mrs. Otto Brown, Amaranth, Manitoba, May 1975.

[50] Spettigue, *Frederick Philip Grove*, p. 91.

[51] *ISM*, p. 384.

[52] Professor Spettigue was kind enough to show me examples of Grove's German work where dots and other devices are used for effect.

[53] Stobie, p. 77.

[54] Phelps to Grove, January 20, 1926.

MARTHA OSTENSO

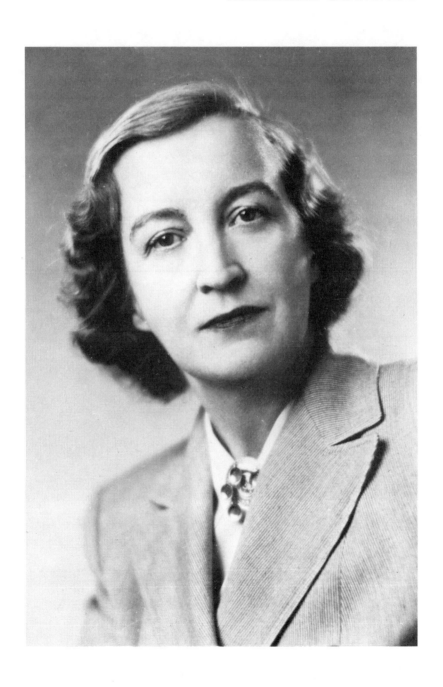

OSTENSO REVISITED

Stanley S. Atherton

In a sense, Martha Ostenso is not a Canadian writer at all. Like the wild geese of her best known novel, she came from and soon returned to the United States; her literary career flourished almost entirely south of the forty-ninth parallel. Born on September 17, 1900 in the Norwegian village of Haukeland, near Bergen, she was taken to the mid-western United States two years later when her parents emigrated. For the next thirteen years, she was to live in a string of "mean yet glorious little towns" in Minnesota and South Dakota, and dream of becoming a writer.[1] Precocious and talented, she was being paid for contributions to the Junior page of the *Minneapolis Journal* by the age of eleven. And soon after the family moved to Brandon, Manitoba at the beginning of the First World War, she had won a prize for poetry in a contest sponsored by the *Winnipeg Telegram*.[2]

As the title of a literary notebook she kept at the time suggests, even as a schoolgirl she enjoyed casting herself in the role of creative writer. "Runaway Rhymes: A Book of Spasmodic outbursts from the cranium of ye youthfull poet Laureate of ye Goldenn Schoole Days" contains entries dating from January, 1915, and includes the only manuscript section still existing of her first novel, *Wild Geese*.[3] On graduation from Brandon Collegiate Institute, she moved to Winnipeg, where she attended classes at the University of Manitoba, taught school and worked as a reporter until she left for New York in 1921.

In New York she found a position as social worker with the Brooklyn Bureau of Charities, and continued to write. She took a course in creative writing called Techniques of the Novel at Columbia University, worked on a novel entitled "The Passionate Flight" she had begun in Manitoba, and began to submit her poems and stories to the magazines. By the end of 1924 she had achieved a modest success, with work appearing in a number of periodicals including the *American Scandinavian Review, Literary Digest, Poetry* and the *Saturday Review of Literature*. And she had published her first book, a collection of poems entitled *A Far Land*.[4]

In 1925 she entered "The Passionate Flight" under the revised title of "Wild Geese" in a competition sponsored by *The Pictorial*

Review, the publishing firm of Dodd, Mead and Company and the Famous Players-Lasky Corporation to find the best first novel by an American author. It won the $13,500 first prize over 1,388 other entries. More than half a century later *Wild Geese* still validates the judges' decision, for it is on this remarkably good novel, more than any of the others which bear her name, that her reputation rests today.

Wild Geese grew out of Ostenso's personal experience. In one of her summer breaks from study in Winnipeg, probably in 1918, she taught in a one-room schoolhouse in the farming community of Hayland, near the Narrows of Lake Manitoba.[5] She boarded with a family named Hay, and modelled one of her characters in the novel, Judith, on the Hay's daughter Aggie.[6] Hayland was to provide her with far more than the setting and a model for one of her principal characters, however. Here in a frontier community, at what must have seemed the edge of civilization, she was able to observe for the first time that special combination of unrestrained human passion and elemental natural forces which could galvanize her peculiar creative imagination.

Clara Thomas has suggested that Martha Ostenso's imagination "did not move toward the heroic, but rather toward the grotesque.'"[7] Whatever the reasons for this imaginative cast of mind — it is intriguing to speculate, for example, on childhood enchantment with the darker aspects of Norse mythology — it is clearly at work in *Wild Geese* and, to a lesser extent, in *The Young May Moon*, the only other novel in which she used a Manitoba setting. The idea of the grotesque suggests the unnatural, the distorted and the absurd, and these elements are all present in her characterization of Caleb, one of the most memorable figures in Canadian fiction. Caleb Gare is at the centre of *Wild Geese*, a mad and monstrous being who terrorizes his wife and children, cheats and bullies his neighbours, and is seen as "a spiritual counterpart of the land, as harsh, as demanding, as tyrannical as the very soil from which he drew his existence.'"[8] The source of Caleb's malevolence is his lust for power, his insensate need to dominate; and it is exercised over his family through the unwilling help of his wife, Amelia, who will do anything to stop Caleb revealing the parentage of her illegitimate son, Mark Jordan. Inevitably the children of Caleb and Amelia become unnatural caricatures, subjugating their dreams and desires to Caleb's will, beaten into passive acceptance of their lot by his unquenchable appetite for power, wealth and land. Ellen, the elder daughter, "reasoned only as Caleb had taught her to reason, in terms of advantage to their land and to him" (p. 96); her twin brother Martin "worked with the bowed, unquestioning resignation of an old unfruitful man" (p. 36). Only one of them, seventeen year old Judith, finds strength to rebel against her father's oppression.

It is in the confrontation between Judith and Caleb that the important issues of *Wild Geese* are dramatized. Their struggle is a contest of individual wills; but it is also a collision between the life-denying forces embodied by Caleb and the life-embracing and affirming forces which Judith represents. The opposition is clearly apparent in their differing reactions to the land. For Caleb the land is something to be owned and dominated. It is above all else "*his* land", and whatever it produced is the "result of *his* industry" (p. 249). Although for him the time of growth in the fields is "a terrific, prolonged hour of passion," it is a passion perverted:

> While he was raptly considering the tender field of flax — now in blue flower — Amelia did not exist to him ... Caleb would stand for long moments outside the fence beside the flax. Then he would turn quickly to see that no one was looking. He would creep between the wires and run his hand across the flowering, gentle tops of the growth. A stealthy caress — more intimate than any he had ever given to woman. (p. 171).

"The land has become a substitute for Caleb's wife," as Laurence Ricou has pointed out, and like Amelia, the land must be bent to his will.[9] It remains an implacable adversary, however, offering him only the perennial challenge "to force from the soil all that it would withhold" (p. 250). Blinded to other considerations, Caleb comes to see the land (even his favoured field of flax) only in terms of profit, as a means to secure ever greater amounts of the wealth and power he obsessively craves. [10]

In sharp contrast, Judith's relationship with the natural world is one of passionate kinship. Early in the novel she lies naked on the warm spring earth, revelling in "the waxy feeling of new sunless vegetation under her," knowing intuitively that she had been "singled ... out from the rest of the Gares" to apprehend the mystery of life, "something forbiddenly beautiful, secret as one's own body" (p. 67). Judith embraces the natural world, literally and figuratively, in a scene that is powerfully reminiscent of D. H. Lawrence:

> ... at the spring ... she threw herself upon the moss
> under the birches, grasping the slender trunks of the
> trees in her hands and straining her body against the
> earth. She has taken off the heavy overalls and the
> coolness of the ground crept into her loose clothing.
> The light from the setting sun seemed to run down the
> smooth white bark of the birches like gilt. There was no
> movement, except the narrow trickle of the water from
> the spring, and the occasional flare of a bird above the
> brown depth of the pool. There was no sound save the
> tuning of the frogs in the marsh that seemed far away,
> and the infrequent call of a catbird on the wing. Here
> was clarity undreamed of, such clarity as the soul
> should have in desire and fulfillment. Judith held her
> breasts in ecstasy. (p. 216)

Judith's openness, her ability to accept and respond to the elemental rhythms of the natural world, stands in direct opposition to the perverted responses of Caleb, who must turn everything he touches to his own unnatural ends.

Physically as well as spiritually, Caleb and Judith are poles apart. Caleb is physically repulsive. His "tremendous and massive head" at first "gave him a towering appearance. [But] when attention was directed to the lower half of his body, he seemed visibly to dwindle" (p. 5). "Broad and bent over," he moves with a "dragging step", "his top-heavy body forming an arc toward the earth" (pp. 262, 269, 270). Other characters in the novel see him as a hypocrite, "too sly for honest people," an insane egoist, and a murderer (p. 286). In extra-human terms he is "demoniacal", "an old satyr", and "the devil himself" (pp. 8, 36, 104). Judith, on the other hand, is a sensual passionate beauty, "the embryonic ecstasy of all life" (p. 35). She is "like some dark young goddess," and sees herself as "an alien spirit ... in no way related to the life about her," unwilling to submit like her mother and siblings to a "meager and warped" life under her tyrannical father (pp. 97, 124, 332).

She defies him openly, denouncing his insatiable demands on members of the family, and clandestinely, in meetings with her lover Sven Sandbo, a young Norwegian "god" from the neighbouring farm (p. 216). When Caleb threatens to beat her into submission, after spying on her love-making with Sven, she flings an axe at him, narrowly missing his head. The scene is superbly drawn, and provides the novel with a memorable metaphor for the fundamental antagonism of the forces Judith and Caleb represent. The confrontation is not climactic: Caleb has yet to provoke the terrible defiance of Amelia. But, it does dramatically reinforce the patterns of conflict — repression and freedom, denial and affirmation — which are at the heart of *Wild Geese*. After the attempt to kill her father, Judith is virtually imprisoned on the farm and Caleb's tyranny seems unassailable. A resolution is achieved when Judith, who is bearing Sven's child, is helped to escape by Lind Archer, the school-teacher who boards at the Gares, and by Amelia, who is unwilling to let Caleb destroy her daughter's life as he had her own. Caleb's death, which swiftly follows Judith's flight into life, is both appalling and ironically appropriate.[11] Frantically trying to save his precious flax from fire, he is trapped in the muskeg that borders it and swallowed up in "the over-strong embrace of the earth" (p. 352).

It has been argued that the resolution of *Wild Geese* is too compressed, that "the suddenness with which the fire follows Amelia's critical defiance and Caleb's moment of 'shame and self-loathing' is inconsistent with the subtle development of the novel to this point."[12] Such a reading fails to take into account the enormity of Caleb's transgressions, which require a retributive devastation of his being that must be swift and complete to achieve the optimum dramatic effect. So it is appropriate that man and nature combine in a single powerfully-drawn sequence of events to annihilate him — spiritually through the knowledge of Judith's escape and the harrowing impact of Ameilia's defiance, physically by earth, air, fire and water. The resolution is artistically consistent with the rest of the novel: there is no place for subtlety here.

It would be foolish to claim that *Wild Geese* is technically flawless. It was, after all, a first novel. There are problems with point of view, as Carlyle King pointed out in his introduction to the New Canadian Library edition.[13] Although much of the story is revealed through the consciousness of Lind Archer, there are frequent forays into the minds of Judith, Amelia and Caleb. Dr. King found these shifts disconcerting, but they are unlikely to bother most readers, since they do provide consistent and credible motivation for the actions of the central characters. Ostenso's unsure control of dialoque is more jarring. It is particularly noticeable in the prissy speeches of Mark Jordon, though there are times when the language of most of the main characters is stilted and unconvincing. On the other hand, dialogue carries much of the burden of characterization in the description of Sigri Sandbo, Sven's mother, and it is splendidly effective:

> "It iss him, upon the vall. And a stinker he vass, too. Good Land, I say, t'ousand times a day, I em heppy he iss gone. Vhat he could drink, that von! Never vonce sober in six years!"
>
> "Was he not kind to you?" Lind asked gently.
>
> "Kind? Him? Good land, I vass a dog under him. Now I live good, not much money, but no dirt from him, t'ank God!" She lifted her eyes up to the photograph, and Lind saw unmistakably a look of wistfulness in them. (pp. 29-30)

There are minor irritants — the heavy-handed treatment of Judith's "secret" pregnancy is an example — but these are rare. More predictable is the pleasure to be derived from Ostenso's mastery of mood, in particular from her ability to capture in a few sure strokes the elements in the natural world which complement and highlight the emotional situation of her characters. One of the finest examples of this is her description of Anton Klovacz' final journey, as Mark Jordan and the farmer's eldest son take his body to the Catholic mission for burial. The passage, too long to quote here, is marked by a mood of great loneliness, and in that sense it offers a paradigm of the entire novel.

For *Wild Geese* is a superb study of isolation: each of the central characters (and many of the minor ones as well) is touched by loneliness and forced in some way to explore its mystery. It is a powerful vision, reinforced by Ostenso's skillful use of the words "alone", "lonely", and "loneliness" in one scene after another to create an effect that is almost incantatory. The reader, caught up in the novelist's fascination with the "unmeasurable Alone surrounding each soul," is left at the end with the indelible, haunting image of the wild geese, whose "cry smote upon the heart like the loneliness of the universe ... a magnificent seeking through solitude — and endless quest" (pp. 57, 356).

Ostenso's second Manitoba novel, *The Young May Moon*, appeared four years after the publication of *Wild Geese*. It is, as Clara

Thomas has observed, "a novel whose seriousness of theme is more satisfyingly matched by its tightness of structure" than is the case in *Wild Geese*.[14] This achievement should not be attributed solely to an improvement in Ostenso's control of her material, however, for there is evidence to suggest it is the result of dual authorship.

It is highly probable that *The Young May Moon* was written in careful collaboration with Douglas Durkin, the Canadian academic and author who became Ostenso's mentor as early as 1919 and her husband in 1944.[15] Durkin's command of narrative technique may be seen in a number of ways: the development of events in this novel is more measured than in *Wild Geese*, the opposition of characters is more carefully balanced, their confrontations are more predictable and controlled, the opening and closing scenes are neatly parallel and echo one another, and so on. It is important to remember, however, that the darkly powerful imagination that informed *Wild Geese* is still at work in *The Young May Moon*, exploring and developing meaningful patterns of isolation and integration, denial and affirmation.

The Young May Moon, set in the fictional prairie town of Amaranth, is the story of Marcia Vorse, the young wife of Rolf Gunther.[16] After a winter of living in "the house of Dorcas Gunther," the dominating, repressive mother-in-law who has hung a sample above their bed with "Repent Ye!" "worked in red wool against a white background," Marcia is reduced to pleading with Rolf for physical love (p. 21). After a passionate argument she impulsively runs away, returning a few hours later to find her husband drowned, a probable suicide. She stays on with Dorcas, partly to atone for the guilt she feels over Rolf's death, and submits to a soul-destroying regimen of domestic and spiritual tyranny.

With the painful recognition that her life has become "dwarfed and twisted under the old woman's blighting intolerance," Marcia is finally able to confess her "responsibility" for Rolf's drowning to Dorcas, and to leave (p. 102). Her departure marks a turning point in the novel. In self-imposed isolation in a ruined house at the edge of town, she wrestles with her special demons, by turns exultant and terrified at what is happening to her. In the end, after a harrowing journey through self reproach, denial, doubt and fear, she comes to terms with herself and her obsession, helped in no small way by the young doctor Paul Brule, who has survived a similar crisis of his own.

The Young May Moon, unlike Wild Geese, was never made into a film, nor was it ever issued in a paperback edition, but it deserves to be better known. Indeed, it is arguable that the two novels should be read in tandem, for The Young May Moon offers an intriguing reversal of the pattern of characterization evident in Wild Geese. In both novels the central characters are obsessed by unacceptable variations of the most basic human events, a birth that is illegitimate and a death that is premature. In coming to terms with their obsessions, the protagonists move in opposite directions on a moral spectrum. Caleb Gare sees himself as a victim and turns into a vengeful, life-denying tyrant, while Marcia Vorse, at first an apologist for atonement, rids herself of ''the recurrent obsession'' and joyously reaffirms life: ''all eternity was [for her now] but a single fierce stroke of rapture'' (p. 298). The treatment of other characters in the novel reinforces this pattern.[17]

Ostenso's influence on other prairie writers has received little attention from contemporary critics, yet it offers a number of avenues for research. The connection with Margaret Laurence, for example, is rich in possibilities. Marcia Vorse would seem to prefigure Rachel Cameron in A Jest of God. Some of the external similarities between Ostenso's own life and that of Morag Gunn in The Diviners suggest that Laurence may have had her in mind when she created Morag. And the imagery of the geese in The Diviners finds an obvious parallel in Wild Geese. There is also an interesting parallel between Amaranth in The Young May Moon and Sinclair Ross's Horizon in As For Me And My House; and it may be that the character of Judith in that novel was suggested by Ostenso's Judith. On a lighter note, one might speculate where Aritha van Herk found the model for her pig farmer, the title character in Judith, bearing in mind that in Wild Geese it was Judith Gare who ''fed the pigs'' (p. 232).

It is demonstrably clear that the Manitoba novels of Martha Ostenso are worth serious critical evaluation. Although the author spent only a short time in Canada, her work represents a significant contribution to Canadian prairie fiction. Like the best work of her contemporaries, her novels ''dramatize the difficulties of affirming life in a world constantly threatened by absurdity, suffering, and death.''[18] It is time we paid her greater attention.

Notes

1 Grant Overton, *The Women Who Make Our Novels* (New York: Essay Index Reprint Series, 1967), p. 247.
2 Manuscript note dated January 12, 1915 beside poem entitled "The Price of War" in Martha Ostenso's notebook.
3 The section consists of eight pages from Chapter III, with minor variations from the published text. The notebook was made available to me through the kindness of Professor Stan Stanko, London, Ontario, Miss Ostenso's literary executor.
4 Martha Ostenso, *A Far Land* (New York: Thomas Seltzer, 1924).
5 Hayland became Oeland in *Wild Geese*. The pronunciation is similar in Norwegian and Icelandic.
6 This information was given to me by Professor Stanko, and has been corroborated elsewhere.
7 Clara Thomas, "Martha Ostenso's Trial of Strength", in Donald G. Stephens, ed., *Writers of the Prairies* (Vancouver: U.B.C. Press, 1973), p. 41. Hereafter cited as Thomas.
8 Martha Ostenso, *Wild Geese* (New York: Dodd, Mead & Co., 1925). All page references in citations are to this original edition.
9 Laurence Ricou, *Vertical Man Horizontal World*: Man and Landscape in Canadian Prairie Fiction (Vancouver: U.B.C. Press, 1973), p. 75. Hereafter cited as Ricou.
10 See *Wild Geese*, p. 311, final paragraph.
11 Judith's escape with Sven is the "passionate flight" which gave the novel its working title.
12 Ricou, p. 79.
13 Martha Ostenso, *Wild Geese* (New York: Dodd, Mead & Co., 1925; rpt. Toronto: McClelland and Stewart, 1961, introduction by Carlyle King.).
14 Thomas, p. 43.
15 This information was given to me by Professor Stanko, who has described published contracts in his possession which link the two writers.
16 Martha Ostenso, *The Young May Moon* (New York: Dodd, Mead & Co., 1929). All page references in citations are to this original edition. Ostenso may simply have used the name of Amaranth, a small town quite near the Narrows of Lake Manitoba, as a substitute for Brandon, whose general topography and possession of a college match the characteristics of the fictional Amaranth.
17 Foils for the protagonists offer an interesting extension of the pattern. Judith Gare's youth and openness oppose Caleb's age and habitual egoism in *Wild Geese*; in *The Young May Moon* Dorcas Gunther's age and puritanical nature oppose Marcia's youth and sensuality.
18 D. G. Jones, *Butterfly on Rock* (Toronto: University of Toronto Press, 1970), p. 8. The quoted passage did not originally refer to Ostenso, but offers a particularly apt description of her work.

MORLEY CALLAGHAN

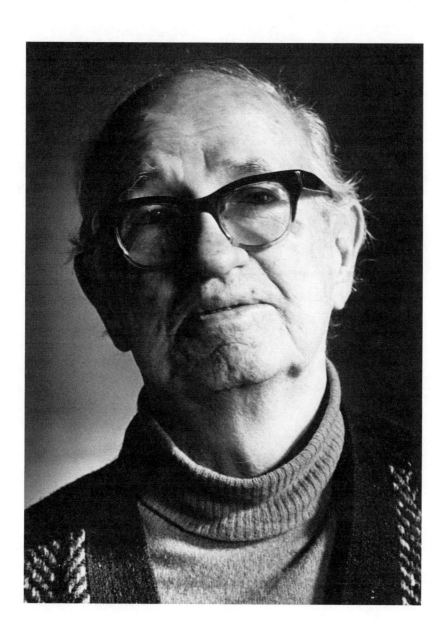

MORLEY CALLAGHAN'S PRACTICAL MONSTERS: DOWNHILL FROM WHERE AND WHEN?

Wilf Cude

"I know why I like you," Carol Finley tells Ira Groome, her lover and the protagonist of Morley Callaghan's latest novel, *Close to the Sun Again*! "You're a monster .... I'll bet you don't throw a shadow when you're walking in the sunlight."[1] Ira Groome is, in truth, a monster — a moral monster, and Callaghan makes us see exactly how he got that way. An imposing figure at fifty-three, a much decorated veteran of the Battle of the Atlantic nicknamed "Ribbons," a dominating presence in corporate boardrooms after the war, Groome seems a most unlikely candidate for monstrosity.

But Carol, assessing him with her "crazy" blue eyes, knows well enough what he lacks. "You've no past," (CSA p. 29) she says simply, touching him on a raw psychological wound. For "Ribbons" Groome, "the Commander" to past and present associates alike, had ruthlessly amputated all memory of his innocent youth in response to one night of trauma during the war: and from that moment on, he forced his way through existence as a dispassionate, even cold calculating, man of reason, masking with a worldly persona the poor emotionally-truncated thing he had elected to become.

Alerted by his mistress to something he had "long ago forgotten," that "before the war he had been another kind of man," he is moved despite himself to muse over his metamorphosis into "this Commander who might never again be able to hear the voices of his own heart" (CSA p. 2). The death of his dipsomaniac wife, Julia; the estrangement from his hippy son Chris; the resignation from his position as Chairman of the Brazilian Power Corporation in Sao Paulo; and his return to Toronto as Police Commissioner; bringing Carol Finley almost casually into his bed: these events free him to confront his self-imposed isolation, to ask the question he has avoided for decades. "Downhill from where and when?" (CSA p. 32). It is a question that informs, not only this retrospective and summational book, but also the entire body of Callaghan's work.

Carol's words only trigger a reaction that had been building in Ira for a long time. His resignation from the Brazilian Power

Corporation came swiftly after he saw his colleagues in a different manner. "These weren't his people," he suddenly understood: "these careful men, these bookkeepers who knew only the tragedies of trivia, and nothing of a beauty born in excess."

Drifting loosely in a daydream, he visualized "lawless men and women, holed up somewhere, nursing passions that made life so real"; and he recoiled almost in pain from a touch to his wound, the unavoidable realization that one such as he could not "feel" anything of "their ruthless passions and their suffering." He was a monster of practicality, and he was hurt by his exclusion from a more vital, important and demanding state of being. "He felt fettered, pushed away, scorned, and doomed to stay where he was and as he was."

His agonized stream of questions "Yet why? What had he done? Where had he done it?" (CSA p. 5). Would it bring him, first to Carol and the restated question, "Downhill from where and when?" and then to the answers he seeks? The process is a complex one, involving the disinterment of memories long ago excised and laid away, memories of Gina Bixby and Jethroe Chone. "Wild ones, weren't they, sir?" (CSA p. 27) asks Horler anxiously, the former navy bosun turned faithful manservant, hesitantly acquiescing in the Commander's probing of a past long repressed and discarded. Wild, indeed. Wild and lawless and yet terribly, awesomely alive, matching in their own excesses even the excesses of the Second World War. They passed in an instant, an instant either to be nurtured or slashed away, for it underscored the dichotomy of Ira's own soul — a dichotomy Callaghan has probed ceaselessly, in one form or another, over the course of his lengthy career.

"Downhill from where and when," within the context of Ira Groome's life in *Close to the Sun Again*, is readily answered: from the moment Ira decided to repress his memories of a Carley float swirling across a frigid moonlit Atlantic, when Jethroe Chone and Gina Bixby vanished before his horrified eyes, eluding his numbed and bloody hands forever. We will return to that; but we should perhaps first determine, within the context of Callaghan's full range of writing, where this central question is anticipated with the greatest clarity and force.

My choice will no doubt surprise most Callaghan enthusiasts: within the pages of *Luke Baldwin's Vow*, the usually-neglected novel intended for young readers, the novel that appeared in shorter form in the *Saturday Evening Post* in 1947, reappeared in full length in 1948, and then — so far as literary analysis was concerned — vanished. Like Jethroe Chone and Gina Bixby, gone without a trace.

And that is something of a pity, since it is here, in the pages of a book written with particular attention to the dichotomy between reason and emotion that sunders each person's soul, that we can trace Callaghan's fascination with the evils of our workaday middle-class world. Or, to rephrase the matter somewhat, if we are ever tempted to wonder whatever became of Luke Baldwin when he grew up, we need only move from the centre of the Callaghan canon to the end. The chances are, I would argue, that little Luke might have turned out perilously akin to Ira Groome — practical monster.

Luke should be of interest, if for no other reason than that he constitutes Callaghan's most unqualified portrait of an innocent. Bereft of his mother when he was an infant and of his father when he was about to enter adolescence, Luke bravely faces, at the novel's opening, a new life with his Uncle Henry and Aunt Helen. He is a sensitive, perceptive and intelligent boy eager to learn from his practical uncle, just as he had promised his dying father he would try to do. Moreover, his uncle and aunt are kindly folk, intent upon making this bright young nephew feel at home.

All should go well, but everything goes wrong, simply because Uncle Henry's practicality renders him monstrously blind to any values other than the economic ones. "In the long run you pay for what you get,"[2] he tells Luke; and, from that pronouncement, Luke works out the essence of the philosophy he is expected to acquire. "A thing that was needed had to be obtained. A thing that was no longer needed had to be tossed aside" (LBV p. 40).

This is a philosophy he cannot accept, for he knows it threatens Dan, the old purebred collie that Uncle Henry intends to destroy. To Luke, Dan is an almost mystical presence, "more than a dog; the collie seemed to have come out of that good part of his life, the part he had shared with his own father" (LBV p. 132). To Uncle Henry, Dan can only be useful one last time, as an example to his too-imaginative nephew of how "you have to do the sensible thing" (LBV p. 148). Luke's desperate struggle to save the dog becomes an outward manifestation of the conflict between the polarities of his own young soul. "You'd wonder, wouldn't you, Dan," he confides to the dog, "that my father and Uncle

Henry could be so far apart on what was useful in the world?'' (LBV p. 109). His father, the quiet and dedicated doctor who read ''fairy stories by Hans Andersen'' to him when he ''was small'' (LBV p. 25), would never destroy a faithful old dog; but his uncle, the hearty and prosperous mill-owner who denounced the ''fairy book'' as ''lies'' (LBV p. 27), could not tolerate the irritation of an animal ''no good even as a watchdog'' (LBV p. 27). Luke loved his father, but he admires his uncle; and, in shielding the dog, he can remain faithful to the one only by opposing the other — choosing emotion and intuition over practicality and calculation. It is a choice Callaghan would have all his innocents make, though the choice is rarely possible and never unequivocal in the benighted money-grubbing world he depicts with such accuracy and distaste.

Even Luke, sustained by his youthful resilience and his awareness of a ''world of strange wonders'' (LBV p. 52) cannot hold aloof from the taint of practicality. Drawn with Dan to the house of Willie Stanowski, a Polish mill-hand who is ''quick and intelligent'' and who has ''eight children,'' he enjoys a taste of life his practical relatives would keep from him. One of the Stanowski children is Tillie, ''a pretty and friendly kid'' (LBV p. 87) of thirteen, a classmate of his; and another is Maria, the eldest at twenty with ''the largest dark eyes'' and hair ''so black it gleamed in the sun,'' the ''prettiest girl Luke had even seen'' (LBV p. 90). Luke and Dan cavort about the old home with the Stanowski brood, until Maria brings the unrestrained romp to a close by playing the piano and singing ''*Alouette.*''

Luke's pleasure with this hearty approach to life, however, is abruptly terminated when Aunt Helen forbids him to associate further with people who ''can't do you any good'' (LBV p. 93). Against his will, he avoids Tillie and stays away from the Stanowski place, ''filled with discontent because all the wild happiness contained in that house was never to be touched by him'' (LBV p. 94). He is tempted one moonlit night to approach the Stanowski place again, listening to the music and the laughter; but, despite Dan's blandishments, he dare not knock and enter. He walks away, knowing that ''for years afterwards the Stanowskis would live in his mind as a fabulous family, and that whenever he heard a piano in the darkness he would remember'' (LBV p. 96).

The poignancy of his loss is driven home to him the very next day, in a wounding encounter with Maria. When she realizes he will not be back, she shrugs her shoulders "contemptuously," and says "I'll see that Tillie doesn't stay around here." She speaks in a soft voice, "as if she had forgotten Luke was there" (LBV p. 97). This is, in effect, banishment from a more passionate world; and Luke is left disconsolate, to reflect that "perhaps God hadn't intended him to be a shrewd and useful man" (LBV p. 98).

Callaghan renders Luke's spiritual failure more apparent by having the boy wander aimlessly in the woods with Dan, seeking in solitude some clue concerning what is happening to him. After eating some raspberries, he notices his hands "were stained as if with blood," and he concludes: "It's blood on my hands from some great wrong I've done" (LBV p. 108). The "wrong" is in fact his acceptance of his uncle's values, no matter how reluctantly and no matter with what justification.

This perception is designed to undermine the otherwise superficial, slick and happy ending, in which Luke saves Dan by making Uncle Henry "a practical proposition" (LBV p. 183). Acting on the advice of old Mr. Kemp, a sympathetic neighbour whose attitude reminds Luke of his father, the boy offers to pay for Dan's keep with the money he will earn by tending Mr. Kemp's cows. Confronted with the boy and dog, shaken by forces he only dimly apprehends, Uncle Henry accepts the arrangement: and Luke is left with his dog, to make in the last paragraph the vow of the novel's title.

> Putting his head on the dog's neck, he vowed to himself fervently that he would always have some money on hand, no matter what became of him, so that he would be able to protect all that was truly valuable from the practical people in the world. (LBV p. 182)

For Luke Baldwin, it could be downhill from there and then. To earn Uncle Henry's respect, he had to fashion himself into a junior version of Uncle Henry; and that, we have already seen from Maria's reaction, converts the triumph over Dan into a Pyrrhic victory at best. Spiritually speaking, Luke has won only by losing; he has moved, with all the commitment of his youthful innocence, further into the world of the practical man — the world that, in Callaghan's view, produces moral monsters.

The relevance of *Luke Baldwin's Vow* to *Close to the Sun Again* should be apparent from the details of the latest novel, since the progression of the young Ira Groome from innocence to monstrosity is more than slightly reminiscent of Luke's movement towards what Uncle Henry termed "the hard bright world" (LBV p. 28) of the practical man. Before the war, Ira was a junior archeologist working "on a dig in the Yucatan" (CSA p. 75), seeking in "a great mound covered with vegetation" some hint of "the life that had been lived there." But he could not shake the eerie sensation that "he was working in a boneyard, a graveyard, and the skulls they dug up, the ruins, the sacrificial stones, told nothing ...."

To ease the sensation, he turned to an ardent relationship with a local girl, an eighteen-year-old named Marina with "black hair" to "her waist," a "simple warmth" and "great dignity." He finds "a strange, terribly heightened feeling of enchantment" (CSA p. 80), one that leads him to taunt his superior with the statement: "You're dead, Dr. Ball." The senior professor, enraged at this insolence from a junior walking off the project, screams "come back here" (CSA p. 81): and the men fight, before Ira leaves. This story fascinates Gina Bixby, the sensual castaway Groome's corvette picks up from a drifting boat during the Battle of the Atlantic. Something of a mystery herself, accompanied even in shipwreck by a polished thug named Jethroe Chone, she is drawn to Ira's account of what he had learned from Marina: that the Mayan vision was "cruel and senseless, a nightmare" and "all we can do is make something beautiful out of the nightmare" (CSA p. 81).

Confiding to Ira her own philosophy, "if we do know in this world, then we should seize the time of knowing" (CSA p. 110), she tells her own wild, inchoate and barely believable tale. The fragile harmony building between them, menaced by the ominous presence of Chone, is shattered when the corvette takes a torpedo — spilling Gina, Chone, Ira and two sailors into a cold and moonlit sea, where they cling for very life to a Carley float. Ira had received a nasty splinter wound in his arm, and "in the dark he could feel the warm blood in his hand" (CSA p. 144).

Like Luke, the still-innocent Lieutenant Groome had encountered two attractive girls, one older and more sophisticated than the other, who introduced him into a world of passions. And, like Luke, the still-innocent Lieutenant Groome was to prove insufficient for that world: he would turn away from it, a sin against the self greater than any other, a sin marked by his own

blood on his hands. For Jethroe Chone, only a day before the corvette went down, had challenged his claim to passionate life with
words suggesting his own taunt to the professor in Yucatan:
"You've got the cold hand, Mr. Groome .... Archeology, my ass.
You're a gravedigger" (CSA p. 128).

Lurching across the frigid night sea, clinging to each other for
warmth, and love, and life itself, the five in the float move towards
the time when Ira will fail as a human being. Chone, hopelessly
wounded, whispers "contemptuously" to Ira, "You were
nothing" (CSA p. 155); and then, renouncing his own claim to
life, slips back into the dark waters. Gina, watching, screams,
"Jethroe, come back here ... come back, you bastard"; and then,
as nobody else moves, she dives after him into those same dark
waters. Ira is left, "bewildered by his stunned moment of indeci-
sion" (CSA p. 156), with numbness spreading up his arm and
his own blood on his hands, gathering the thoughts that will later
convince him "he had been betrayed" (CSA p. 164). His response
to those thoughts, when he recollects them aboard the rescue
packet that lifted the survivors out of the sea the next day, is to
seal his soul off from all but the practical, immediate, tangible
world:

> ... he lay down and shut his ears to the moaning wind,
> and shut his heart to his wonder about Chone, and to
> the voices in his own heart, and thought instead about
> tomorrow and about being dressed and out on the
> deck. He concentrated on seeing himself in his lieute-
> nant's uniform .... (CSA p. 165)

Downhill from there and then. At that moment,"Ribbons"
Groome was born, the man of prudence replacing the wide-eyed
innocent questing after passion. But, as "Ribbons" himself comes
to conclude decades later, "prudence in the heart makes cowards
of us all" (CSA p. 48). The echo of Hamlet applies to him, to Luke,
to all the other innocents who sell themselves into practicality in
the Callaghan canon.

Nowhere in Callaghan's writing is this complex of themes en-
twined in a more accomplished manner than in the short story
"Getting on in the World." Henry Forbes, piano player at the
Clairmont Hotel on his last two weeks of work before an indefinite
lay-off, is joined as he is playing one evening by the kid sister
of a former friend. Jean Gorman is a beautiful and impressionable

eighteen-year-old, convinced by her brother Tommy's stories that Harry must be "a pretty glamorous figure," a man of the world who "knew everybody in town."[3] Harry is naive enough to be convinced, in his turn, that this must indeed be so, since this lovely young girl takes it to be evident.

Over the next few days a romance blossoms between the two, marred slightly for Henry by his feeling that "the pair of them looked like a couple of kids on a merry-go-round." He would have preferred a girl "like some of the smart blondes" with "that lazy, half-mocking aloofness"; (GW p. 42) but he comes to see Jean anew when Eddie Convey, "who just about ran the city hall and was one of the hotel owners, too" (GW p. 40), asks him to send Jean to a party as his place. Jean is reluctant to accept the offer, until Harry persuades her to oblige by blurting out the truth: "It looks like I'm through around here. Unless Convey or somebody like that steps in I'm washed up" (GW p. 40). After delivering Jean to Convey's apartment, he returns to his piano and scrutinizes the audience:

> ... his heart began to ache, and he turned around and looked at all the well-fed men and their women and he heard their deep-toned voices and their lazy laughter and he suddenly felt corrupt. (GW pp. 44-5)

He returns to Convey's place, but cannot nerve himself to go in. Instead, he waits until all the guests leave, and then he waits some more. At four in the morning, Jean finally comes out, no longer looking "worried," but rather "blooming, lazy and proud" (GW p. 45). He accuses her of staying with Convey, "just like a tramp"; and she replies by slapping him, "appraising him contemptuously," and dismissing him with a sudden laugh. "Get back to your piano," she orders. He mutters: "I'll show you ... I'll show everybody"; and the story closes with him "watching her go down the street with a slow, self-satisfied sway of her body" (GW p. 46).

In my estimation, and making due allowance for the difficulties of a comparison with a work in translation, the story is fairly ranked as an achievement with Anton Chekhov's "At Sea — A Sailor's Story." The Chekhov tale is narrated by a sailor, who tells how he and his father won by lot the privilege of viewing the interior of a passenger's cabin through two covert peep-holes cut by the crewmen in the cabin walls. The cabin was usually occupied by honeymooning couples, and the present occupants seemed especially promising, "a young pastor" and his bride, "a very beautiful, shapely young woman." What the voyeurs witnessed, however, was not the amorous coupling of two attractive people; instead, they watched in a revolted fascination as the pastor sold his bride's favours to a monied elderly tourist. The older sailor, "that drunken, debauched old man," pulled his son away and said: "Let's go away from here! You shouldn't see that. You're still a boy."[4]

The Chekhov tale, in its brevity and precision, constitutes a classic treatment of violated innocence; and the reader is left to ponder the question, with all its convolutions, of just who in the tale was the innocent. We encounter similarly classic elements, executed with a comparable economy and force, in the Callaghan story. Harry, the would-be sophisticate, materializes as a hopelessly naive young man crushed by his own callow ineptitude. And Jean, the archetypal ingenue, the stereotyped girl from the small town come wide-eyed to the city, metamorphoses in a few hours into the knowingly chic sort of woman a man like Harry will lust after in vain. Who, here, was really the innocent? And how could it be that any seeming innocent can fall so readily into the trap of "Getting on in the World?" Callaghan's work, in this story, is unmistakably of enduring value.

It would appear I have come to endorse Edmund Wilson's still controversial dictum that Callaghan is an author "whose work may be mentioned without absurdity in association with Chekhov's ...." Indeed, in the instance of "Getting on in the World," I take the assertion as valid; however, with respect to the entire body of Callaghan's writing, I am not so sure the generalization holds. The scope of this essay prevents me from pursuing the issue further, but this at least in fairness should be said: one work of demonstrable excellence is warrant enough to search for more.

Callaghan's themes are of continuing interest in a materialistic world; his execution of those themes across the full range of his writing should therefore be considered with care, in order to determine exactly to what extent he might be reckoned a figure of world literature. That this process has not already started, at the culmination of decades of recognized and often-praised artistry, is no reflection on Callaghan; it is, rather, yet another indication of the reluctance of Canadian critics to attempt the most fundamental of aesthetic functions — honest evaluation.

78   MORLEY CALLAGHAN

Notes

1 Morley Callaghan, *Close to the Sun Again* (Toronto: Macmillan, 1977), p. 29. All subsequent references to this work will be given in parentheses in the text.

2 Morley Callaghan, *Luke Baldwin's Vow* (Toronto: Macmillan, 1974), p. 39. All subsequent references to this work will be given in parentheses in the text.

3 Morley Callaghan, "Getting on in the World" in John Stevens, ed. *Modern Canadian Stories* (New York: Bantam, 1975), p. 40. All subsequent references to this work will be given in parentheses in the text.

4 Anton Chekhov, "At Sea — A Sailor's Story," *Anton Chekhov: Selected Stories*, trans. Ann Dunnigan (New York: Signet, 1960), pp. 33-6.

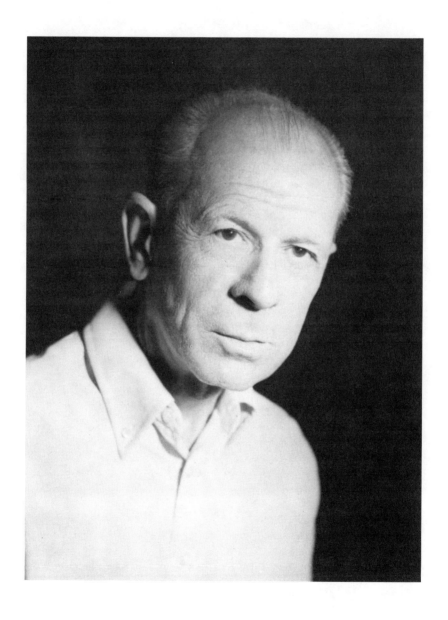

MRS. BENTLEY AND THE BICAMERAL MIND: A HERMENEUTICAL ENCOUNTER WITH *AS FOR ME AND MY HOUSE*.

John Moss

Virtually all the criticism that has been written about *As For Me and My House* holds in common the intent to explain, to interpret the narrative as if it were a portion of real life, somehow isolated by the author through an act of genius or grace. Critics have offered diverse readings of Sinclair Ross's novel, some of them intriguing, and yet the novel remains remarkably opaque. As much as I enjoy the commentaries by Wilf Cude, Lorraine McMullen, W. H. New, David Stouck, Sandra Djwa and others, I am no closer for reading them to comprehending the nature of Ross's achievement. They have told me about life, a bit about style and about voice, less about form, but (and I have been among them in writing towards meaning) they have not illuminated the novel itself. They have moved with their readers away from the text, towards explanation, rather than into it, towards understanding.

Mrs. Bentley's world is a contained reality generated by a text, manifest in the minds of its readers. Yet rare is the critic who resists offering a resolution to the novel as if it were a problem to be solved, or a map to be decoded in order to see where it will lead. Of critics I am familiar with, only Morton L. Ross in his essay, "The Canonization of *As For Me and My House*", avoids this textual fallacy, possibly because his concern is more with criticism of the novel than with the novel itself.

A more appropriate analogy for the text of *As For Me and My House* would be a labryrinth. There are two things to remember about labyrinths: you have to get in, and you have to get out again. To do so you need guides and markers. These cannot be drawn from the text, for the nature of a labyrinth is to mislead. They must come from outside the novel, specifically from other texts where they have already been summoned into coherence out of the chaos of abstract thought and actual experience. They need not be works which might have influenced the author. He had other guides and markers: you do not build a labyrinth and explore it in the same way.

The most useful work to me in this regard was the novel *Badlands* by Robert Kroetsch, published long after I first became familiar with *As For Me and My House*. In considering Kroetsch's novel, recently, I came to recognize the unusual possibilities of representing opposing concepts of reality in terms of male and female gender. Kroetsch does not develop a struggle between two factions within his narrative, but two narratives — the man's, a quest for meaning; the woman's, an escape from meaning. The novel as a whole describes a dichotomy based on current critical theories of structuralism and phenomenology. Kroetsch's chief male protagonist articulates a phenomenological world, and embodies precepts of contemporary existentialism. His female protagonists, both called Anna, occupy a structuralist reality and, then, at the novel's close, animate a deconstructionist vision which seems to inform Kroetsch's subsequent work.

In the arcane textual strategies of postmodern criticism, the reader and critic are set free to be, to exist. The text alone is incomplete, a script for a play to occur in theatres of the mind. The sources of my own limited knowledge of these strategies are of no particular interest to the present exploration. Critical thought associated with Claude Levi-Strauss and Martin Heidegger, whose works inform the extremes of structuralism and phenomenology, and the hermeneutical responses to literary texts modelled on the work of Frank Kermode, are for the most part as obscure as they are illuminating — like a luminescent fog. The freedom they allow within the text and beyond it, combined with their opacity makes them useful here, without them being considered further in themselves.

In postmodern novels like *Badlands* and, even more, in John Fowles's *The French Lieutenant's Woman*, the relations between text and reader are wilfully exploited. The author, as a trickster-god, intrudes, manipulates, lays himself and the machinery of his art exposed, all to free the imagination of the reader from the tyranny of the text as an alternative reality continuous with our own. It is all an illusion, insist both Kroetsch and Fowles: see, they say, this is how it's done. But, of course, such revelations are themselves illusion. That is the anomaly of postmodernism.

As For Me and My House is a modern novel, not postmodern. Ross is nowhere to be found in his text. His novel is of its time, and he is out of it. All that we receive as readers is the product of Mrs. Bentley's mind. Nor does she enact a drama devised by the author's will against a carefully extolled background of nature and society. Such is the mode of nineteenth-century realism.

Rather, in the best tradition of modernism from Joyce to the present, reality and consciousness share mutual boundaries. While the surrounding world and the mind alive within it are not equivalents, each reflects the condition of the other, each exists at the other's pleasure. The author is not to be seen; the proposition essential to the modernist is fostered that he does not exist.

In one sense, the reality of the novel is entirely subjective, originating as it does with Mrs. Bentley. In another sense, it is entirely objective, the created world of Sinclair Ross. But Ross defers to Mrs. Bentley. What we receive, in the final analysis, is neither subjective nor objective but a fusion of the two. To filter them, one from the other, in a critical quest for clarity, insults the structural integrity of the text and denies the author's prerogative to be absent from it. To consider Mrs. Bentley unreliable is an evasion. Mrs. Bentley observes and interprets the world and that same world she lives in, occupies, often revealing far more of it than she intends. Sometimes her observations are objective and reliable, her commentaries fair and perceptive, while the world revealed appears a sham. At other times, she is unreliable indeed, and the world appears a solid separate place.

The dualities, dichotomies, polarities that fibrillate throughout the text like random static charges can all be traced to the mind in which they seem to originate. There are not two realities in this novel, but a single world perceived from the same perspective, Mrs. Bentley's, in two distinctly different ways. It is as if the text articulates the interaction between two sides or, more accurately, two chambers in Mrs. Bentley's mind, roughly corresponding to the two hemispheres of the human brain, or two legislative bodies in a single parliament. I have no intention here of acceding to the extravagant arguments of Julian Jaynes in his book *The Origin of Consciousness in the Breakdown of the Bicameral Mind*, but its principal concept offers a revealing model for understanding the textual anomalies of *As For Me and My House*.

Mrs. Bentley's mind, as text, is bicameral. One side is dominated by words and meaning, by linearity, logic and progression. This is the side conventionally associated with the masculine, and its ascendancy, with existentialism and phenomenology. The other side is dominated by form and pattern, by intuition and discontinuous connections. This, by convention, is deemed the feminine side, and is associated with structuralism. Both exist, side by side, as parallel functions of the mind, sometimes competing, sometimes complementary. In Kroetsch's novel, gender determines the reality of the moment. Narrative reality in *As For Me and My House*, however, cannot be reduced to a simple arrangement of antitheses based either on gender stereotype or the ambivalence of gender in the mindtext itself.

Badlands offers a useful paradigm to work from, in considering the labyrinthine complexity of *As For Me and My House*. Kroetsch's novel quite clearly differentiates between masculine and feminine conceptions of reality. Kroetsch depicts male reality as an existential search for continuity and historical relevance. Dawe's journey down the Red Deer River in pursuit of dinosaur bones which will give him fame and redeem his name for a time from oblivion, is an archetypal quest for meaning through experience; a male quest. Anna Yellowbird watches from the riverbank, occasionally connecting in a random pattern with the different males, and withdraws to watch with Anna Dawe, some fifty-six years later, the Dawe account re-enacted as their common dream. The female presence in the narrative, both structurally and thematically, is spatial not temporal, embodying not progression but discontinuity and transformation. Between them, Anna Dawe and Anna Yellowbird represent escape from myth and language; freedom from meaning.

Kroetsch is doing more in *Badlands* than fleshing out an argument, but there is little question that the informing dialectic of his novel originates in the philosophical bases of current and opposing schools of critical thought. One conception of reality in his novel is existential; one is structuralist. The existential, following empirically unfounded convention, is associated with the male; the structuralist, with the female. Truth, with the success of his narrative as proof that truth is a possibility, lies in the shared configuration of the two within the text. The text is truth, but the way to truth is through the pact between author and reader to rise above the text, to agree that only by rejecting both conceptions of reality at work in the novel will the truth be revealed.

The artist in Kroetsch's fiction subsumes opposing philosophies to his purpose, and the method of his art elevates the receptive reader to share the heady sensation with its creator. Ross, as much of his own age as Kroetsch of his, remains concealed behind his fiction, but he allows the same antitheses to work within it. Ross, as the creative source of his novel, to all intents and purposes, ceases to exist in 1941 when it was published. Kroetsch, the postmodern, refuses to stay behind — through arrogance or humility (the two are inseparable) he remains within the text of *Badlands* in the present presence of his reader's mind.

Ross, as the source of his fiction, generates from his experience of the world and himself a text as labyrinth. Having given us the labyrinth, we are set free of Ross, by Ross, to make our own way. Critics to date have tried to lead us out by the shortest routes conceivable. But it might be more appropriate to a labyrinth to move inwards, away from meaning, towards the centre, towards an appreciation of the enigmatic and anomalous form we find ourselves within. Such a procedure will, at the very least, leave the labyrinth intact.

....

Mrs. Bentley needs desperately to see her husband as an existential hero; a man who turns inwards to himself alone, each time he enters his study; a man in search of consolation within, for the indignities of his personal history, for abandoning Christianity, for his failure to be "manly"; consolation through solitude, and most of all, through art. Yet he is a failed hero, because in her estimation he has not the sufficient requirements of his gender to sustain the existential role she imposes on him. She is the victim of her own sophistry. She needs to see him as an artist-hero in order to make sense of her own life, to make the mean conditions of their lives yield meaning. She must build a myth out of his past and personality which will in effect justify her continuing existence. But this myth depends on Philip's masculinity, his function as the heromale, and this function she repeatedly usurps. To build the myth, she must shape the man; and in shaping the man, she destroys the myth.

Only a few instances need be drawn from the text to affirm the point. As the novel opens, Mrs. Bentley allows, "today I let him be the man about the house."[1] A short time later she suggests that there are times "when I think he has never quite forgiven me for being a woman" (p. 24). And she surmises that his art "can only remind him of his failure, of the man he tried to be" (p. 23). She revells, that he "manfully" refuses convalescence for a cold (p. 34), and later that he displays "masculine aloofness" (p. 82), even though she is its object, but she repeatedly sneers that his "useless hands" cannot accomplish manly tasks as Paul's can, and that he lacks the set of mind of "other men". In a fit of pas-

sionate self-pity she derides Philip, the "sensitive, fine-grained
... genuine man" as "a poor contemptible coward" (p. 86). The
paradox momentarily becomes clear, to us at least, while they are
visiting Paul's family:

> ... perhaps ... years ago, trying to measure up intellec-
> tually to Philip, I read Carlyle too impressionably, his
> thunder that a great man is part of a universal plan,
> that he can't be pushed aside or lost .... Perhaps had he
> been stronger he might not have let me stop him. He
> might have shouldered me, gone on his own way too.
> But there was a hardness lacking. His grain was too
> fine. It doesn't follow that the sensitive qualities that
> make an artist are accompanied by the unflinching,
> stubborn ones that make a man of action and success.
> (p. 103)

Her winning his affection seems, ironically, the proof of Philip's
failure as both an artist and a man.

Mrs. Bentley's identification with her own gender is no more
stable than that which she allows her husband. This instability
in turn undermines her estimation of herself at the centre of what
amounts to a structuralist world, the complement in a bicamerally
conceived reality to the willed presence of her husband at the centre of an existential world. She watches herself with a mixture
of exultation and despair caught up in a mounting struggle to
seize control of the myth, born of Philip's childhood, or her
perception of it, which sees them together repeating endlessly
the mean achievements and petty failures of his past. She com-
forts herself against the squalid condition of their domestic life
by envisioning in the patterns of their shared experience the
possibility of a transformation, wherein they will remain
themselves, yet be changed. A move to the city, a new career,
a child to call their own, such changes will redeem their fallen
lot. The myth will be subsumed by history of Mrs. Bentley's
making.

She does not recognize that such a transformation is merely
the illusion of change. The very act of bringing it about as an expression of her will ensures the perpetuation of their same relationship: she will possess Philip, control his destiny, as it were,
in order to submerge herself within him, in order to be somebody,
to take possession of herself, to be free, to be. Such irony is not

a projection beyond the text: the pattern of their lives together within the text declares, there will be no change without progression. The baby, to be called Philip, is a bastard child as Philip was. The man whose failure as a minister was assured by his lack of conviction before he took a church, this man who failed, also, as a writer will now sell books, with his wife as much a force behind this career as the last. Mrs. Bentley plans to stay away from the store, maybe in the fall to give a recital: against his awkwardness in the practical world, she sets her art. She assures the structure of their lives together will remain the same, even while planning out and extolling the virtues of change.

Structural transformation such as Mrs. Bentley envisions is based upon a fixed notion of gender, wherein the female nurtures and creates the conditions for change, while the male provides the force and knowledge that make changes come about. But her ambivalence in regard to her own gender, as well as her husband's, precludes the possibility of transformation. Repeatedly she ascribes to herself the characteristics of weakness and passivity accorded by convention to her sex. Yet time and again she defies the very stereotype she holds to be true, and then cowers with shame or exults, depending on whether her breach of convention is public or in private. Their poverty, the mark of Philip's failure as a traditional provider, she wears in public as a burden, but at home she wields as a weapon against his self-respect. She understands too well what society demands of her as a woman, and not at all what Philip needs of her, not what she as a woman needs of herself.

Mrs. Bentley proclaims, in her journal entry for *Tuesday Evening, March 5*: "I've fought with myself and won at last" (p. 154). She has decided to adopt Judith's baby: outsiders will see it as a gracious and maternal gesture; she sees it as the transformation of shame to triumph; for Philip, it is a humiliation in which his identity will be virtually overwhelmed. In winning because, as she says, "I want it so" (p. 165), she loses.

This is one side of the world, born out of Mrs. Bentley's bicameral mind: the male is a failure as an existential hero; the female's structuralist reality threatens to collapse. This is one way of seeing things, and the text offers numerous motifs to affirm its viability. Two in particular stand out for their compatibility with gender stereotypes: the horse and the garden. Neither motif is static; both develop in parallel with the narrative. Horses are early in the text associated with coming to manhood, and then with masculine sexuality. At the Kirby farm they become an emblem of infidelity, quite literally, and eventually horses come to represent Philip and his affair with Judith, while in one particular scene the string of broncos in a sketch admired by Mrs. Bentley and Paul casts over their relationship, in Philip's eyes, at least, an ominous cloud of suspicion. It is in the unforgettable image of the frozen carcasses, however, that Philip's affair with Judith and its aftermath are brought into chilling focus: the two horses stand where they died, "too spent to turn again and face the wind" (p. 153). Philip, as his wife declares in naming the child of his indiscretion after him, means "lover of horses". The association and its implications are difficult to ignore.

For Mrs. Bentley, the garden is an emblem of gender, as ambivalent in her regard for it as she is in respect to herself. She relates to it with a sort of plaintive desperation that recalls to her an earlier garden and its associations with the child she lost (p. 44). Her struggle to make that garden yield an array of flowers, not food but beauty, was a link with Philip's struggle to write: and its failure both echoed the death of their child and parallel - ed Philip's failure as a writer. Still, she determines to seek refuge in another garden. Inevitably these flowers die as well, in the wind and the dust and sun, and she gives up on it. She has work- ed against proprieties of gender to water, weed and care for her garden, doing men's and women's labour both, and her garden withers; and with it, her connections with the earth, with mater- nity, natural beauty and her husband's existential being. She has invested her garden with so much of herself that its failure seems her own.

. . .

It is in the ambiguities of gender sustained by the text that op- posing ontologies are freed of a fixed association with one char- acter or another, one sex or another. Mrs. Bentley places herself in what amounts to a structuralist cosmology, and sees her hus- band as the existential protagonist in a phenomenological con- text. But the text affirms her own existential function, and insists that Philip is at least as readily accommodated by a structuralist context. The bicameral mind of Mrs. Bentley sustains either set of extremes, and a multiplicity of possibilities between. While Philip's gender and his wife's demands on him push him towards the existential, his own nature, experience and desire insist that he more comfortably inhabits and animates a structuralist reality. And Mrs. Bentley, contrary to the impress either of gender or wilfull intent, is a far more convincing existential protagonist than her husband.

Philip's consciousness of the world is dominated by form, in spite of what his wife may think or wish. There is little continuity between his experience, as a minister or as a man, and his values. For him, the church provides a sustaining structure to his life, but no meaning. His chosen text for his first sermon, *"As For Me and My House We Will Serve the Lord"*, is not a declaration of faith, as Mrs. Bentley takes it, but a statement of purpose. The theological, social and domestic mythologies associated with the ministry give shape to the Bentley's presence in Horizon, but within the strictures of his function serving community and church Philip leads a separate life as an artist and solitary man.

We are never given the words of his sermons, and rarely their subjects. Yet numerous works of his art are described in detail. Words do not express Philip's condition in the world, nor his understanding of it. He is the antithesis of Paul, the philologist, a marvelous figure in whom words are reduced to meaning alone, without context or syntax, so that meaning becomes meaningless. He is far more like Judith, whose purity of voice lifts the words she sings to soar beyond their meaning. Significantly, Judith responds to drawings of herself with an exclamation on the quality of their likeness, then with silence. The affinity between Philip and Judith is reinforced by their similar defiance of gender conventions, while still being fully representative of their sexes, a point made manifest in their eventual affair. Paul, when he sees Philip's art, interprets it, reduces it to explanation. Paul, like Mrs. Bentley, relates to reality through words; Philip, like Judith, in spite of them.

At one point, and the context is irrelevant, Mrs. Bentley says of Philip, "I took my place beside him, and as he groped for words began explaining the situation as it really was" (p. 73) There is no break for her between how things seem and how they are. Words, her words, declare the continuity between experience and reality: they mean what they say. For Philip, words are a barrier. To penetrate it and make the way things are accessible, is only possible through perceptions of form. In models devised within his art, he searches out the hidden meanings of reality. The real is in the shape of things, not the things themselves. The real is in relationships, structures; in the syntax, not the words. Mrs. Bentley tries to understand his art, but succeeds only in understanding its content, and cannot see the function of its form. In the following passage, both the struggle for Philip's art to emerge from a welter of words, and the struggle of Mrs. Bentley to reduce it once again to words, are in striking evidence:

> He had been drawing again, and under his papers I found a sketch of a little country schoolhouse .... You see it the way Paul sees it. The distorted, barren land-scape makes you feel the meaning of its persistence there ... suddenly like Paul you begin to think poetry, and strive to utter eloquence.
>
> And it was just a few rough pencil strokes, and he had it buried among some notes he'd been making for next Sunday's sermon.
>
> According to Philip it's form that's important in a pic-ture, not the subject or the associations that the subject calls to mind; the pattern you see, not the literary emo-tion you feel; ... A picture worth its salt is supposed to make you experience something that he calls aesthetic excitement, not send you into dithyrambs about humanity in microcosm. (p. 80)

Here quite clearly Philip's structuralist conception of art is shown in confrontation with his wife's phenomenological perception of things. Herein lies the crucial conflict of the novel — not a dialec-tic, but the struggle between two mutually exclusive conditions of mind; and ultimately the mind containing both is Mrs. Bentley's.

Mrs. Bentley insists on her guilt for having forced Philip to aban-don his art for the ministry. She willingly accepts responsibility, as the proof of his affection. She readily accepts blame for the instability of their lives, since each new move seems evidence to her that Philip "still must care a little for his dowdy wife" (p. 10). Because her guilt is the measure of her husband's love, she cultivates the tawdriness and improprieties that cause it. This ac-counts for her acceptance of the discrepancy between her estima-tion of his love and his expression of it. When finally the discrepancy cannot be reconciled with experience, Mrs. Bentley seizes control of their lives, determined to change reality.

Working against Mrs. Bentley's will to change, however, is the pattern of Philip's existence; a series of transformations, a story repeated with variations but without fundamental change or progression. He was a bastard child; the natural son of a preacher who belongs in young Philip's mind to the escape world of imagination, and a drab woman who embodied for the boy his sordid surroundings. Philip's adopted son Steve is an outcast in Horizon. His real son, the first one, dies. His other son is a bastard child as well. As a boy, his father's books gave Philip scope to imagine in life more of value than experience allowed, but crushed him by forcing him to realize his personal insignificance. So too with his writing; so too with his art. The ministry at least gives his life structure and purpose; if not meaning. The painful gap between interior and external worlds that characterized his childhood, that recurred with variations at university, is sustained by his role and function as a minister. In her proposed changes, Mrs. Bentley makes no provisions to bridge this gap — which she, tragically, is incapable of recognizing. In an urban bookstore, Philip's ideal world of the imagination will be no closer to the surrounding conditions of his life than it has ever been.

Philip remains locked into a highly structured and discontinuous existence by the text, although his wife would by choice have him otherwise. She, in turn, remains the existential protagonist in a phenomenological continuum. The form of the text as a journal, self-consciously written, is proof enough that she occupies and animates a world in which explanation is everything, in which things mean what they are said to mean. She equates appearance with reality: thus, it is she, in fact, not Philip, who is so concerned about what everyone thinks of them, of her. And it is she, not Philip, who is so concerned about the continuity a child will provide: "It's going to be a boy, of course, and I'm going to call him Philip too" (p. 158). Even her art, her music, has value to her for what it does, and means, as much as for itself. She plays to win Philip, to win Steve; she plays for Paul. She uses music, by her own admission, not to transcend ordinary experience or to elevate it, but to draw it into coherence, into her control.

Mrs. Bentley writes to interpret lives; she yearns towards meaning. She tries desperately to submerge herself in her husband's mythology, while trying as desperately to lift him out of it. She manipulates to gain control of his life, in order to yield control of her own; to gain possession of both. The creation of her journal is from an existential perspective an act of self-creation. What she writes, the text, however, is beyond her will. In it, both structuralist and phenomenological conceptions of reality converge. It is the literal embodiment of her bicameral mind. With the end of the text, the Bentleys end as well. The novel, however, remains intact, a perpetual presence in the reader's mind.

Notes

1   Sinclair Ross, *As For Me and My House* (New York: Reynal, 1941; Toronto, McClelland and Stewart, 1969), p. 3. This and all subsequent references in parentheses within the text are to the Toronto edition.

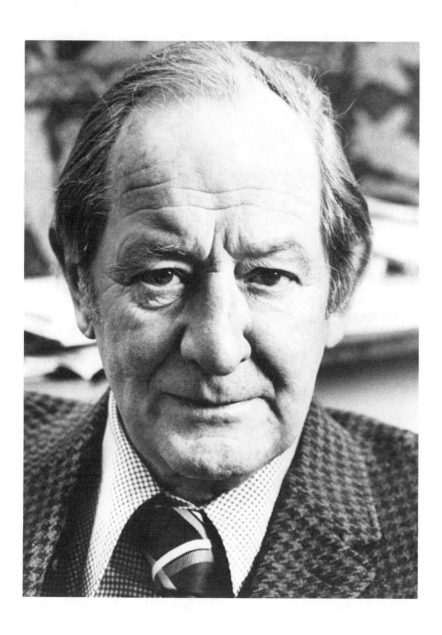

CANADIAN NATIONALISM IN SEARCH OF A FORM: HUGH MacLENNAN'S *BAROMETER RISING*

David Arnason

Hugh MacLennan published his first novel, *Barometer Rising*, in 1941. Since that time, he has become the "grand old man" of Canadian novelists, an assessment that has little to do with his age or the quality of his achievement, but is rather an acknowledgement that the development of a Canadian consciousness is paralleled in the development of his work.

Success did not come easily or quickly to MacLennan. He wrote two novels, *So All Their Praises* (1933) and *Man Should Rejoice* (1937) which were never published. Both were concerned with broad international issues. It was only when MacLennan narrowed his scope and turned to a Canadian subject that he did succeed. That success was marked by the publication in 1941 of *Barometer Rising*, the first novel written in Canada, by a Canadian, in which a peculiarly Canadian consciousness manifests itself.

Since that time, MacLennan has continued to expand his vision of Canada and Canadian consciousness. At the same time, his importance has been recognized, and a growing body of critical study of his work is available. Unfortunately, certain critical clichés have prevented a balanced assessment. The first of these is that MacLennan has, in some incomprehensible way, suffered "a failure of imagination," and the second is that he is a sociologist in disguise. Neither of these views will stand close scrutiny.

A reassessment of *Barometer Rising* must begin with MacLennan's second novel, *Two Solitudes*. In it, he has created his vision of the artist as a young man, in the person of Paul Tallard. Though Paul Tallard comes from a very different background than Hugh MacLennan, he is the young artist who discovers the difficulty of dealing with broad world themes, and turns back to his Canadian roots. The insights, values and ideas that Paul gains in *Two Solitudes* mirror MacLennan's aesthetic and ethical views.

For instance, in *Two Solitudes*, Paul gains an insight into the problem of writing a Canadian novel:

> ... he realized that his readers' ignorance of the essential Canadian clashes and values presented him with a

unique problem. The background would have to be
created from scratch if his story was to become intelligi-
ble. He could afford to take nothing for granted. He
would have to build the stage and props for his play,
and then write the play itself.[1]

It is an insight which MacLennan himself shares with his
character, and it accounts, in part, for some of the successes and
some of the failures of MacLennan's work.

The basis of Paul's insight is an assumption that the reader will
be ignorant of things Canadian. Who then is this hypothetical
reader? Obviously, he is not a thinking modern Canadian, or else
he should know something of the "essential Canadian clashes
and values" and the kind of stage-business that Paul envisions
would be superfluous. Is he then some outsider, some American
or English, or non-Canadian-Canadian literary creature to whom
the author offers his work with built in apologies? This appears
to be the case and many of the excesses in MacLennan's work
spring from an assessment of his audience that is parallel to the
assessment that Paul makes. Why else would a man suffering
from shell-shock, obsessed by thoughts of revenge and desperately hungry for love be permitted by his artistic creator to think:
"The Citadel itself flew the Union Jack in all weathers and was
rightly considered a symbol and bastion of the British Empire."[2]

Why else would a wounded alcoholic doctor, seconds before
he is to deliver a proposal of marriage be permitted to pause and
contemplate irrelevantly that

"... Halifax, more than most towns, seemed governed
by a fate she neither made nor understood, for it was
her birthright to serve the English in time of war and to
sleep neglected when there was peace. It was a bondage Halifax had no thought of escaping because it was
the only life she had ever known; but to Murray this
seemed a pity, for the town figured more largely in the
calamities of the British Empire than in its prosperities,
never seemed able to become truly North American."
(BR p. 33)

These examples are typical, and they are by no means isolated
instances. Throughout both *Barometer Rising* and *Two Solitudes* action is continually interrupted by contemplations about Canadian
society, Canada's place in the world and the forces that operate

in Canada. Usually, these thoughts do not arise as any consequence of the action and seem to exist purely as apologia to the un-Canadian reader. Sometimes they seem to be meretricious interpolations on the part of the author, a difficulty in form that arises from MacLennan's inability to handle his narrative with skill.

In part, though, MacLennan's insight is a valid one. At the time of his writing *Barometer Rising*, there were not many people in Canada who thought of themselves as essentially Canadian, and so some of the stage business is not so superfluous as it might first appear. Now, thirty years later, when people can refer to themselves as Canadians without feeling that there is something embarrassing or pretentious about the use of the word, MacLennan's self-consciousness seems particularly clumsy. In retrospect, any battle that has been won seems disproportionate to its causes. Today, we wonder whether Canada, as a nation, can survive. Thirty years ago the problem was not whether Canada survived, but whether it existed at all.

Since MacLennan is very much concerned with ideas, it is necessary to examine some of the ideas that he considers important. That is to say, since MacLennan is building ''the stage and the props for his play,'' it might be worthwhile to examine them before we look at the play itself.

First, MacLennan's conception of Canada's possibilities seems to be based on an idea of corporate spiritual energy invested in the state. The wars in *Barometer Rising* and *Two Solitudes* are testimony to the expended energy of the Europeans. The First World War, MacLennan feels, will leave only madness, contempt, despair and an ''intolerable burden of guilt'' in Europe, because the war is the ''logical result'' of the Europeans ''living out the sociological results of their own lives.'' Canada's role in the future will be to ''pull Britain clear of decay and give her a new birth'' (BR pp. 200-201). MacLennan is a bit less overtly didactic and somewhat more dramatically convincing in his treatment of European decadence in *Two Solitudes*. First, the reader is given a picture of a cultured, wealthy, Parisian woman, the carefully wrought product of an European civilization caught, fascinated, waiting for a brutal German to debase her sexually. It soon becomes apparent, as MacLennan moves toward the lecturer's tone in which he is most comfortable, that she is an analogue for one part of Europe and the brutal porcine German is an analogue for the other. As Paul retraces in his mind the progress of his novel *Young Man of 1933*, we find that an effete, wasted civilization that has abandoned itself to machines and cities and has forsaken God is powerless to resist the resurgence of totemism, magic and brutal atavism, in fact, the whole *danse macabre* that "had burst out of the unconscious" (TS p. 338) and found its focus in Hitler.

Speaking for MacLennan, Paul says "the same brand of patriotism is never likely to exist all over Canada. Each race so violently disapproves of the tribal gods of the other, I can't see how any single Canadian politician can ever imitate Hitler — at least, not over the whole country" (TS p. 362). MacLennan clearly feels that the future is Canada's. In *Barometer Rising* he confidently and optimistically foresaw Canada as "the central arch which united the new order" (BR p. 218). A trifle more subdued in *Two Solitudes*, he sees Canada acting "out of the instinct to do what was necessary" taking the first steps to self-knowledge, aware that she is "not unique but like all the others, alone with history, with science, with the future" (TS p. 412). This view of Canada is not, however, as chastened as it may first appear. The war is leading the rest of the world to self-destruction while it leads Canada to self-knowledge.

Against this backdrop of historical inevitability, MacLennan sets his props: his own ideas and attitudes, and his impressions of what are typically Canadian ideas and attitudes. MacLennan clearly distrusts certain aspects of progress. In *Barometer Rising* his characters deplore the mass production of ships, and regret deeply the passing of honest craftsmanship. In *Two Solitudes* Paul sees the machine behind Hitler, "the still small voice of God the Father no longer audible through the stroke of the connecting rod" (TS p. 339). Angus Murray in *Barometer Rising* has a theory that "... this war is the product of the big city" (BR p. 50). Paul Tallard in *Two Solitudes* sees "the new city-hatred (contempt for all things but cleverness)" (TS p. 339) as the foundation for anti-semitism, class warfare and economic jealousy. The conscienceless American engineer of *Barometer Rising* is the typical product of the city.

On the other hand, MacLennan clearly feels a deep emotional attachment to certain aspects of the old order. The simple, God-fearing farmer-fishermen of Cape Breton epitomize for him the enduring values. Tied both to the sea and the land, governed by the natural rhythms of the earth, they are honest and noble. Alec MacKenzie of *Barometer Rising* and Captain John Yardley of *Two Solitudes* function as archetypal figures, symbols of human potentiality against whom the other characters may be measured.

This is not to say that MacLennan is opposed to change. Indeed, there are many things about the old order that he resents — the desperate and cold materialism of men like McQueen, the aristocratic conventions of people like Colonel Wain and the Methuens which lead them to debase the country in which they live and which gives them their living, and the narrow religious bigotry of Alfred Wain and Father Beaubien. Change offers not only the hatred of the cities and the brutality of the machine, but also the possibility for growth and renewal, for the fulfilling of destiny and the achievement of self-knowledge. The drastic and accelerated changes occasioned by the war are the flames from which Canada will arise, Phoenix-like, to take its rightful place in the world.

Canada, as MacLennan sees it, and presumably as Canadians themselves think of it, is the product of two cultures. On the one hand, it is tied to England and "a world without England would be intolerable" (BR p. 54). On the other hand it is tied to the United States by "a frontier that was more a link than a division." Uniquely, it partakes of the two cultures. MacLennan clearly sees a dialectic at work, and Neil Macrae expresses it: "... if there were enough Canadians like himself, half-American and half-English, then the day was inevitable when the halves would join and his country would become the central arch which united the new order" (BR p. 218). The same kind of dialectic functions in *Two Solitudes* in which Paul Tallard becomes the synthesis of the French-Canadian and English-Canadian cultures. Here, though, the symbolic form of the dialectic functions against MacLennan's thesis that the cultures are in fact solitudes and must co-exist rather than merge. The title of the novel is from a poem by Rilke, and is part of a definition of Love, another example of MacLennan's incurable optimism.

There is one more significant idea that must be mentioned, and that is the sense of geography that MacLennan feels is part of the Canadian vision and which becomes, in his novels, an important device. In *Two Solitudes*, Heather paints a picture and asks Paul to comment on it. When he sees it, he (or else the author — there is some confusion) notices "... she had missed the vastness of such a scene, the sense of the cold wind stretching so many hundreds of miles to the north of it, through ice and tundra and desolation" (TS p. 307). It is an error that MacLennan has no intention of making. The sun that sets on Halifax makes long shadows in Montreal, glints on the prairies and beams down from high noon on Vancouver. MacLennan seems determined to create a vision of Canada as at least a geographical reality if not a social one, and he loses no opportunity to tie a description of a particular place into a vision of the whole continent.

A set of ideas provides the stage and the props for MacLennan's play: the background is an historically inevitable achievement of destiny and self-knowledge by a young and vigorous country pulled from the outside by two cultures and from the inside by two cultures, caught between the old and the new. The props are certain attitudes and representative characters. Against this is to be set a play which will be an artistic whole, and which will utilize this stage and these properties. Obviously enough, since a nation is a composite of its individuals, the play will concern itself with the achievement of individual destiny and self-knowledge.

It is fashionable to claim that the failures in MacLennan's novels are the result of a failure of imagination. This is not an adequate assessment. The failures that occur are usually the result of a failure to handle with skill the technical form of the novel and sometimes the result of the misapplication of an unbalanced talent.

First, every novel must have a voice, a presumed narrator who tells the story. In the case of *Barometer Rising* the voice is that of an omniscient author who sees everything, who can move about at will and permit the reader to share the thoughts, feelings, and vision of various characters. At times, he exists independently of any character and observes and comments for himself. Like the characters themselves, he is limited to a present and retrospective vision, and none of the unfortunate dramatic ironies of the "dear and gentle reader" school of omniscient author intrude themselves. When the voice speaks for itself, and when it operates at some distance from the characters, it is observant, acute, and incisive. When it moves closer, though, it runs into problems. Too often we begin with the description of a character's thoughts, and find that the anonymous voice has taken matters out of their hands and is commenting itself. For example, on page 67 of

Barometer Rising we discover Wain contemplating Alec MacKenzie. "Wain puffed a lungful of smoke against the windowpane"; at this point the anonymous voice is watching from outside. "MacKenzie was the only man in the world capable of upsetting his apple-cart, of cancelling out all the patient work he had done in Halifax since his return from France" — now we have moved into Wain's mind and are observing his thought. "But the big man had no notion of this" — so far, so good. "When he had accepted the job and brought his wife and family to Halifax he had never guessed that it had been Wain's motive to make him a dependent." By this point there is some considerable doubt as to whether Wain is thinking or the narrator has taken over.[3]

The result of this unsureness in the handling of point-of-view is that the characters are blurred. At times the thoughts of the characters are authentic and individual; at other times they are not. Penny, for instance, is distinctly feminine much of the time, but when she contemplates the Nova Scotian scene, an anonymous voice intrudes. She could be Neil Murray or anybody else:

> Her eye wandered back to the freighter sliding upstream: a commonplace ship, certainly foreign and probably of the Mediterranean origin, manned by heaven knew what conglomeration of Levantines, with maybe a Scotsman in the engine-room and a renegade Nova Scotian somewhere in the forecastle. The war had brought so many of these mongrel vessels to Halifax, they had become a part of the landscape. (BR p. 17)

Besides blurring the identity of the characters, the authorial voice also blurs the action and interferes with the dramatic power of the narrative. MacLennan's chief skill lies in his ability to write sustained passages of descriptive narrative. This is obvious in his powerful description of the events leading to the explosion and the chaotic action thereafter. He chooses to dissipate this power by his refusal, in the first half of the book, to sustain his focus on any action. As the action approaches a climax, the focus shifts and the dramatic tension created is lost. To be sure, this shifting focus is obviously intentional. The unfulfilled nature of the characters calls for unfulfilled action, and provides a striking contrast to the sharp decisive nature of the action in the latter part of the book, as the cathartic effect of the explosion impels the characters to self-knowledge and the fulfillment of their destinies. In theory, it is a fine idea, and as an outline for a novel it has a compelling symmetry. Unfortunately, in practice it is unsatisfying, and even more unfortunately, MacLennan is incapable of supplying any richness of imagery and metaphor to make up the deficiency.

It is frequently pointed out that the explosion in *Barometer Rising* operates as a kind of *deus ex machina* which dispenses an arbitrary, though poetic justice. It interferes with the action, and prevents the confrontations that the early development of the book would seem to demand. For instance, Neil does not encounter Geoffrey Wain until he is safely dead, and the triangular relationship between Neil, Penny, and Angus creates none of the difficulties inherent in the situation. This is quite simply explicable, though, in terms of MacLennan's aesthetics. Just as Canada itself must work out its destiny in terms of individual self-knowledge, so must each of the characters in the novel.

Confrontation leads to victory or defeat, but not to the kind of self-knowledge that MacLennan wants to delineate. The explosion prevents Neil from confronting Colonel Wain and Angus from confronting Neil. Instead, it makes each confront himself and learn to understand himself. At the end of the novel, each of the characters is oddly isolated and self-contained. There has been no development of relationships; but then, that is not what the novel is about. Though Penny and Neil are reunited physically as they ride together on the train, each is completely separate and distinct; that is to say, no communication goes on between them. Neil does not even know that he is a father when the novel ends.

This argument does not absolve the novel of weakness in its close. The process of self-discovery is not particularly convincing, and MacLennan's refusal to permit relationships to grow and change limits the novel and is frustrating to the reader. The argument does absolve MacLennan of much of the charge that his imagination is limited. He does not fail to develop interpersonal relationships because he cannot envision them, but because he chooses to concentrate on the individual's relationship with himself.

Another defect in the novel occurs as a result of MacLennan's use of characters in his novel both as props in his stage setting and participants in the action. The characters are too obviously symbolic. Colonel Wain and Alec MacKenzie represent two facets of the old order, Angus Murray represents the transition and Neil and Penny represent the new order. MacLennan makes the mistake of overestimating the obtuseness of his readers, and to make sure that nobody has missed the point, he allows Angus Murray to sum up the symbolic action in a neat little précis:

> There was Geoffrey Wain, the descendent of military colonists who had remained essentially a colonist himself, never really believing that anything above the second rate could exist in Canada, a man who had not thought it necessary to lick the boots of the English but had merely taken it for granted that they mattered and Canadians didn't. There was Alec MacKenzie, the primitive man who had lived just long enough to bridge the gap out of the pioneering era and save his children from becoming anachronisms. There were Penny and Neil Macrae, two people who could seem at home almost anywhere, who had inherited as a matter of course and in their own country the urbane and technical heritage of both Europe and eastern United States. And there was himself, caught somewhere between the two extremes, intellectually gripped by the new and emotionally held by the old, too restless to remain at peace on the land and too contemptuous of bourgeois values to feel at ease in any city.

All in all though, struggling under the symbolic load they must carry and with their thoughts continually being wrenched away from them by the author, the characters do remarkably well for themselves. Angus Murray is not a very convincing alcoholic, and is perhaps a bit too clear sighted, but he does seem motivated by genuine concerns, and his responses are convincing. Penny Wain does not convince us of her brilliance, but does convince us of her femininity. Colonel Wain, though a megalomaniac is not much more a parody than many real-life colonels. Alec MacKenzie, though a bit too good to be true, is acceptable. Neil number one is indecisive and paranoid, and his actions confirm this. Neil number two is smugly selfish and competent, as is shown by his handling of things after the explosion. The difficulty is that it takes an unusually powerful ability to suspend disbelief to be convinced that the two are one, and that is a chief flaw in the book. We have seen no flashes of the old Neil or the Neil to come in the shuffling character of the first part of the book, and so we are not convinced at his change. The peripheral characters — Aunt Maria, Roddy and the rest who have escaped the symbolic load and who don't do much thinking are all quite delightful.

Style is as much an aspect of form as it is of thought and it is in respect of style that the novel has its chief virtues and its chief faults. MacLennan's greatest strength is in pure narrative description. His point-by-point description of the Halifax explosion is as good as anything of its kind in Canadian literature, or any other literature, for that matter. His description of the details of the landscape are deft and sure and he can characterize people with swift, sure and precise detail. Where he is weakest is in his handling of metaphor, and his novel loses strength from his inability to make vivid and animate comparisons. His ear for dialogue is not particularly good. The speech of his characters is a bit bookish at best, and collapses at moments of deep emotional stress, as may be seen by the stilted conversation between Neil and Penny at their first confrontation. John Yardley's accent in *Two Solitudes* is chiefly the result of his inability to pronounce the "a" in "that," though he can pronounce the same sound well enough in other words. Finally, a tendency to prefer latinate forms, possibly as a result of his training in the classics, leads MacLennan at times to such infelicities of expression as "she welcomed the lassitude as an anodyne to thought" (BR p. 11).

In the end, a novel is not judged by weighing its strengths and weaknesses and drawing up a balance sheet. It must stand on its own, apart from the author's intent and its significance as a philosophic document. On these terms, *Barometer Rising* is a limited success. MacLennan has taken the subject of national consciousness in Canada and given it a form that is convincing. Unfortunately, the novel is weighed down by a lot of stage business that reduces its immediacy and vitality. The clutter is in part a weakness in MacLennan's writing, but another part of it is sheer historical necessity. An evolving Canadian consciousness found its first firm voice in MacLennan, and if that voice is a bit self-conscious, surely that is understandable.

In a conversation between Margaret Laurence and Robert Kroetsch in a book called *Creation*, an interesting passage occurs:

L: You know, I read Kipling, and what the hell did Kipling have to do with where I was living? And that isn't to say that we shouldn't read widely, but it is a good thing to be able to read, as a child, something that belongs to you, belongs to your people. And you and I might have sort of subconsciously had a compulsion to set down our own background.

K: I've suspected that often. We want to hear our story.[4]

Laurence and Kroetsch speak of "our people" and "our story," and unselfconsciously regard themselves as Canadians. I don't think it is too much of an overstatement to say that their easy acceptance of the Canadian fact owes something to the ground broken by Hugh MacLennan.

Notes

[1] Hugh MacLennan, *Two Solitudes* (Toronto: MacMillan of Canada, 1969), p. 365. All further references to the novel will be indicated by the abbreviation TS.
[2] Hugh MacLennan, *Barometer Rising* (Toronto: McClelland & Stewart, 1969), p. 6. All further references to the novel will be indicated by the abbreviation BR.
[3] See pages 133-134, page 197, and pages 200-201 for similar examples.
[4] Robert Kroetsch, ed., *Creation* (Toronto: New Press, 1970), p. 63.

OF CABBAGES AND KINGS: THE CONCEPT OF THE HERO IN *THE WATCH THAT ENDS THE NIGHT*

Elspeth Cameron

In November 1952, MacLennan made the sweeping statement, "As Hemingway goes, so goes writing in our time."[1] It was the publication of *The Old Man and the Sea* which prompted this remark, but it was not in any way tossed off glibly as a book reviewer's means of drawing attention to his subject; it was, and had been for some time, a deeply held belief of MacLennan's. "To those like myself who discovered Hemingway at the end of the 1920's," he would later recall, "English prose as they had known it seemed suddenly stale and dull ... reading Hemingway was pure excitement. He was so fresh then, he so perfectly combined poetry with meticulous accuracy of fact, that for a time he overwhelmed the literary world."[2]

MacLennan's view of Hemingway as "the bell-weather of our flock these past twenty-five years"[3] was of crucial importance in the emergence of the novel he had begun two years earlier in the fall of 1950 — a novel that would not ultimately see publication until 13 February 1959 — for it was through his struggle to define his personal relationship as a writer to the fiction of Hemingway that his unique concept of the hero would emerge in *The Watch that Ends the Night*.

Hemingway did "overwhelm the literary world," as MacLennan observed, by speaking directly to the young men and women growing up in the shadow of the First World War. But not every reader of Hemingway was affected as intensely as MacLennan was. He was utterly enthralled by *The Sun Also Rises* (1926), *A Farewell to Arms* (1929) and *For Whom the Bell Tolls* (1939), novels that were appearing at the very point at which he himself turned from writing "modern" romantic poetry to attempt fiction in the late twenties.

In many ways. MacLennan was exceptionally ripe for the kind of impact Hemingway's fiction was making. His situation virtually guaranteed identification with the youthful North American expatriates Hemingway depicted. As a student at Oxford from 1928-1932 travelling during his "vacs" on the Continent, he fancied himself an "internationalist", observing and comparing the customs of other nations, picking up a smattering of French and much more than a smattering of German, acquiring drinking habits that openly transgressed the teetotaller ethics of his Nova Scotia background. In fact, Hemingway's characters provided ready models for what would soon develop into outright rebellion against the excessively Victorian upbringing he had endured.

His subject at Oxford was classical literature, a study he had pursued under the direction of an overbearing father since boyhood. Not that MacLennan disliked the Classics; on the contrary, Greek and Latin myths had nurtured his early notions of the heroic and Homeric adventures had prepared him to accept their modern counterparts with ease. Now, in Hemingway's bull-fighters and soldiers, he saw classical exploits brought to life in contemporary terms; the First World War, of which he had vivid memories from boyhood himself, was a welcome replacement for the Trojan War as a stage for life's important conflicts.

Furthermore, for a young man in his early twenties existing in what he himself called the "monastic"[4] world of Oxford, Hemingway's women must have seemed delectable. Above all, perhaps, the zeal with which he was throwing himself into rugger and tennis year round as an outlet for his various frustrations as a student, offered a perfect entrée to Hemingway's world of sport and violent activity. This was a heady mixture for MacLennan, and he drank down Hemingway's works in draughts so strong that they became the model outright for his first novel, begun in 1921.

That novel — "So All Their Praises"[5] — was never published, partly because of the effect the Depression had on publishing in general, but also because MacLennan unwittingly had chosen as a model a writer with whom he was at odds in a fundamental way. The rejection of his novel by several publishers forced him to re-assess his talents and begin the process of defining his own theories of fiction. By March 1935, in the midst of a second novel "A Man Should Rejoice"[6], he over-reacted to Hemingway with a disapproval as forceful as his initial idealization: "Inside a few years," he wrote to a friend, "the Hemingway school will be a back number. It is now in process of apotheosis, which is evidence for my statement. The apotheosis of Shaw took place around 1928, and now he is a joke. I believe that by the time we are fifty the Hemingway crowd will be studied as examples of stupidity and derangement." Indeed, he extended his indictment to include all American writers who were, in his opinion, "swimming up

and down sewers saying how tough they were." American fiction seemed to him to be unduly concerned with "the succulence
of mortified flesh."[7] These were strong words from a writer whose
main character in "So All Their Praises" had claimed
Hemingway-style that "bawdiness and art are inseparable."[8]
Since traces of Hemingway's influence persisted well into
MacLennan's second novel (to such a degree that the novel's ending is strongly reminiscent of A Farewell to Arms), his diatribe
in 1935 probably owed more to anger at not finding a publisher
than to any well-reasoned evaluation of Hemingway. It would
be a long time before he could free himself of the spell Hemingway's work had cast over him. Nonetheless, as even the title
of his second novel — "A Man Should Rejoice" — suggests, Hemingway's profound disillusionment with what he called the
"obscenity" of abstract words like "honour" and "duty" (in a
passage which especially intrigued MacLennan)[9] did not jibe with
his own sense of the modern world.

    The borderline rejection of MacLennan's second novel in 1937
was traumatic. In his painful recognition that something was
seriously amiss, he hit on an insight that was to pave the way
to success with his third manuscript, Barometer Rising. Publishers'
reports had indicated that there was considerable confusion over
the novel's point of view; it seemed neither British, nor American,
yet it was English. Where had it come from? Eventually, MacLennan realized that his "Canadianness" (or rather the absence of
any recognizable "Canadian" tradition of fiction to prepare the
way for his work) was an obstacle. As a Canadian attempting to
imitate Americans (and in his second novel he had branched out
to include Sinclair Lewis's Babbitt as a model), he was running
against the grain. As he would later describe it, "Suddenly I
realized that no matter how hard they may try, few writers can
escape their own environment. They are stuck with their own
country whether they want it or not .... Hemingway may have
used Italy, Spain or Cuba for most of his settings; but ... Spain
and Italy are always seen through American eyes."[10] Once
Barometer Rising was published in 1941, he was convinced that
he had been right to give up attempting to become "a Canadian
Hemingway."[11] Nonetheless, he had not entirely laid the ghost —
or rather the all-too-alive presence — of Hemingway to rest.

    How did MacLennan's sense of the modern world differ from
Hemingway's? He worked this out in a series of essays and ar-

ticles written in the fifties while he was working on *The Watch that Ends the Night*. He agreed with Hemingway that the First World War had been a cataclysmic turning point in history. But whereas for Hemingway (as for the majority of so-called "modern" writers and painters between the wars) the War marked a total disillusionment with the Victorian ideals which had fostered it, to MacLennan it represented the ultimate expression of those ideals in a form so extreme that a new age was called for. The post-war years of the twenties and thirties, in MacLennan's eyes, had been "the most prolonged and violent transition human society has suffered since the fall of the Roman Empire,"[12] a transition which had held him "prisoner".

Specifically, these years had been "transitional" in his personal life. Especially between 1932 and 1935, when he had endured a great misery and frustration complying with his father's ambition that he get a Ph.D. from Princeton, MacLennan had felt like a "prisoner". So great had been his despair that the thought of suicide had occurred to him. Eventually, however, the Second World War, which for Hemingway and others would simply spawn further disillusionment, marked the regaining of balance for MacLennan: in 1949 he claimed that there had been "a crystallization of the spirit which possessed England in the summer of 1940 (later he would date this specifically as 10 June 1940[13] when Neville Chamberlain resigned and Churchill took over)" by which he meant generally the rallying speeches in which "Churchill used great words like duty and honour, staked his life on them and restored them to dignity."

In clear opposition to the leading writers and painters of the day, MacLennan went on to state, "the world at large was not as supine or infected as T. S. Eliot and the avant-gardists thought it was. It did not end with a whimper, and those who tried to end it with a bang suffered the greatest military defeat in history."[14]

These observations helped MacLennan identify those aspects of Hemingway's work with which he could not agree. Although he was willing to grant that Hemingway was "a concise, polished craftsman" who, being sensitive, quite rightly had portrayed a violent reaction to the trauma of World War I, he could not condone "his total, his almost nihilistic pessimism." "His desire for honesty," MacLennan explained in an essay called "Changing Values in Fiction", "made life appear worse and more sordid that it actually is."[15] He used a novel by Tom Lea called *The Brave Bulls* to illustrate how the romantic realism of Hemingway was now developing away from nihilism toward an affirmation of life more representative of the times. In contrast, he mentioned Norman Mailer's *The Naked and the Dead* as a deplorable example of the impasse which could result when Hemingway's "nihilism" was taken to extremes.

A decade older than when he first read Hemingway, and happily married to Dorothy Duncan, MacLennan now found Hemingway's women inadequate: "they are almost never real women: they are at best lyric emotions."[16] Indeed, to MacLennan "the history of literature never saw a period in which women were treated with a more incredible contempt and indifference than they were by the best writers of America   between the years 1920 and 1940."[17]

Thus, by 1950 when he began writing *The Watch that Ends the Night*, MacLennan had clarified his position on Hemingway without entirely dispensing with him. There remained an emotional attachment to the first contemporary writer to strike his imagination that he could not shake off. Long before Hemingway committed suicide, he seemed "unbalanced" or deranged to MacLennan, who somewhat clumsily dragged in Freudian references to "the death-wish" to describe Hemingway's most fundamental drive. His ambiguous feelings about Hemingway centred on the passion in Hemingway's work: on the one hand, it was moving, even thrilling; on the other hand, it was dangerous, undoubtedly destructive. As he wrote in 1948, "Canadians might enjoy the books of Hemingway and Faulkner, but we couldn't help regarding them as extreme; and, in the bottom of our hearts we felt that both men were unsound because they both so obviously lacked commonsense."[18]

It is evident from a long letter MacLennan sent to his friend and editor at Macmillans, John Gray, that almost as soon as he had begun drafting scenes for *The Watch that Ends the Night* late in 1950, the whole question of the nature of the hero perplexed him. One aspect of his musings — which had arisen naturally out of the service his previous fiction had done for the growth of Canada's national identity — centred on the relationship between the nation and its citizens, particularly its important citizens or leaders. "It is a fact today," he argued,

... that the destinies of millions of people are not affected by their own characters at all, but by the policies of nations. The novel of civil life, one might say, becomes indistinguishable from the novel of the private soldier in the army. And this theme — the soldier as victim of a huge, blind, inhuman organization — has been done to death.

On the other hand, where individual character was destiny before, national character seems to be destiny now. I have felt this deeply for a long time, ever since before World War II began. And it was this feeling, probably more than anything else, which was responsible for the nature of at least two of my novels before *Each Man's Son*. People who don't feel this way about national character naturally have thought that a book like *The Precipice* was cold and intellectual. At any rate it was a relative failure.

But if you look back on the great dramatic characters — Oedipus, Faust, Hamlet, Lear, Othello, Macbeth — only Hamlet is credible today, assuming Hamlet to be a modern man. No modern man could ignore so blindly the warning signs of impending danger as did the others unless he were mad, in which case he would not be tragic. The last great tragic heroes were Capt. Ahab [*Moby Dick*] and Rubashov [*Darkness at Noon*], and it is significant that Rubashov was not so much the symbol as the incarnation of communistic intellectualism. But any other man intelligent enough to be a great general (Macbeth and Othello), or a great king (Oedipus) would inevitably have enough sophistication, enough knowledge of society and psychology, to withhold his decisive actions until he had verified the evidence. At least, any modern civilized man would so act.

On the other hand, this is not true of nations. Nations are apparently as incapable of heeding warning signs as were primitives like Othello and Oedipus. Nations succeed or fail according to their characters, and in the case of nation after nation, the indirect tragic flaw has brought them to visible ruin before your eyes. Germany was Faust (the ablest and blindest of all the tragic heroes). The flaw in France is *La peur d'être dupe* – the overtrust in the intellectual which enables France as a nation to be satisfied

if she can analyze a situation in such a way to uphold her intellectual vanity even at the cost of her existence. The flaw in the United
States is the flaw of adolescent pride, which is constantly at war
with the good side of that same adolescent who has received a
very moral upbringing and can't understand why everyone
doesn't like him, who doesn't want to grow up and – oh, God,
the United States is so complicated and yet so transparent!

But a country like ours, at least up to the moment, is at best
a sort of Horatio to Hamlet – though the U.S.A. is not much
of a Hamlet.[19]

Behind these remarks hovered the Korean War which for the
last six months had been much on everyone's mind. To MacLennan, it had special significance because it threatened to disprove
his theory that the Second World War had marked a strenthen-
ing of moral optimism and that a new (and better) age was imminent. Judging from his literary comparisons, he was now ignoring Hemingway (possibly because Hemingway's *Across the
River and Into the Trees* had attracted critical scorn that year) and
turning instead to Shakespeare (whose tragedies had been held
up by both his father and his Oxford friends as supreme example of the heroic) in his search for models. Certainly his own personal experience had militated against his accepting any notion
that character is destiny: a wilful father, the Depression and two
world wars — to mention only the salient examples which might
have sprung first to his mind — had moulded his life regardless.
What he groped for, as if in the dark, was a hero that would both
be as "great" and "tragic" (and as "famous") as Shakespeare's
heroes, but who also would reflect the modern age more accurately than most so-called "modern" protagonists. "It is no accident," he maintained to Gray, "that the best contemporary
novels have narrowed the field so that they deal with only a few
individuals and probe the depth of those characters, yet have,
on the whole, been unable to make the claim that these characters
are "great" enough to be genuinely "tragic."[20]

To complicate matters, after getting his knuckles rapped by
Canadian critics for straying south of the border in his third
published novel *The Precipice*, he was more convinced than ever
that he must write out of and reflect the Canadian scene if he
was to be successful. That meant that his hero must also be

quintessentially "Canadian". Since Canada seemed to him (in that comparison suggested by an image from a poem by Douglas LePan, "Coureurs de bois" (1948)) much more like the minor character Horatio than the flamboyant hero Hamlet, the dilemma seemed impossible to resolve. Overlooking Horatio's sterling qualities for the simple reason that he was not centre-stage, MacLennan wrestled with the contradiction he saw between the need to create a modern hero of real stature and the necessity of reflecting a national character that was far from heroic.

Fortunately, the new job he took up at McGill in the fall of 1951 gave him the security he needed to ponder these issues. Gone was the insistent desperation with which he had churned out *Each Man's Son*, a novel which had, in his opinion, "become narrow, cloistered and bitter"[21] in the writing. Teaching courses on the history of English prose and modern fiction, both of which included Hemingway, were just what he needed to allow his mind free range on literary matters and to give time a chance to pass.

Six months later, he looked once again at the world in general and at Canada and literary matters in particular and put forward his views in an address for the University of New Brunswick called "The Present as Seen in its Literature".[22] Although he spoke of the artist at large, his remarks were highly personal:

> The literture of doom and despair - its eloquence and sombre beauty has filled our minds and interpreted our emotions from 1914 to the present time. And now, quite suddenly, its mood has been fractured. Any one who writes books today feels as if he were in the unnatural calm which lies in the cone of a typhoon. The hour is midnight and all around him the winds are whirling. He knows they are there, but suddenly he can't hear them, he can't guess what their direction will be when they strike again. Since the atom bomb fell on Hiroshima; more particularly since the world split into two opposite camps between east and west; the shape of things to come has been obscured. The artist, like everyone else, feels the iminent presence of tremendous events. But what their nature will be — above all what direction these events will take — the artist cannot even guess. Not only are signs lacking. Familiar symbols have become inadequate .... Since 1945, most of our literature has lost the power to use the symbols of its

trade to mediate between men and the corrosive force of their undefined emotions .... It may very possibly mean that the moral climate has changed for the better.[23]

With reference to Hemingway, T. S. Eliot, Faulkner, Mailer and others, MacLennan described the literature of the first half of the twentieth century as one of "frustrated heroism", the high point (or rather the low point) of which was "the suicidal mood of the 1930's"[24] best represented by Hemingway. MacLennan singled out a novel by the South African writer Alan Paton, *Cry, The Beloved Country*, as an example of what he thought was a shift from nihilism to affirmation: like Hemingway, Paton "shrinks from nothing," but his hero, the black parson Stephen Kumalo, is a "symbol which will have, for later writers, a power of attraction greater than that of any hero of Hemingway" because he demonstrates that love is "more enormous" than hate.[25]

And what of Canada's potential role in this moral edification? MacLennan rose to rhetorical heights as he expressed his renewed faith in a Canada that had been changing apace: "Canada has been uniquely fortunate in the past forty years. She entered this century as narrowly innocent as a puritanical adolescent .... She, too, has undergone prodigious psychological changes, but instead of being ground down into the mud, she has only been splashed with it by passing cars. She has lost her innocence and with its loss the symbols of childhood have lost their power and use .... More and more we are becomng a nation of city-dwellers. More and more have we become involved directly and past recall in international affairs."[26]

As MacLennan indicated here, Canada was evolving into a position that would render her *especially suited* to represent the spirit of the new age. Canadian writers and painters alike, according to him, were already busy exploring "in their own quiet way" the "frontiers of the spirit." Gone was Canada's earlier Victorian notion of "virtue" as equivalent to "good" (a subject he had treated in *The Precipice*; at last the time was ripe for the treatment of evil in relation to love. With new confidence, MacLennan baldly claimed, "I predict that twenty-five years from now the literature and art of Canada will have developed so far that it will be recognized as an integral part of the literature and art of the English-speaking world."[27]

Within a year, he had refined these ideas into the single statement that was to be the bedrock of his aesthetic theory from then
on: that the artist had the responsibility "within a framework of
truth to make compensation for the human predicament."[28] In
other words, great art must show that good triumphs over evil,
that the force of love is more powerful than that of destructive
hate.

Although this speech shows that MacLennan had resolved national matters for his own purposes as a writer, it reveals that
he was still having difficulty settling on a hero. "The mercury
is still wavering in the glass," he admitted. "The compasses are
still swinging in wild and contradictory directions."[29] A scan of
the many articles and essays he wrote for journals during the
1950s suggests the crux of his problem: he was torn in his notion
of the "heroic". On the one hand, he greatly admired sheer
physical strength, but on the other hand, he respected moral
strength, a strength of character which might be termed stoic.
The former arose directly from his boyhood love of boxing, tennis, sailing and other sports and was reinforced in much of the
literature he enjoyed — Homeric adventures or the Boys Own Paper
and Chums escapades; the latter resulted from his admiration of
his father who set his son an example of stoicism by his great
powers of endurance which MacLennan — especially in completing the long education his father chose for him — imitated
through the habit of self-denial, an attitude also reinforced by
literature, mainly explicitly Christian.

These two concepts of the "heroic" were not entirely compartmentalized for MacLennan — his father encouraged his tennis,
for example — but for his purposes as a writer, they were not
easily reconciled. His articles during the decade frequently concerned athletic heroes: baseball stars like Ty Cobb,[30] hockey
players like Maurice "Rocket" Richard,[31] tennis champions like
William Tilden[32] and sailors like Joshua Slocum[33]; a fascination
which culminated in an essay called significantly "The Homeric
Tradition" (1955).[34] In this piece, MacLennan admitted that his
favourite writers (judged at least by the amount of time spent
reading) had been the sports columnists in the newspapers. He
confessed at once that the "celebration of champions" in modern
sports columns was exclusively male fare, but went on to justify
his enduring interest by tracing the genre right back to Homer's
Iliad. Such heroes display "enough physical, mental and moral

capacity to offer a real challenge to destiny." For most readers, he concluded, "physical prowess, the perfect control of the nervous system, the body and the mind, the absolute dedication to performing a difficult action supremely well, is worth any man's life-time effort." Successful athletes provide modern men with "a larger-than-life" hero.

Although MacLennan stoutly defended this view of the "heroic" with some consistency, and even claimed that it put demands on the intelligence that equalled the physical, he knew better. The truth was that the kind of intelligence he saw in sports was closer to the cunning of Ulysses than to any civilized wisdom. "The better an athlete is," he said elsewhere, "the less he knows about what he is doing .... His performance rushes right out of his subconscious so that he seems possessed by a power greater than his own."[35]

The instinctive man of action, he knew, had limitations: too often such men could degenerate into mere brutality. Shakespeare's heroes, he observed in contrast elsewhere, Hamlet in particular, represented man as "noble, like an angel, the paragon of animals,"[36] since heroes like Hamlet were more likely to think and debate than act. MacLennan, intellectually at least, was more likely to agree that Shakespeare's heroes were more truly "great" and "tragic" than Hemingway's. Emotionally, though, his attraction to the heroic splendour of men of action persisted, not least in his continuing admiration of Hemingway.

In an essay that obliquely throws considerable light on this matter, "Modern Tennis — A Study in Decadence",[37] he defined decadence in sport by referring to Hemingway's description of the development of bull-fighting in Spain: "decay sets in when an art, once satisfying, begins to magnify certain aspects at the expense of the activity as a whole." His argument eventually carried over into the realm of writing. Just as he saw tennis being destroyed by the "mania for speed," so also he saw that Hemingway's need for "immediate and constant tension"[38] had chipped away at the integrity of the "hero": Hemingway's "heroes," he was saying by 1954, "are generally monosyllabic primitives in search of dream girls and combat for the sake of the muscle-flexing and excitement it gives them"; they are "incomplete ... as human beings."[39]

If MacLennan saw so clearly the limitations of the physical hero, if he really believed that the heroes of most modern literature

(Hemingway's in particular) were adolescent, incomplete, even decadent, and if he truly wished to opt for the quiet maturity he considered representative of the new era in general and of Canada especially, why did his attachment to the physical style of heroism persist? One simple answer might be that he had not entirely outgrown those adolescent fantasies he claimed to deplore. But there is another reason more important to his craft as a writer. Although he did not see it fully himself, he sensed that the physical hero demanded fast action writing, and that fast action writing was more dramatic and interesting for readers of fiction. To put it another way, ever since his success with the powerful description of the Halifax explosion in *Barometer Rising*, he had felt most at ease writing about violent action. Physical conflict had always called forth his best talents. And it was this that he continued to admire in Hemingway. The master's heroes might be brutal goons, but the descriptive prose their antics elicited was matchless.

By 1954, by which time he was well into the writing of his own novel, he was finally able to separate Hemingway's content from Hemingway's style. In "Homage to Hemingway", the only original essay in the collection *Thirty and Three* which Dorothy Duncan assembled that year, MacLennan praised "the morning freshness of his style," the power of his language and his fidelity to the world of the five senses.[40] "The undeniable fact remains," MacLennan maintained, "that each time we encounter the prose of Hemingway himself (divorcing it from any ideas we may expect it to convey) we recognize it as the work of a master in its ability to move us and expand our perceptions."[41] But that parenthetical qualification was crucial:

> Since his interest is to make us feel, he can seldom allow us to think. He dare not use characters who are thoughtful men, for if he did they would ruin the bare perfection of his style by speaking in a dialogue full of abstract words .... Thoughtful men cannot help living on mental levels that are distinct from physical ones. They are too rational, or too engrossed with the need of earning a living, to go to Africa to shoot lions or to Spain to watch bulls being killed. Liquor is apt to dull their perceptions instead of heightening them, as liquor seems to do for Hemingway's heroes. Rational men discuss their own neuroses, they are interested in

science, they become involved in a multitude of activities for which the Hemingway style lacks an adequate vocabulary. They argue about communism and
democracy, are concerned with the high cost of living
and getting on in their jobs, they worry about their
children's education and the danger of another depression. They show an interest in women as personalities,
not as mere embodiments of a sensual dream. Their
sexual lives are not ritualistic. In short, their minds,
their ambitions, their awareness of themselves as
coherent, complex personalities involved in a mundane
existence makes them entirely unsuitable as catalysts for
Hemingway. Such men are even apt to wonder at times
how they can save their souls.[42]

Because Hemingway had reduced men to the level of animals and
influenced others to do the same, MacLennan judged him "to
a considerable extent responsible for the unhappy condition of
the novel at the present time."[43]

By the spring of 1955, this view of Hemingway had firmed into a doctrinaire stance: "Hemingway's very genius," he told a
gathering of the Royal Society of Canada, "has put him in a strait-
jacket .... Educated men do not talk like Hemingway
characters."[44] From now on, MacLennan would associate Hemingway with derangement by using the image of the "strait-
jacket" to describe what his style did to content. "The novel must
return to people again," MacLennan confidently asserted in what
was implicitly a description of his own contrasting aims with his
current novel, "must prove its power to celebrate and judge their
lives, must believe in their value, and must respect the
audience."[45]

To whom could MacLennan now turn for models of "heroism"?
Shakespeare, as we have seen, had been lurking in the back of
his mind since 1950 in relation to his theory of the "tragic flaw"
in nations. In his letter to John Gray, he had decided that among
Shakespeare's heroes, he could imagine only Hamlet taking part
in any modern dilemma. It seemed since then that he had abandoned them as models, but now, five years later, he re-read
twenty-two plays of Shakespeare with some view to evaluating
those heroes once again.

To his astonishment, he found that "more than any writer who
ever lived, Shakespeare took it for granted that decent men are

dull. Worse still he assumed they were all dupes. He does not offer a single truly religious person in the whole folio, none who is at once steadfast, intelligent and competent."[46] Like the heroes of Hemingway, Shakespeare's men seemed incomplete to MacLennan; like Hemingway, Shakespeare seemed to know "that ... even an attempt to tell the whole truth about his characters would spoil the fine theatrical effects he wanted"; like Hemingway, Shakespeare was foremost a "magician" skilled at "incantation".[47]

The only thoughtful heroes MacLennan could locate in contemporary literature were those of the British novelist C. P. Snow who seemed to have appropriated the authority of science for the world of fiction,[48] but somehow — although they commanded his respect — Snow's novels left MacLennan a little cold: "But what of books like these?" he wrote to John Gray. "Is knowledge and insight and analytical power enough? Somewhere the soul rebels .... Reading Snow reminded me of the passage in Lucretius about the joys of standing on a promontory and watching the sailors struggling in the sea."[49] Ultimately, MacLennan abandoned the search for a model hero, and turned instead to Conrad and Tolstoy for inspiration in the realm of theme and form. He would have to work the matter out on his own.

In an essay exploring this quandary, called "The Death of the Hero"[50], MacLennan continued to chart the direction he himself must take. Neither in life nor in literature were there heroes to emulate: "With the resignation of Winston Churchill from active life," he wrote, "it has become a time without heroes above the level of the sports arena .... The few literary heroes remaining, Eliot, Hemingway, Faulkner, are tired old men .... There are no heroes any more, either in books or in the world of letters itself." Recognizing that "heroes can exist only when men have some fairly clear idea of what they think life ought to be," he concluded that "literature ... must continue to nudge closer and closer to the truth of life, deal with more reality and less magic and the incantation of words."

Considering that MacLennan had been struggling hard to work out his own theory of the heroic at the same time he was incorporating those notions into his novel, and that he had already created heroes in four previous novels, it must have irked him to read in a learned journal "that Canada has produced no great writers because ours is a country without a single literary hero

— the argument being that greatness in a literary man depends on his ability to create characters."[51] This remark prodded him into further action, however. Two months later, in an essay called "The Transition Ends" (1955), he appears to have considered and accepted this premise and to have focussed many of his previous thoughts about the present situation in literature:

> If it is in the character of the fictional hero that an age reveals its inner meaning, it seems to me the best proof that the temper of society has changed is that these solitary, neurotic, haunted heroes of the past fifty years are already beginning to look like historical characters. What manner of man the new hero will be cannot yet be seen, but it is almost certain that he will be more intelligent than the haunted men of the transition, less desperate, less neurotic, and more willing to accept life as it is. As it is with men, so it is with nations. Only by accepting their own limitations can they become wise; only by facing their own fears can they be happy. [52]

"The world of art," he maintained in an image from his earlier speech about watching the "typhoon" of the modern world, is "barometric"[53], since it reflects society. Because "the conditions which produced the attitudes of 'modernists' like Eliot, Picasso, James Joyce, Proust, Dos Passos and Hemingway have changed out of all recognition," a hero more typical of the "quiet accents" of the "new age" is called for. As MacLennan now saw it, the "ferocious neuroticism" that characterized the heroes of the age of transition "developed into the psychoses of fascism, communism and naziism" with the result that "the literary heroes of the transitional age became increasingly more desperate and still more solitary." For examples he referred to Andre Malraux's *La Condition Humaine* and Arthur Koestler's *Darkness at Noon*. It was now the ordinary man, the "little man" [as in *Little Man, What Now?* by Rudolf Ditzen] that typified that 1950s. In an article only three months later, "Will TV Produce a New Breed of Canadian Hero?"[54] he concluded that the absence in Canada of "hero-worship" for any Superman (which he dismissed as "the oldest recurrent dream of the mentally ungrown") signalled national maturity. As for Canada's adulation of athletes, he excused this on grounds that it provided a healthy "emotional safety-valve" for man's innate aggression.[55]

Although MacLennan's deliberations about the nature of the hero were not the only problems with which he was wrestling during the first half of the fifties (considerations of form, time and theme also plagued him), it was primarily of his own heroes that he was thinking when he confessed to John Gray in 1954, "I'm still hoping to get the novel ready for a fall publication in 1955, but this is one book I simply can't afford to rush. Which doesn't mean the writing — that in itself is no longer a problem to me — but grasping the meaning."[56]

Grasping the meaning of casting an ordinary man or "little man" as his hero was indeed difficult. As he recognized, "it is not the new age, but the transition to it that stirs the passions."[57] How was he to make a quiet, little, ordinary man as interesting as those shocking, even scandalous heroes of the transition had been?

The resolution of this challenge came gradually through the merging of an opinion MacLennan had long worked on independently and the theories of psychology which had by now filtered into common parlance. As far back as 1949, MacLennan saw the use to which psychology might be put in the service of fiction. Neither television nor movies, he argued, could "probe deeply below the surface of the individual mind .... The inner scene of a novel — the one that counts — is more private than a confessional box, for it is both the conscious *and* unconscious of the individual character .... The more public our outer lives are, the more private our inner lives have become .... It is to this privacy, this solitude within the apparently uniform crowd, that the novelist of today addresses himself."[58]

By 1956, that vague "search for the frontiers of the spirit" which had been the keynote of his address at New Brunswick in 1952 had become much more precise. "In the human subconscious," as everyone these days is supposed to know," he wrote, "sadism and masochism are constantly at grips. Between the hunter and the hunted, the slugger and the slugged, the subconscious bond is profound."[59] The truly dramatic conflict of the mid-twentieth century for MacLennan as he worked through this theory was the one that took place within every individual between the contradictory impulses that made man the unique creature he is. Fascinated as he had always been at the tension between man's urge to create and his compulsion to destroy — a concern that lay behind the best essay he wrote during these years "Joseph

Haydn and Captain Bligh"[60]—MacLennan absorbed the popular psychology of his day and created for his fourth published novel a protagonist whose response to inner conflict illustrated his heroic mettle.

With George Stewart in *The Watch that Ends the Night*, MacLennan illustrated his theory of the hero. A man of no extraordinary talents, not even possessed of that "life-force" he envies in both his friend, the surgeon Jerome Martell, and his own wife, the painter Catherine, George embarks on a heroic odyssey of the soul. The circumstances of his life compel him to respond, and he does so with innate nobility. Like Marlow in Conrad's *Heart of Darkness*, one of the books MacLennan was teaching at McGill and which in its psychological theme was one model for his own book, George plumbs the depth of human despair and feels every lust and murderous impulse of which man is capable. He travels down into the evil in his own soul, knows chaos, and, despite the temptation to commit suicide in the face of nihilism, chooses form, morality and love. At the novel's climax, George faces the crippling knowledge that Catherine must die — and fairly soon — of the embolisms caused with increasing frequency by her weak heart. Furthermore, he must come to grips with this under the enormous stress of knowing that Jerome, the man Catherine has passionately loved and married before himself, although long thought dead, has returned and visited her in his absence. "Then," as George puts it, "comes the Great Fear .... There was no discharge in this war. There was only endurance. There lay ahead only the fearful tunnel with nothing at the end. Could I or could I not — could she or could she not — believe that this struggle had any value in itself?"

For a time, George weakens and yields to the destructive impulses in himself, an experience which is mirrored by MacLennan in one of the very few passages that approach stream-of-consciousness in his work:

> My subconscious rose. The subconscious — the greedy, lustful, infantile subconscious, indiscriminate and uncritical discoverer of truths, half-truths and chimaeras which are obscene fusions of foetal truths, this source of hate, love, murder and salvation, of poetry and destruction, this Everything in Everyman, how quickly if it swamps him, can it obliterate the character a man has spent a lifetime creating!

Then a man discovers in dismay that what he believed to be his identity is no more than a tiny canoe at the
mercy of an ocean. Shark-filled, plankton-filled, refractor
of light, terrible and mysterious, for years this ocean
has seemed to slumber beneath the tiny identity it
received from the dark river.

Now the ocean rises and the things within it become
visible. Little man, what now? The ocean rises, all
frames disappear from around the pictures, there is no
form, no sense, nothing but chaos in the darkness of
the ocean storm. Little man, what now?

The resolution comes from deep inside himself; somehow he finds
the strength to cope:

... And the earth was without form, and void; and
darkness was on the face of the deep.
... And the spirit of God moved upon the face of the
waters. And God said: *let there be light*: and there was
light.
Here, I found at last, is the nature of the final human
struggle. Within, not without.[61]

Although it is possible to criticize MacLennan for casting his
hero's revelation in words from the Bible rather than his own,
or to fault his artistry for leading us up to this tremendous insight only to admit that he finds it impossible to describe such
a struggle in words, his representation of a type of heroism suited
to contemporary times is clear. And it could not be further from
Hemingway. Indeed, it is a total rejection of those "greedy,
lustful, infantile" impulses that, according to him, motivated his
former idol's heroes. As George comments elsewhere in the
novel, "there it was, the ancient marriage of good and evil, the
goodness of this day and compulsive evil people must see and
know, but the sky dominated in the end. Pale and shining, it told
me that our sins can be forgiven."[62] As the novel's original title
— "Requiem" — suggests, MacLennan intended to pay tribute
in a way more appropriate to the 1950s to his own "lost
generation."[63]

The extraordinary thing about *The Watch that Ends the Night*
seems to be MacLennan's inclusion of a character such as Jerome
Martell in a novel that relegated Hemingway and his heroes to
the back seats of modern fiction. At first glance Jerome is a hero

remarkably similar to Hemingway's men: physically strong, animalistic and instinctive, full of that "explosive" life-force that more often than not causes chaos, a man attracted to war (even to the Spanish Civil War in which Hemingway's Robert Jordan had fought), his essence seems to be caught in the name he has taken from his adopted parents — Martell "the hammer". According to MacLennan, he flowed directly from a dream into his imagination in the winter of 1956, complete with the episode (so reminiscent of Hemingway) in which he escapes down-river in a canoe from a man bent on destroying him. In fact, he would later single Jerome out as "the key figure of the novel:"[64]

> By what strange guidance was he nameless? Why that scene in New Brunswick .... Ostensibly he had no part in the novel I was blundering along with, but some force caused me to know this was integral, and I spent a winter on it.[65]

For MacLennan, the character Jerome had come to him as a flash-back to "the prehistoric origins of original sins"; "if the public," he could later claim, "can't feel any sympathy or pity for Martell, all I can say is that they refuse to look into their own souls."[66] Tracing Jerome's revolutionary tendencies right back to the first rising of man against the father, MacLennan created a character who seems to be taken wholesale from Hemingway.

However, although Jerome is portrayed in much the same way as a Hemingway hero, and is manifestly a protagonist of what MacLennan called the "transition", he is fundamentally different from Hemingway's men: the great "spirit" in him that expresses itself destructively also shows itself in the *creative* drive to heal others through his extraordinary powers as a surgeon. Ultimately, it is Jerome whose mere presence in her hospital room calls Catherine back from the brink of death: "He is," MacLennan would later explain to John Gray, "in some ways, a great man. The same force which gives life also destroys it, and then rebuilds it."[67] The hammer is not only a weapon, it is also a *tool*; the Biblical Jerome may have been militant, but he was also a soldier *of God*. It is true that MacLennan emphasizes Jerome's destructive capacities, but it is important to note that he illustrates that it is *circumstances* beyond the control of the individual (in this case that "transition" of the thirties which included the Spanish Civil War) that are responsible for this. It is man's prerogative, however, within any particular arena, to choose the direction his energies take: every man has the opportunity to resolve within himself the great conflict between his destructive urges and his creative powers.

Jerome is not a Hemingway-style hero; he is simply George Stewart writ large. Both men share with all men and women[68] the same dilemma, and to MacLennan that dilemma was the fundamental nexus of the human condition. Circumstances might vary from one person to the next and the inner strength of one individual would never be exactly the same as that of another, but for MacLennan, as he described it in a CBC talk later published as "The Story of a Novel"[69], "somehow I was going to write a book which would not depend on character-in-action, but on spirit-in-action. The conflict here, the essential one, was between the human spirit of Everyman and Everyman's human condition." This, he explained, meant rejecting both Shakespeare's external action (as both "inaccurate and inadequate") and the heroes of modern novels (who were "outcasts ... men excessively primitive ... excessively criminal").

In *The Watch that Ends the Night*, MacLennan managed to have his cake and eat it too. Not only did he create in George Stewart a hero who was truly representative of the modern age, whose inner conflict seemed both "great" and "tragic", but he managed in Jerome Martell a "larger-than-life" hero who could be represented in Hemingway-style fast action prose without endorsing Hemingway's "pessimistic nihilism." MacLennan portrayed the variety of "Everyman's human condition" by showing these two men side by side. For George, a cruel personal fate imposes itself from without; Jerome is swept up on the wave of mindless passion that war had always seemed to MacLennan. Each of them pits that "human spirit of Everyman" against his own particular "human condition", but the struggle is at heart the same. And the resolution is the same: the power of good (or the creative drive) ultimately triumphs over the power of evil (or the destructive drive). Why? Because for MacLennan the will to survive is stronger than despair.

From his personal experience, MacLennan was predisposed to view the world this way. Not only did his intensely Christian upbringing have its effect, but his own struggles to overcome despair[70] — both in the 1930s at Princeton and again in the 1950s when his wife's existence hung teetering in the balance — also marked him. The aesthetic philosophy of affirmation which he developed theoretically during the fifties and incorporated into *The Watch that Ends the Night* reflected a temperamental necessity.

As he wrote his novel, his choice for a personal hero, as described in his essay "Triumph: the Story of a Man's Greatest Moment" (1957)[71], was Handel. An unlikely choice at first glance, but the pattern was the same: a life that was a sequence of disasters, temporary despair, forbearance derived from Christian revelation, a drying up of artistic inspiration, despair; and then, in a burst of glory, the creation of the *Messiah*. Overcoming the urge to destroy oneself, faith that life is worth living, patience while waiting for creativity to flare up again — this was for MacLennan the truly heroic enterprise of man, and one which he was watching firsthand during this decade while his wife — like Catherine — fought for her very life as a series of embolisms broke her strength but not her creativity. Despair might haunt the darkest watch that ended the night, but the rising sun of affirmation was sure to follow.

In dramatizing the "subconscious bond" between the creative and destructive aspects of man, MacLennan's fiction took a giant step forward. In *Each Man's Son* he had tried to illustrate each of these impulses in separate characters: the brutal prizefighter Archie MacNeil and the humanitarian doctor Daniel Ainslie. But even in those two characters there were hints that personality could not be that simple. Despite MacLennan's confidence in the almost god-like powers of doctors, Ainslie has more than a touch of granite in his will; and Archie somehow enlists our sympathy in a way no outright goon ever could. In *The Watch that Ends the Night*, these undertones blossomed into full understanding. Through battling with the theory of a hero for modern times, MacLennan had seen that all of us are potential bullies and possible healers; the two were never mutually exclusive.

MacLennan used the work of Hemingway as a springboard to launch a hero he thought reflected the new age. George's maturity would represent a development beyond those adolescent heroes of the twenties; his "quiet accents" would replace the "ferocious neuroticism" that had characterized the "suicidal" thirties; above all, his inner battle to overcome the destructive demons called forth by despair would transport readers across the frontiers of the spirit. Although the splendid Jerome might seem remote from the lives of average readers because his particular "human condition" was unusually dramatic and his "human spirit" remarkably strong, George Stewart was a man with whom any reader could imaginatively trade places in order to see the importance, the depth and even the beauty of the age-old pattern.

Notes

1   H.M., "The View from Here", *Montrealer* (Nov. 1952), p. 58.
2   H.M., "Hemingway, Hunter and the Hunted", A Writer's Diary, *Montreal Star* (21 Sept. 1963), p. 4.
3   H.M., "The View from Here", *Montrealer* (Nov. 1952), p. 58.
4   H.M., letter to his mother, 4 Dec. 1929, property of Frances MacLennan.
5   H.M., "So All Their Praises", unpublished ms., McGill Collection, box 3, part 1, folders 1-2.
6   H.M., "A Man Should Rejoice", unpublished ms., McGill Collection, box 3, part 2, folders 3-9.
7   H.M., letter to George Barret, 5 March 1935, McCord Museum, Montreal.
8   H.M., "So All Their Praises", p. 147.
9   This passage, found in *A Farewell to Arms*, is quoted and analysed at some length by MacLennan in "Changing Values in Fiction", *Canadian Author and Bookman*, 25, No. 3 (Autumn 1949), pp. 13ff.
10   H.M., "The Discovery of Canada as a Literary Scene", unpublished address, University of Rochester (1935), McGill Collection, box 1, part 1, folders 3, 1-9. See also "Literature in a New Country", *Scotchman's Return and Other Essays*, (Toronto: Macmillan, 1960), pp. 140-1.
11   H.M., "Culture, Canadian Style", *Saturday Review of Literature*, 25 (28 March 1942), p. 18.
12   H.M., "Fifty Grand", *Montrealer* (May 1957), p. 38.
13   H.M., "The Present World as Seen in its Literature", Founder's Day Address, University of New Brunswick (18 Feb. 1952), p. 8.
14   H.M., "Changing Values in Fiction", p. 14.
15   *Ibid.*, p. 13
16   H.M. probably took this idea directly from an essay on Hemingway by Edmund Wilson in 1941; see "Hemingway: Gauge of Miracle", *The Wound and the Bow* (London: Methuen, 1961), p. 199, where the lovers in *A Farewell to Arms* are described as "the abstractions of a lyric emotion."
17   H.M., "Changing Values in Fiction", p. 15.
18   H.M., "The Future Trend in the Novel", *Canadian Author and Bookman*, 24, No. 3 (Sept. 1948), p. 5.
19   H.M., letter to John Gray, 7 Dec. 1950, Macmillan Collection.
20   *Ibid.*
21   H.M., letter to John Gray, 5 Jan. 1953, Macmillan Collection.
22   H.M., "The Present World as Seen in its Literature", Founder's Day Address (18 Feb. 1952).
23   *Ibid.*, pp. 5-6.
24   *Ibid.*, p. 7.
25   *Ibid.*, p. 11.
26   *Ibid.*, p. 12
27   *Ibid.*
28   H.M., "The Artist and Critic in Society", *Princeton Alumni Weekly*, 53 (30

Jan. 1953), p. 91.

29 H.M., "The Present World as Seen in its Literature", p. 11.

30 H.M., "The View from Here", *Montrealer* (May 1952), pp. 58-9.

31 H.M., "Cinerama 'Nightmare'; Spirit of Hockey", *Saturday Night* (26 Feb. 1955), pp. 9-10.

32 H.M., "Modern Tennis — A Study in Decadence", *Montrealer* (Nov. 1953), pp. 54-5.

33 H.M., "A Great Story Reborn", *Montrealer* (May 1953), pp. 54-5.

34 H.M., "The Homeric Tradition", *Montrealer* (Sept. 1955), p. 21, p. 23.

35 H.M., "The View from Here", *Montrealer* (May 1952), pp. 58-9.

36 H.M., "The View from Here", *Montrealer* (Nov. 1952), pp. 58-9.

37 H.M., "Modern Tennis — A Study in Decadence", p. 54.

38 H.M., "Changing Values in Fiction", p. 15.

39 H.M., "Homage to Hemingway", *Thirty and Three* (Toronto: Macmillan, 1954), pp. 86-7.

40 *Ibid.*, p. 86.

41 *Ibid.*, p. 87

42 *Ibid.*, pp. 94-5.

43 *Ibid.*, p. 95.

44 H.M., "The Challenge to Prose", *Transactions of the Royal Society of Canada*, 49, Series 3, Section 2 (June 1955), p. 53.

45 *Ibid.*, p. 55.

46 H.M., "Shakespeare Revisited", *Montrealer* (May 1955), p. 23.

47 *Ibid.*, pp. 23-4.

48 H.M., "Death of the Hero", *Montrealer* (June 1955), p. 25.

49 H.M., letter to John Gray, 21 Dec. 1951, Macmillan Collection.

50 H.M., "Death of the Hero", *Montrealer* (June 1955).

51 H.M., "The Homeric Tradition", *Montrealer* (Sept. 1955), p. 23.

52 H.M., "The Transition Ends", *Montrealer* (Nov. 1955), p. 27.

53 *Ibid.*, p. 25.

54 H.M., "Will TV Produce a New Breed of Canadian Hero?" *Liberty* (Feb. 1956), pp. 32-3, 52, 54.

55 This was an idea he explored elsewhere, notably during the same year in "Confessions of a Wood-Chopping Man", *Montrealer* (Nov. 1956), pp. 22-4. Characteristically, he saw his own athletic endeavors as serving the same purpose.

56 H.M., letter to John Gray, 6 July 1954, Macmillan Collection.

57 H.M., "The Transition Ends", p. 25.

58 H.M., "Changing Values in Fiction", *Canadian Author and Bookman*, p. 25, No. 3 (Autumn, 1949), p. 18.

59 H.M., "Will TV Produce a New Breed of Canadian Hero", *Liberty* (Feb. 1956), p. 54.

60 H.M., "Joseph Haydn and Captain Bligh", *Montrealer* (July 1953), pp. 50-51.

61 H.M., *The Watch that Ends the Night* (New York: Scribners, 1959), pp. 342-3.

62 *Ibid.*, pp. 168-9.

63 "The title came to me the other day, and the requiem is only incidentally for Dorothy. As I see the novel, it is for our whole generation." (H.M., letter to John Gray, 15 June 1957).

64 H.M., letter to John Gray, 28 Jan. 1958, Macmillan Collection.

65 H.M., letter to John Gray, 4 Feb. 1958, Macmillan Collection.

66 H.M., letter to John Gray, 9 March 1958, Macmillan Collection

67 *Ibid.*

[68] Although this paper deals only with MacLennan's male heroes, the same truths are demonstrated in Catherine who is both creative painter and "spiritual vampire".

[69] H.M., "The Story of a Novel", *Canadian Lit.*, 3 (Winter, 1960), pp. 35-9.

[70] H.M., "Fifty Grand: A Semi-Centenarian Takes Stock", *Montrealer* (May 1957), pp. 37-41.

[71] H.M., "Triumph: The Story of a Man's Greatest Moment", *Montrealer* (March 1957), pp. 53-6, 58.

ELISABETH SMART

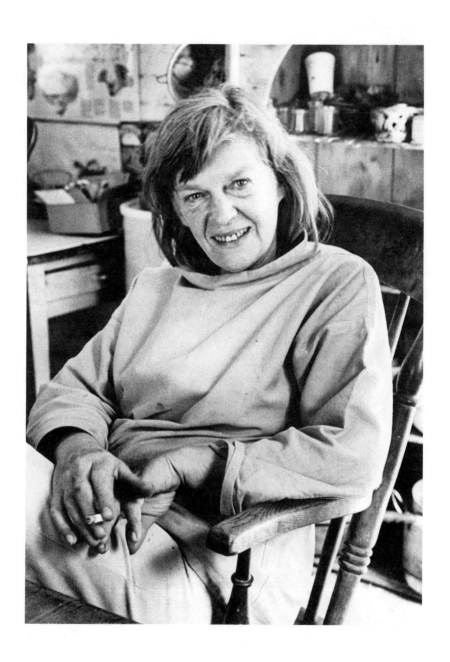

ELIZABETH SMART'S LYRICAL NOVEL: *BY GRAND CENTRAL STATION I SAT DOWN AND WEPT*

Lorraine McMullen

Elizabeth Smart's *By Grand Central Station I Sat Down and Wept* is an unusual novel. Closer in many ways to a symbolist poem, an impressionist painting, or a piece of music than to the traditional novel, it is most aptly termed a lyrical novel.

When pieced together, events of the novel strike us as ordinary, perhaps even mundane. A young woman falls in love with a married man and has a brief affair with him; he returns to his wife and she finds herself alone and pregnant. Magazine racks are filled with stories of such unhappy love affairs, but the classics, too — Shakespeare, Ovid, Euripides, Wagner — all give us tales of ill-starred romances. The mode of expression, not the plot line, dictates whether a work is a world classic or pulp magazine fiction. Elizabeth Smart is aware of the paradox that what may appear sordid and disreputable in one form may appear lyrical and magnificent in another. She is aware also that the experience which is central to her novel encompasses the sordid and the marvellous, the sacred and profane; and her language is devised and structured to reflect these polarities.

Smart has divided her novel into ten short parts. The first three, set in California, encompass the meeting of the lovers and the consummation of their love, complicated by the presence of the lover's wife and the sense of guilt her presence engenders in the narrator-protagonist. In Part Four, the lovers are stopped by police at the Arizona border and questioned about their relationship. In Parts Five and Six, the woman returns to her Ottawa family and acquaintances, all of whom prove unsympathetic. In Part Seven, she travels to New York to meet her lover and finds him hospitalized after attempting suicide. In Part Eight she awaits his hoped-for return in a dingy New York hotel room. In Part Nine, she is once more on the west coast, now alone, pregnant, in growing despair. In Part Ten, in New York, facing her desertion, she awaits the birth of her child.

The novel begins with the first meeting of the protagonist with her future lover and ends with her realization that the affair is ended. While the novel involves a circular journey tracing a path from west to east, north to Canada, south to New York, west again and once more east, it is also, and more importantly, a voyage of mind and heart, which traces the complex graph of the protagonist's emotions throughout the affair. The novel is created of this emotional voyage. While we have come to expect a novel to concern itself with events and character development, in this lyrical work, events and character are subordinate to effect. Using words less as a language of communication than as an expression of emotion, the novel directs itself to rendering the texture of experience. "I was trying to say that this is how it is,"[1] the author explains. "How it is" — the inner reality — is the focus of this work.

As a lyrical novel, *By Grand Central Station* is something of a hybrid, combining aspects of two genres. Time, place, character, and event still exist: events occur within the space of a year; setting shifts from west to east and back; three characters interact. At the same time, much as in lyrical poetry, incantatory rhythm, lyrical and evocative language, daring and extravagant imagery heighten emotional expression. While novels are associated with storytelling, and the reader expects to find a character with whom he can identify and a plot in which he may become involved, in this novel emotional experience rather than external experience or individual character is central. The skeleton of barely identifiable events exists so that the resulting emotional effects can be expressed. Narration is subordinate to lyricism. Because it is the voice of the unmarried woman protagonist that we hear, from her perspective that we enter into experience, and her emotions that we share, the fictional world of the novel is her internal world. Events and individuals become aspects of the poetic vision, raw material for imagery. The protagonist shapes the world she sees to the expression of feeling. Objects, scenes, characters exist as images within the protagonist's lyrical subjective point of view, while the underlying plot fuses the array of disjointed images. Intensely emotional and lyrical, hence romantic in expression, the language of feeling is never out of control. Analogies and conceits, however exaggerated and even startling, are never ill-conceived or inappropriate. Literary allusions link the love affair with expressions of love throughout the ages, and biblical allusions underline its essentially sacred and eternal nature.

Interior monologue can be used to present realistic details filtered through an individual consciousness. To some extent this is what Smart does in seeking to describe "how it is". But because the reality she seeks to present is the protagonist's sensibility, the point of view is lyrical and confessional. A design of images and motifs takes form from the loose, disjointed series of events, recollections, conversations, displacing the external world or shifting from the external to the internal world to reveal the protagonist's mind and heart. Her emotional journey becomes a quest in which she abstracts impressions from the concrete world and refashions them into the texture of lyric poetry.

Characters exist to serve the lyrical intentions of the novel. The protagonist is the lyrical "I", as in a lyric poem; others are image-figures with which she interacts. Neither the protagonist, nor her lover, nor his wife, is named: all three remain shadowy figures in the lyrical acting out an archetypal pattern. Nor is any of the three described except for a few evocative details. On first meeting, the wife is seen first by the waiting protagonist, before the husband, as indication of how she is to continue to stand between the two. As the traditionally-termed injured party, the wife is portrayed as trusting and vulnerable, appealing in her very helplessness. It is her eyes that first strike the protagonist and which come to represent her innocence: "But then it is her eyes that come forward ...: her madonna eyes, soft as the newly-born, trusting as the untempted."[2] She is compared to a nymph: "... she leans over in the pool and her damp dark hair falls like sorrow, like mercy, like the mourning-weeds of pity" (p. 25). In a technique of reversal, not uncommon in this paradox-filled novel, this married woman, compared to a madonna and a nymph, appears virginal. She is associated with the fragility and innocence of flowers and birds. Her innocence is both childlike and saintly: "... the gentle flowers, able to die unceremoniously, remind me of her grief ... more angels weep for her whose devastated love runs into all the oceans of the world" (p. 27); "... her pathetic slenderness is covered over with a love as gentle as trusting as tenacious as the birds who rebuild their continually violated nests" (p. 25); "She knows nothing, but like autumn birds feels foreboding in the air ... but less wise than the birds whom small signs send on three thousand mile flights, she can only look vaguely over the Pacific ..." (p. 29).

When first seen, the protagonist's love "... fumbles with the tickets and the bags, and shuffles up to the event ..." (p. 17). "Shuffle" and "fumble" are hardly the action verbs one associates with a long-awaited romantic hero. Nor does he ever prove to be particularly heroic. This man is even more imprecisely described than his wife; in fact, he never becomes more than a silhouette or a shadow. Neither his appearance nor his personality is important. What is important is his effect on the protagonist: "... he, when he was only a word, was able to cause me sleepless nights and shivers of intimation" (p. 20). The ambivalence with which the lover is viewed is a reflection of the conflicting emotions with which the protagonist experiences her love affair, an affair she anticipates from its beginning will bring sorrow as well as joy, "I do not beckon to the Beginning, whose advent will surely strew our world with blood..." (p. 22), she says, saying at the same time of her future lover, "His foreshortened face appears in profile on the car window like the irregular graph of my doom, merciless as a mathematician, leering accompaniment to all my good resolves." The word "shadow" recurs insistently: "When his soft shadow which yet in the night comes barbed with all the weapons of guilt, is cast up hugely on the pane, I watch it as from a loge in the theatre, ..." (p. 22). As he takes her hand in the darkness of the car, she says, "... but now that hand casts everywhere an octopus shadow from which I can never escape" (p. 23). From the protagonist's lyrical point of view, the lover appears as a spectral, fateful, and often threatening figure.

The protagonist herself is passive. Her own personality is even less clearly drawn than that of her lover or his wife. Like them she is a figure in a drama which she watches unfold. She, too, serves the lyrical intention of the novel. The closer to the heart of the experience, the less concretized the individual. The protagonist remains only a voice.

Setting takes on the texture of imagery. Like the characters, it is mirrored through the eyes of the protagonist as an adjunct to emotional expression. The lush California setting presides over the lover's apotheosis, imaging its eroticism, its ecstasy, and its dangers. Like the protagonist's love, the setting appears excessive, larger than life: "Up the canyon the redwoods and the thick-leafed hands of the castor-tree forebode disaster by their beauty, built on too grand a scale" (p. 19). Menace is hidden within the beauty of the landscape: "But poison oak grows over the path and over all the banks, and it is impossible even to go into the damp overhung valley without being poisoned. Later in the year it flushes scarlet, both warning and recording fatality" (p. 19). The description underlines the sensuousness of the surroundings: "Round the doorways double-size flowers grow without encouragement: lilies, nasturtiums in a bank down to the creek, roses, geraniums, fuchsias, bleeding-hearts, hydrangeas. The sea booms. The stream rushes loudly" (p. 19). As the lush and sensuous flowers grow without encouragement, so does emotion, and it is in the lush and sensuous, and at the same time menacing, valley that the love is first consummated, a love which is to contain at least as much agony as ecstasy: "And I lay down on the redwood needles and seemed to flow down the canyon with the thunder and confusion of the stream, ..." (p. 26).

In similar, though less lyrical, fashion, the Canadian winter mirrors the response of family and acquaintances, "... how sympathetic the frozen Chaudière falls seem under the December sky, compared with these inflexible faces. ... They, who talk of a greater love, what is under the long cold of their look?" (p. 68). "Remember Ottawa in New Year's Eve sulking under snow" (p. 69). Finally, the all-night café at New York's Grand Central Station, a hangout for derelicts, where the novel ends is equally appropriate. Here the protagonist sits alone, deserted: "These tables are topped in leather on which the blood has never dried" (p. 119).

A lyrical novel is itself a paradox in its combination of features of two genres, its use of elements of the novel for lyrical purposes. In *By Grand Central Station* the aesthetic arrangement of the traditional elements is designed to express the pleasure and pain of love in a paradoxical structure, with motifs and symbols designed to show the existence of the polarities of joy and sorrow. The protagonist sees the world and experience in terms of paradox. While joyously embracing her experience, she is always aware of its dangers and of the inevitability with which sorrow follows happiness. She accepts love as "a happiness which, like birth, can afford the blood and the tearing" (p. 26).

The first words of the novel create oppositions which mirror the dialectic within the mind and heart of the protagonist. Awaiting her first meeting with her future lover, she says, "... all the muscles of my will are holding my terror to face the moment I most desire." By linking the two seeming contraries, "terror" and "desire", she sets the stage for the continuing paradoxical structure of the novel and her own ambivalent, sometimes contradictory, emotions. In the next sentence, with the words,

"Apprehension and the summer afternoon keep drying my lips
....," she links emotion with physical sensation, fusing the two
worlds, the emotional and the physical, as she will continue to
do throughout the novel.

All elements of the novel contribute to the tension of opposites
within the experience. As the effects of love and joy, of grief,
ecstasy, and despair, birth and death are the opposites to which
the narrator returns obsessively, so blood and water, the central
symbols to which she returns insistently, are paradoxical. Blood,
while associated with birth, is also linked with passion, suffering, sacrifice, and death. Water, most often linked with life and
creativity, is also associated with death.

Love is viewed by the protagonist as a flood on which she is
borne, by which she may be swept away, and in which she might
drown. "I thought [love] would be like a bird in the hand, not
a wild sea that treated me like flotsam" (p. 41); "I flow away in
a flood of love" (p. 41); "Where are we all headed for on the
swollen river of my undamned grief?" (p. 118); "I am going to
have a child, so all my dreams are of water, across which the ghost
of an almost accomplished calamity beckons. But tonight the child
lay within like the fated and only island in all the seas" (p. 118).
Through the water image, the child is linked with love.

Blood, associated with sorrow and death, is also linked with
birth: "Will there be birth from all this blood, or is death only
exacting his greedy price?" (p. 34). "Lucky Syrinx, who chose
legend instead of too much blood!" (p. 26). "He also is drowning in the blood of too much sacrifice" (p. 127); "Not all of the
poisonous tides of the blood I have spilt can influence the tidals
of love" (p. 41). The association of blood with "tidals of love"
fuses the two central images, blood and water as do the words,
"But the sea that floods is love, and it gushes out of me like an
arterial wound. I am drowning in it" (p. 118), an image which
at the same time links love with death. The flood of love on which
the protagonist is borne does become the flood in which she
drowns: "The drowning never ceases. The water submerges and
blends, but I am not dead. I am under the sea. The entire sea
is on top of me" (pp. 118-19). The emotion which carried her to
ecstasy carries her to despair.

Birth as a motif is linked with love from the novel's beginning.
"Will there be a birth from all this blood, or is death only exacting his greedy price?" "Is an infant struggling in the triangular

womb?'' (p. 34) the protagonist asks as the affair begins. The birth motif embraces several kinds of birth, linking three levels of experience: the birth of a passionate love affair, the birth of a child, the creation of a lyrical work.

The narrator turns to the classics and the Bible for analogies and symbols adequate to express her passion. She makes of herself and her love archetypal figures acting out their love in the world of myth and legend. Their experience and emotions rise above the temporal and parochial to become constituents of the eternal and the infinite. By their association with gods and heroes, the lovers are mythologized. The protagonist links herself with others loved by gods: ''O lucky Daphne, motionless and green to avoid the touch of a god'' (p. 24), of the nymph transformed into a bay tree to escape Apollo; ''Jupiter has been with Leda, I thought, and now nothing can avert the Trojan wars,'' she says of their first union (p. 27). Implicit in the classical allusions is recognition of the inevitability of the protagonist's acceptance of love and of the unhappiness, even disaster which will be its inevitable result. She associates herself with other women involved in tragic love situations, such as Ophelia and Isolde. When deserted by her lover, the protagonist associates herself with Dido, the queen of Carthage who committed suicide when deserted by Aeneas: ''By the Pacific I wander like Dido, heaving such a passion of tears in the breaking waves, that I wonder why the whole world isn't weeping inconsolably'' (p. 108). With this analogy, the narrator also lends cosmic significance to her experience, a significance amplified by association of herself with the natural world and translation of her experience into hyperbolic and dramatic metaphor and symbol: ''I am the same tune now as the trees, hummingbirds, sky, fruits, vegetables in rows. I am all or any of these. I can metamorphose at will'' (p. 45); ''Take away everything I have, or could have, anything the world could offer, I am still empress of a new-found-land, that neither Columbus nor Cortez could have equalled, even in their instigating dreams'' (p. 47); ''... but can I see by the light of a match while I burn in the arms of the sun?''(p.28).

Along with the cosmic significance which such metaphors, analogies, and classical allusions lend to the love affair, there are important religious overtones. The biblical cadence of the novel's rhythms contributes to the love's apotheosis. The most dramatic of the biblical allusions underlining the religious dimension is the use of verses from the Song of Solomon which, in the voice of the protagonist, are counterpointed with the crude questioning of the police who stop the couple at the Arizona state border. This counterpointing of voices points out the dichotomy between the two ways of looking at the experience: for the protagonist, her love is sacred and lyrical; for the police, as outsiders, it is adulterous and sinful.

The interweaving of the lyrical, cadenced biblical language with the direct and brutal words of the interrogators also recalls to the reader the inextricable link between the sensual and the spiritual; the sensual is not denied but made transcendent, the marvelous is shown to exist within the corporeal. In her use of the Song of Solomon, Smart comes full circle: the lyrically erotic language which in the Old Testament was transposed to express a divine love, to image a transcendent world which can only be express-ed through the concrete, now is turned back, still carrying its sacred implications, to add to an erotic experience the resonance of the spiritual, to underline one of the main paradoxes of the novel, that to be human is to be both flesh and spirit, human and divine.

The intermeshing of the spoken words of the police with the silent discourse of the protagonist is achieved by the use of paren-thesis for the silent discourse. In the conjunction of the exterior dialogue (which is actually a dramatic monologue, since only one side of the conversation is given) with the interior monologue, the impression is created of the spoken words entering the pro-tagonist's consciousness, the dialogue entering the monologue frame. An ironic tension is created and developed between outer appearance (the words of the police) and inner reality (the pro-tagonist's recitation from the Song of Solomon). While to some extent the effect may be compared to that of an aside in drama, the emphasis remains with the interior monologue. The opposi-tion of the views expressed by the two voice levels underlines the impossibility of communication:

> Did you sleep in the same room? (Behold thou art fair, my love, behold thou art fair: thou hast dove's eyes).
> In the same bed? (Behold thou art fair, my beloved, yea pleasant, also our bed is green).
> Did intercourse take place? (I sat down under his

shadow with great delight and his fruit was sweet to
my taste). (p. 51)

As the grilling is continued by a police matron, the protagonist's
reaction remains the same:

> The matron says: Give me your bracelet, no jewelry
> allowed. (My beloved —). At once. And your ring. (My
> beloved —). And your bag ....
> The eyes of the jealous world peer through the
> peephole in the door, in the eyes of the keeper. But still
> the only torture is in his absence. (p. 52)

While such other voices impinge upon the consciousness of the
lyrical "I" through whose sensibility the world is filtered, we
never hear, directly or indirectly, the voices of the lover or his
wife, the two other figures central to the lyrical experience.
Distanced from the reader, they remain shadowy figures in the
experience of the narrator-protagonist, acting out their parts in
an elemental pattern. Other voices heard directly are those of
secondary figures, largely unsympathetic, acting as a kind of
chorus. These voices express an attitude and a reaction antithetical
to hers. Through them, the world in general is shown to be unsympathetic, capable of viewing the affair only from the most
superficial level, but capable, nevertheless, of passing judgment.

Brief comments of family and acquaintances, directly reported
as scattered bits of conversation recalled by the protagonist, tend
to isolate her further: " 'Love? Stuff and nonsense!' my mother
would say, 'It's loyalty and decency and common standards of
behaviour that count' " (p. 67); "... the well-meaning matrons
who, from their insulated living say, 'My dear, I think you would
regret it afterwards if you broke up a marriage, ... when you
felt it about to happen the right thing would have been to have
gone away at once,' 'If he needs money why doesn't he get a
job?' 'What does he know of Love that lets his country down in
her Hour-of-Need?' " (pp. 67-68). The clichés spoken by these
observers reflect the conventional and unthinking views of
onlookers to any adulterous affair.

For the most part, the novel consists of the present tense
discourse of the lyrical "I" which is overheard by the reader. Ver-
balization is synchronized with action or experience. In the course
of the interior monologue, the lyrical "I" conveys to us what she
is doing and what is happening to her, and what she is feeling.

Present-tense discursive language lends a sense of directness and immediacy as the reader overhears the lyrical "I" in the act of responding to her situation.

There are times when the monologuist addresses her thoughts to others, human or divine. When considering her feelings of guilt at injuring her lover's wife, she addresses God: "God, come down out of the eucalyptus tree outside my window, ..." (p. 33). After her recitation from the Song of Solomon, she addresses Solomon in language ironically more appropriate to her crude interrogators: "Get wise to yourself, Solomon, lay off all that stuff. Join a club. Get pally with the gang" (p. 54). She apostrophizes the angels, "What was your price, Gabriel, Michael of the ministering wing?" (p. 38). Travelling to rejoin her lover she addresses him as "you" (pp. 74-77). Such make-believe communication further underlines her loneliness and isolation.

While most of the novel is narrated in the present, that present shifts in its mode of operation. We think of the present in its most common use, expressing immediate action, emotion, or response, but there are times when the present becomes a timeless present shifting to the expression of a generalization, as in these thoughts of the monologuist:

> And over the fading wooden house I sense the reminiscence of the pioneer's passion, and the determination of early statesmen who were mild but individual, able to allude to Shakespeare while discussing politics under the elms. No great neon face has been superimposed over their minor but memorable history. Nor has the blood of the early settlers, split in feud and heroism, yet been bottled by a Coca-Cola firm and sold as ten-cent tradition. (p. 63)

At times too, the present modulates from instant present to habitual present to indicate a repetition or a longer duration. Such uses of the present contain, at least implicitly, such adverbs as whenever, sometimes, always, never. The monologuist says, for example, "Like Anteus, when I am thrust against this earth, I bounce back recharged with hope" (p. 62); of her lover's wife, she says, "I see she can walk across the leering world and suffer injury only from those she loves" (p. 18); and "How can she walk through the streets, so vulnerable, so unknowing, and not have people and dogs and perpetual calamity following her?"

In keeping with these varied modes of present tense, are the paradigmatic scenes, which, while they are in themselves individual scenes, are representative of other similar scenes. Such a scene occurs in the home of the Wurtles, a couple with whom the lovers stay for a short time:

> When we tear ourselves out of the night and come into the kitchen, Mrs. Wurtle says, "Romance, eh?" but she smiles, she turns away her head, and when we kiss behind her back as we help her dry the dishes, she says, "Oh, you two love-birds, go on out again!"
>
> What is going to happen? Nothing. For everything has happened. All time is now, and time can do no better. Nothing can ever be more now than now, and before this nothing was. There are no minor facts in life, there is only the one tremendous one.
>
> We can include the world in our love, and no irritations can disrupt it, not even envy.
>
> Mr. Wurtle, sitting on the sofa late at night, says, with a legal air, "Then I have it from you there is such a thing as Love?" I lean upon the cushion, faint from this few hours separation, but I sigh, "Yes, oh, yes, ..." (p. 43)

Here the present tense shifts from a brief scene in the instant present to expression of a generalization in the timeless present, and shifts back to another instant moment in another brief scene. The impression created is that of the lyrical "I" speaking to herself while involved in these scenes.

While the present tense in its various modes is used most, a recurrent feature of this monologue is the manner in which from time to time shifts are made to other tenses. For example, while the protagonist's thoughts remain in the present as she travels home, the next episode, in which she considers the unsympathetic and uncomprehending attitude of family and friends, takes place in the past tense. This section begins: "As I sat down in the swivel chair in my father's office, with his desk massively symbolic between us, I realized that I could never defend myself" (p. 67). Recollected words of others are then interjected in present tense direct discourse in a dramatization of recollected attitudes. In such a situation, present experience giving way entirely to a remembrance of incidents and attitudes, the narrator's monologue becomes a memory monologue. In similar fashion, the episode with the police, which begins with the counterpointing of interior and exterior voices, continues in past tense narrative. When the past tense is used, it is never simply to narrate what has occurred but rather to comment upon past situations as in the episode with the police, and as earlier, when the protagonist recalls her feelings for her lover before they met, ''... he, when he was only a word, was able to cause me sleepless nights and shivers of intimation, ...'' (p. 20).

In the final and most emotionally wrought part of the novel, the monologue shifts rapidly from present to past to future in a surreal structure. Bits of action and event are interwoven with lyrical effusions, and the protagonist shifts from speaker to listener to speaker, and from interior to exterior, in a kaleidoscopic shifting of scene and tense:

By Grand Central Station I sat down and wept:

I will not be placated by the mechanical motions of existence, nor find consolation in the solicitude of waiters who notice my devastated face. Sleep tried to seduce me by promising a more reasonable tomorrow. But I will not be betrayed by such a Judas of fallacy: it betrays everyone: it leads them into death. (p. 117)

I race disaster down Third Avenue. It shimmers in the Hudson River. When I dare to look up for a sign of comfort the neons flash relentlessly.

No, no one will pity you here where failure is the same as shame, and tears anachronisms, out of place even in cinemas.

''Sure, kid. We all got troubles. Buck up. Take it on the chin.''

If you can smile now you might become a great success in the advertising business. Brave little woman Quite a gal. Her saucy repartee conceals alluring tragedy. Once she could feel, she could weep. Once she too was human. But you see what can be done? Why, she's making $15,000 a year. (p. 120)

In its handling of voice and language By Grand Central Station is a remarkable accomplishment. Even more remarkable is that it is the first novel of a very young woman, and was written in 1941. In 1941, Canada's best known writers were Frederick Philip

Grove, Hugh MacLennan, Morley Callaghan, and Mazo de la Roche, then still writing her Jalna series. That year Sinclair Ross's *As For Me and My House*, published in the United States, received scant attention in Canada.

Equally remarkable is the history of *By Grand Central Station*. Appearing first in England in 1945, during the last months of the war, it was an underground success, but was not widely known until 1966 when it was republished with an introduction by Brigid Brophy hailing it as one of "half a dozen masterpieces of poetic prose in the world" (p. 5). It was still almost unknown in Canada. It is said that Elizabeth Smart's family blocked its importation into Canada. The first North American publication, the Popular Library edition in 1975, finally brought the novel to attention in Canada. Now at last *By Grand Central Station* joins the list of Canadian classics.

Notes

1   "Psalm of Love," Radio Times, December 1978, p. 19
2   Elizabeth Smart, *By Grand Central Station I Sat Down and Wept* (London: Edition Poetry, 1945; rpt. New York, Popular Library, 1975), p. 17. Page references in parenthesis are from this edition.

AN APPETITE FOR LIFE: THE LIFE AND LOVE OF ELIZABETH SMART

John Goddard

A pair of black doors with frosted windows block the midday driz-
zle and workaday world from the French House pub, cramped
hang-out of the offbeat literati in the heart of London's Soho. Inside, the air is blue, and rife with raucous babble — a witty put-
down of a new play, a smutty anecdote from a late-night party.
The patrons share a vaguely artistic air, but each is distinctive:
an arch young man with deep-set eyes and pointed shoes; a lo-
quacious woman with shredded hair, dyed pink at the ends; a
thin man of shy demeanour wearing a pale-green bow tie.

At one end of the bar is Elizabeth Smart, nursing a Bloody Mary
and waving a cigarette as she talks. Her hair, slightly flattened
by the rain, is still honey-blonde and thick, belying the years that
show on her face. Her accent is compromised by forty years
abroad — the r's and h's still distinct but the o's elongated, the
a's softer. "Why don't we go somewhere else?" she says after
breaking off the conversation with the others. "It's far too noisy
in here."

She was born in Ottawa in 1913, lived among the Establishment and next door to William Lyon Mackenzie King. Then she
rebelled. She made love to a woman to defy her mother, lived
on a commune in Big Sur long before the beatniks, had four
children by British poet George Barker (who was married to someone else), and, when the going got rough, wrote her slim
classic, *By Grand Central Station I Sat Down and Wept*, the story
of a self-defeating passion that is smouldering still. She has spent
the past fifteen years in a remote cottage in Suffolk, a wild spot
one hundred and sixty kilometres east of London, accessible only through a gravel pit and cow pasture. Now, belatedly free of
maternal responsibilities, she is back in circulation, reading at
poetry festivals, going to parties, and "looking in" at the French
House when in London. Soon (August 1982), she is to end the
long estrangement from her native country by becoming writer-
in-residence at the University of Alberta in Edmonton.

"I feel terribly excited about going back to Canada," she says,
settling down on the sofa in her son's flat, away from the French
House din. "It has always been on my mind to return." She had

lost touch for a while, to the point of not knowing that modern Canadian literature existed. But when *Grand Central* was republished by Popular Library in 1975 and made available in Canada for the first time, Canadian writers began seeking her out, sending her books in thanks for her hospitality. "I was much amazed when I read these, mostly women actually: the Margarets, Alice Munro, and even earlier books like *The Double Hook*. I felt a total kinship with them. Even the rhythms of the sentences and so on. It's something I don't understand, why Canadians are Canadians and Americans are Americans. Is it something about the wind blowing over the prairies or something?"

She still considers herself very much a Canadian and has set her new novel in the Canada of her childhood, a novel she plans to complete in Edmonton, adding to a collection of three slim books: *Grand Central* in 1945, a book of poems; *A Bonus*, in 1977; and another novel, *The Assumption of the Rogues and Rascals*, in 1978.

"And we *did* have a wonderful childhood," one paragraph of the new work reads, as it appeared recently in *Harper's & Queen*, a London magazine, "thrilling to the frothing surf on the bland sea of Brackley Beach, Prince Edward Island; or making leaf houses in the woods by the lake at Kingsmere; going for walks with Daddy, begging to be thrown into flat round juniper bushes, just prickly enough for ecstasy; finding enchanted flowers in Flower Ben on early cold picnics; taking the adventurous first trip up to the cottage, wondering if we could get there, because of the congealed snow on the road, packed down in old drifts, and patches of ice. Then we roared with joy and spring. How we must have driven our patient father frantic, bellowing out of tune, loud, excited, *A Hundred Blue Bottles*, from one hundred relentlessly down to one."

Her father was Russell Smart, a pioneering patent-and-trade-mark lawyer who was "retained by Coca-Cola and Kellogg's to fight Pepsi-Cola and Shredded Wheat, things like that." He was a kind, patient, generous man who continued to send Elizabeth a monthly allowance long after she left home, and who sponsored twenty-two boat trips to Europe during her adolescence. "One would think up a project and if it were reasonable he would finance you. I would say that I wanted to study music, and my sister would say she wanted to study sculpture." And off they would go, with a governess in the early days, later by themselves. Her mother was an engaging hostess who kept perpetual open house, or so it seemed. In winter the parties were at home in Ottawa, where Elizabeth met young Mike Pearson and diplomats who later helped her in London when, pregnant with her second child, she fled the man she loved. In summer the activities moved to the cottage at Kingsmere, next to Mackenzie King's estate, where as a child she played in the leaves with Eugene Forsey and as a young woman, provocatively beautiful in photographs, she drew the attention of young men: "I was one of three sisters, lively girls and, you know, men were always sort of nosing around the way they do."

But casting a shadow on the frivolity was the other side of her mother's character. "I loved her very much, but ..." She was bossy, domineering and reproachful. She tolerated the trips abroad but stopped the girls from going to university, keeping them dependent while the son studied law. Elizabeth wanted to be free.

On one trip to England, while browsing in the little magazine and book shops on Charing Cross Road, she got an idea. "There was a wonderful shop called Better Books; I think that is where I found George Barker's and I thought they were marvellous. By that time I knew a few people, and I'd say, do you know George Barker, because I'd like to meet him and marry him. I didn't know he was married you see."

By that time Barker was on his way to becoming known. He'd been singled out by W. B. Yeats as promising, and was a close friend of Dylan Thomas and David Gascoyne — the three of them generally considered to be the best British poets of their generation. But Elizabeth and George didn't meet for another two years. She returned to Ottawa in 1938, to a job on the Ottawa *Journal* against her mother's wishes: "Every morning my mother would say, 'Stay in bed today, don't go in,' and she'd bring me breakfast in bed."

After six months Elizabeth did quit, fed up because the *Journal* wouldn't pay her a living wage — only $2.50 a week because she lived at home. She went to New York, slept on her sister's sofa, worked in art galleries, and tried to sell the manuscripts she had been writing since age ten. "I had written a novel by then and lots and lots of poems. I sent them to an agent and she thought they were very shocking. She sent them back with a reproachful note. The novel was about male impotence and, you see, those things were not discussed in those days. It wasn't explicit like *Fear of Flying* or anything, it was just a little too frank.'' It was never published.

Elizabeth also sent poems to London and Paris and struck up a correspondence with Lawrence Durrell. From Durrell she learned George Barker was broke and willing to sell his manuscripts to collectors. She wrote to Barker and he sold her one, but the correspondence ended there. She went to Mexico City, then to California, had a lesbian affair, and wrote a novel about it called *Dig a Grave and Let Us Bury Our Mother*. It, too, was never published.

In 1940, while she was still in California, Barker sent her an urgent message. He was teaching at Imperial Tohoku University in Japan and sensed war coming. Could she send him money for passage to California — for two passages, one for him and one for his wife — and get immigration papers? She sent him savings she had earned as a maid and some borrowed money, but the documents were more difficult to come by, requiring sponsorship from a millionaire. She engaged the help of Christopher Isherwood, who was working for MGM in Hollywood at the time and knew Barker's work. Finally all was set. Barker and his wife sailed to California and took a bus to Monterey. Elizabeth was waiting for them, as she describes in the opening line of *Grand Central*:

> I am standing on a corner in Monterey, waiting for the bus to come in, and all the muscles of my will are holding my terror to face the moment I most desire.

The book is not straight autobiography, she says. She has trouble remembering now which were the true events and which the fiction. But she found a wooden hut for them at Big Sur, a virtual wilderness in 1940. She thought the three of them could all just be friends but, as the book describes, the inevitable happened: ''Under the waterfall he surprised me bathing and gave me what I could no more refuse than the earth can refuse the rain.''

The triangle broke up after a few months. Barker and his wife left for New York; Elizabeth retreated to an abandoned school house in Pender Harbour, British Columbia — pregnant — where she wrote sequences of *Grand Central* in longhand, out of order, building the edifice brick by brick: ''I wrote the border incident last,'' she says of the passage she most often reads to an audience.

It is a fictionalized account of how she and George are detained at the California-Arizona border and charged under the Mann Act — a law ostensibly prohibiting couples from crossing state lines to fornicate but also a ruse for police in those days to detain suspected gangsters and spies. The passage has a rude American cop interrogating the heroine, who replies with verses from the *Song of Songs*: "Did intercourse take place? (I sat down under his shadow with great delight and his fruit was sweet to my taste)."

"At the time I wrote it, I was terribly pregnant," she says, "and I remember, oh, the boredom of it and looking up the Bible to get the bits I wanted. I didn't feel like doing research but I wanted to get the book done in case I died in childbirth. Well, people used to you know."

She didn't tell her parents she was having a baby — they were already against her for not helping in the war effort — but George knew. He visited her briefly. When he tried to visit a second time, he was stopped at the border. Elizabeth's mother "had harangued the ambassador or something" to keep him out of Canada. To be near him, Elizabeth used her former Ottawa ties to get a job at the British Army Office in Washington.

"I was still in love. I was pretty much in love for about nineteen years, really, but I saw early on, I mean I really started trying to leave him early on, because I saw it wasn't a working proposition. I never expected him to be of any help because I wouldn't have been so silly. I saw there wasn't anything he could do and I didn't expect him to. I just thought I could do it. I was working as a filing clerk and had the lowest salary you're allowed to have in America, and George would say that his wife had gone away and we were going to go to Reno and then, I don't know, there were all sorts of excuses, all very, very, very believable stories. Then I'd get suspicious and look in his pockets and I'd find a laundry list with her writing on it. So then I'd say, Go, I'm not seeing you again, and he could always make jokes and get around my resolution and then I'd let him in again. This went on for ages. But then it was too horrible and awful so I decided to get myself to England."

In 1943, in wartime, pregnant with her second child, she waited three weeks in New York for a ship and crossed the Atlantic in a convoy. Three of the ships went down. She didn't leave a forwarding address, "but of course he got himself over and found me and there we were." They had a third and fourth child, but

he had no money. He lived with his mother and went on to have
more children by other women. *Grand Central* was published but
in a printing of only 2,000 copies. An Ottawa book store imported
six of them; Elizabeth's mother bought them all and burned them,
using her influence again to prevent more copies from coming
into the country.

The book circulated in New York, however, and was praised
by the beat poets. Jay Landesman, now head of Polytantric Press
in London (Elizabeth's publisher), was editor in the late 1950s
of the underground magazine, *Neurotica*. "*Grand Central* is an
historic book," he says, "way ahead of anything written at the
time. It was a forerunner of Kerouac's *On the Road*, and Elizabeth
and George were the forerunners of that kind of living. They
broke down traditions completely, broke down the standards of
morality. Kerouac and those guys broke it down in the 1950s
when it was easier. Elizabeth and George did it in wartime, that's
the exciting thing. They were in pajamas when the rest of the
world was in uniforms."

Landesman first met Barker in New York in the late '50s at a
gathering of beat poets. "Allen Ginsberg was at George's feet.
They were in awe of him. They were aware of what Elizabeth
and George had done." Inspired by such meetings, Landesman
wrote a musical that played on Broadway in 1959 called *The Nervous Set* about Kerouac, Ginsberg, Barker, and a few others.
Kerouac was played by Larry Hagman — the J.R. of *Dallas*.

Grand Central influenced a new generation after Panther Books
published it in paperback in Britain in 1966. "It was one of the
cult books," says Helen Dennis, professor of American literature
at the University of Warwick. "The late '60s was a time of great
optimism among young people, a time to break social and political
conventions, and this book seemed to be an expression of that
spirit."

British novelist Brigid Brophy called the book "a masterpiece
of poetic prose" in her introduction to the 1966 edition: "*By
Grand Central Station* is one of the most shelled, skinned, nerve-
exposed books every written ... a cry of complete vulnerability
... transformed into a source of eternal pleasure, a work of art."

For all its anguish and torment, however, the book is ultimately hopeful and forgiving. "Inspiring, truthful and very feminine,"
says Ann Barr, features editor at *Harper's & Queen*, and a close
friend of Elizabeth's. "It's one of the books everyone has read,

more so than *Ulysses*, which everyone only says they've read.''
Everyone in her circle might have read *Grand Central* but the book
did not attract a mass readership, possibly because, like poetry,
its dense, lyrical style demands concentration.

Meanwhile, Elizabeth had to make a living — for herself, her
two boys and two girls. She got jobs on various women's
magazines, as a music editor and fashion writer, and later worked in advertising. Bob Johnson, now production manager at
Harper's & Queen, shared a cubicle with her in the mid-1960s when
the magazine was called simply *Queen*. "She always seemed to
be at least half on the way to being smashed," he says. "She
needed something to keep her going all the time, what with four
kids, getting older, the whole George Barker thing, and just the
business of getting through life. In the absence of anything else
she would grab a can of Cow Gum (layout paste). She's the first
person I ever heard of sniffing glue.''

At *Queen* she wrote book reviews, but her main job was laying
out fourteen pages of fashion, writing the intros, and making the
captions fit. ''She was tremendous at it,'' says Ann Barr. ''Her
pages were like concrete poetry. When she went into advertising she was the highest-paid copywriter in London.''

But her literary career was in limbo. She regrets her skimpy
output as a writer, but babies, she says, are part of being in love.
''It's a natural feeling to want to have a baby when you're really
in love. Every woman feels it and I think men do too when they're
really involved. A woman is a man with a womb, that's what
the word means. It's not a man without something, its a man
with something and that something is a womb. I wanted these
female experiences.''

At age fifty, with her children grown, she was ready to start
writing again seriously. But problems she doesn't like talking
about obliged her to raise two infant grandchildren. She retreated
to a cottage in Suffolk, channelling her creative energies into a
one-acre garden, cultivating a wilderness that must have resembl-
ed in some ways her childhood playground at Kingsmere. There
was some literary activity. She continued to write the occasional
newspaper and magazine piece and in 1977 published *A Bonus*
— forty-four pages of poetry collected over the years. The book
isn't available in Canada, although Deneau Publishers is interested in it. Deneau also plans to publish a hardcover edition
of *Grand Central* in late 1982. *The Assumption of the Rogues and*

Rascals was published in 1978, a slim book of 120 pages. The reviews in Britain were favourable, but the book never attracted the following of her first. Eleanor Wachtel, reviewing *Rogues and Rascals* for *Books in Canada*, called it ''an elliptical novel, a gathering of reflections, stories, bits of memoir, journal entries and so on that ... lacks the first's drive, just as survival seems somehow less forceful than love.''

After the grandchildren in her care had more or less reached adulthood, Elizabeth was in danger of great-grandmother problems and decided enough was enough. At a poetry festival in Cambridge she met poet Patrick Lane, writer-in-residence at Edmonton for 1981-82. He suggested she succeed him, and the university later sent her a formal invitation.

By the time I heard Elizabeth Smart's life story, I had spent time with her at her son's flat, in restaurants, in cafés, at parties, at her cottage, and at poetry readings, including one she gave at the opening of the cultural centre at Canada House in London. She revealed herself as a warm, kind, giving person. But what was George Barker like? What made him worth pursuing so? Elizabeth alternately describes him as fascinating, selfish, interesting, badly behaved, and a marvellous poet. The nicest thing most of her friends had to say was that he was cruel. ''He'll charm you,'' said Ann Barr.

I phoned him and was invited for Saturday night to his home in Norfolk, near the sea. Elizabeth phoned Saturday morning to say she would be there — they were still in touch, meeting occasionally at poetry readings. I was first to arrive — after dark by train, bus, and taxi — at an Elizabethan stone building said to be haunted by a little girl in the study and by an old sea captain upstairs. Saturday night, it turned out, is drinking night, and George was in the drinking room.

''Come in young man,'' he said, beckoning with one hand. At sixty-nine he retains luminous blue eyes, is lean and tall despite a slight stoop of the shoulders, and, yes, sexy-looking in a turtleneck sweater, blue jeans, and dirty white running shoes — cliché garb for a poet except that he probably invented the look. We talked about the weather for fifteen minutes, a conversation his wife, Elspeth, thought silly. She is a soft-spoken, forty-year-old Scot anyone would at once call beautiful, even in Wellington boots and country woollens. She has been with George for nineteen years, has five children by him, the youngest aged seven, and is considered George's fifth wife, counting Elizabeth. George has fourteen "conspicuous" children, as Elizabeth puts it, though he has boasted as many as thirty-five, she says.

Elizabeth arrived with a friend via three pubs. More drinks were poured, then the fireworks began.

"You cow," George said to Elizabeth in his gravelly voice. "Your face looks like the back of Auden's hand. I love you."

"I love you too but that's irrelevant."

"You loathsome Canadian. You're like something out of Ibsen, horrible. You have no versification."

"I know."

"It was I who taught you the word *eye* is spelled with one letter."

"I know."

And so it went.

Elspeth took me aside to balance the effect, speaking softly. "He's shy. He's a wonderful person and I love him. We sit up in bed sometimes in the early morning, propped up on our pillows, in our own particular darkness, drinking tea, with the light from the windows and the electric fire flashing off the posts and the knobs of the brass bed. He becomes so articulate and poetic."

To quiet the others down, Elspeth read Matthew Arnold's "Dover Beach" to the group, hauntingly, until George complained she read like a waitress. Someone phoned to invite us all to a party and we were off, shouting at each other, singing Presbyterian hymns and getting lost along the way. We finally arrived at an old stone country house that seemed to be full of well-dressed women in their late twenties, and George soon had a clutch of them around him.

"What's his magic?" I asked.

"He's sixty-nine and still very sexy," said one.

"He's just very special," said another.

"He's so overt in his rudeness, he challenges you," said a third. "You keep coming back for more."

"What's your opinion of *Grand Central*?" I asked Barker at one point.

"The best thing since *Wuthering Heights*," he said. "And I hate *Wuthering Heights*. Women don't have souls."

It was clear that Barker and Elizabeth still have strong feelings for each other. It was also clear the encounter was painful for them

— certainly for Elizabeth, who showed pain on her face, in her voice, and in her submissive responses. "So much pain," she said late one night in Soho, in a slightly different context. She had been eating with friends in an Oriental restaurant on Frith Street, talking, joking, by all appearances having a good time, when she abruptly got up, said goodnight, and walked out. Intercepted on the street, she said something ambiguous about pain being hard to bear.

But pain is a prime motivator, a key tool, for Elizabeth Smart the writer. Brigid Brophy touches on the point when she says *Grand Central* is a cry transformed into a work of art. Elizabeth, in fact, has developed a theory about the relationship between love, pain, and art. She wrote about it in the February issue of *Woman's Journal*, in a piece called "How to Mend a Broken Heart" in which she gives advice to spurned lovers. "Pain is, can be, useful," she writes. "But only if you use it. You have to be willing to suffer. You have to accept it … because if you fight against pain you augment it …. So say: Come dear pain. Come, be welcome. Please overwhelm me …."

"Examine yourself," she advises. "Perhaps it was the bastard in him that triggered your susceptibilities. It looked like glamour, then, and you only saw the shiny side. You responded joyfully …. And now you have the beginning of wisdom: the price of love is pain."

She warns against bitterness: "It was a rich experience. Don't deny it. Don't denigrate it. Don't say If Only. Suffer. If bitterness comes creeping in, nip it in the bud. A bitter person has failed as a human being …. A consenting adult cries in private, takes the pain, acknowledges it, praises the experience, blames nobody.

"A consenting adult moves on."

ETHEL WILSON

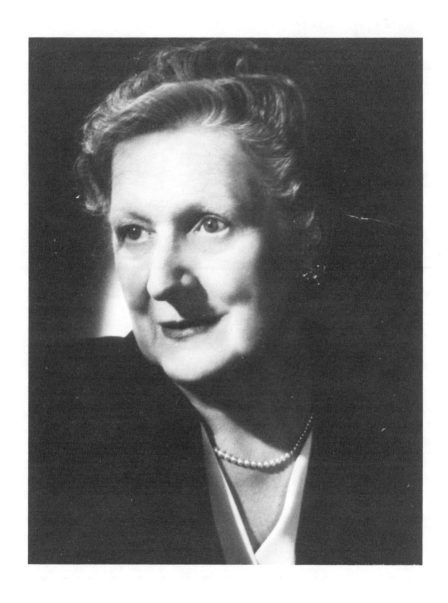

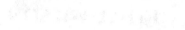

MAGGIE'S LAKE: THE VISION OF FEMALE POWER IN *SWAMP ANGEL*

Donna E. Smyth

In the hands of Nell Severance, the Swamp Angel gun is a dangerous, beautiful, wicked, wonderful thing. Nell has been a juggler and an artist who, in retrospect, describes her performance:

> ... when I think how I used to be able to keep them moving so fluid and slow — how you had to work to get that timing! ... and then the drums beginning, and faster and faster — all timed — and the drums louder and louder — a real drum roll ... and I'd have the three guns going so fast they dazzled, one behind my back and one under my elegant long legs (such lovely legs!), and one out as if out towards the audience and then crack-crack-crack and the audience going crazy and me bowing and laughing like anything ... how I loved it.[1]

For Nell the gun is a charged symbol, an iconic link between herself, the past and Philip Severance. She fondles and strokes it when she needs comfort. She uses it to deflect Eddie Vardoe's murderous anger when he discovers that Maggie has left him. She sends it to Maggie when she can no longer be the guardian of the gun.

In the end, Maggie, as the new guardian, can throw the gun into "her lake" because she has no need for it. She knows she is performing "a rite of some kind" (p. 156) and she throws it, like Excalibur, in a great arc:

> It made a shining parabola in the air, turning downwards — turning, turning, catching the sunlight, hitting the surface of the lake, sparkling down into the clear water, vanishing amidst breaking bubbles in the water, sinking down among the affrighted fish, settling in the ooze. (p. 157)

Restored to the great reservoir of symbols from whence it was derived, the gun, as an object, has played its part. Yet its name dominates the book. Something angelic, full of light, growing out of the muck, out of a swamp. What is potentially destructive becomes energy used to create a human community.

Before Maggie can manifest this vision, she must find herself. Her first act is a refusal. To say No, as Camus knew, is the beginning of rebellion.[2] In Maggie's case the refusal is a rejection of a loveless marriage, and it means she must find a way to make her own living. She has to step outside the traditional women's culture, and unpaid work, into the male preserve of sport fishing. "Brought up from childhood by a man, with men" (p. 30), Maggie, in fact, is an artist in her own right. She ties fishing flies, creating out of bird feathers and a hook, something beautiful and deadly.

From the beginning, Maggie is associated with fishing; she is a Fisher Queen on a quest for self-knowledge and self-healing. The end of that quest is restoration of harmony, not only for herself but for her community.

Maggie times her escape carefully. In her unholy marriage with Eddie, time has been "out of sync", space has shrunk to the prison of a house. Driving away in the taxi, "She exulted in each small sight and sound, in new time, in new space, because she had got free" (p. 23). She takes her own symbols with her: her fishing rod and the yellow Chinese bowl;[3] wand and grail receptacle, male and female, yin and yang, balanced as they are in Maggie's hands. As a grail symbol, the yellow bowl connects several levels of the novel. Yellow is a sacred colour and is related to its Chinese origins, not only on the religious level, but as part of the Chinese connection which is an important link for Maggie between herself and her vision of human community. When she looks at Joey, her taxi driver, "She thought that she understood him ... in a way that seemed open to her" (p. 27). This balance between an old culture and a new, between East and West, is essential to the founding of Maggie's small Utopia in the Canadian wilderness.

Once Maggie has left Eddie, she gains a new name, or rather, her old, true name is restored to her. Maggie Vardoe becomes Maggie Lloyd. It is clear from Maggie's memories that her first marriage to Tom Lloyd was a holy one: that is, mutually loving and balanced. The old, new name is part of the restoration.

Her first stop-over on her flight from Eddie and the City is a small motel cabin at Chilliwack. Here she is "as free of care or remembrance as if she had just been born ..." (p. 34).

Reborn, Maggie passes through the portentously named but real town of Hope on her journey to the interior of British Columbia. The narrator comments:

> Make no mistake, when you have reached Hope and
> the roads that divide there you have quite left Van-
> couver and the Pacific Ocean. They are dispropor-
> tionately remote. You are entering a continent, and you
> meet the continent there, at Hope. (p. 36)

Maggie's own interior journey is subsumed within the geographical framework. Her next step is to restore the harmony between herself and nature symbolized, for her and Ethel Wilson, by fishing. She retreats into isolation by the river where she is one element in the cosmic picture as is the doe who comes to gaze at her without fear. Maggie fishes: "In the pleasure of casting over the lively stream she forgot — as always when she was fishing — her own existence" (p. 38). Forgetful of self, she also struggles with remorse and guilt but, through meditation in Nature, is restored:

> ... the scent of the pines, the ancient rocks below and
> above her, and the pine-made earth, a physical languor,
> her solitude, her troubled mind, and a lifting of her
> spirit to God by the river brought tears to her eyes. I
> am on a margin of life, she thought, and she
> remembered that twice before in her own life she had
> known herself to be taken to that margin of a world
> which was powerful and close. (pp. 39-40)

Maggie remains at the Similkameen cabins for three days and nights, the mythic time for death and rebirth. At this point, the narrator is quite explicit:

> These days had been for Maggie like the respite that
> perhaps comes to the soul after death. This soul
> (perhaps, we say) is tired from slavery or from its own
> folly or just from the journey and from the struggle of
> departure and arrival, alone, and for a time — or what
> we used to call time — must stay still, and accustom the
> ages of the soul and its multiplied senses to something
> new, which is still fondly familiar. (p. 40)

Three Loon Lake is Haldar Gunnarsen's dream which Maggie, through her strength and healing powers, makes possible and manifest in this world. The fishing lodge is a way of living gent-ly off the land and with the land. It integrates the human and the natural. It depends on human love and hard work.

The germ of potential destruction is present in Vera Gunnarsen who is not happy in the wilderness and whose strength is taxed almost to breaking point by the lodge. Vera becomes jealous of Maggie and Haldar, not understanding that Maggie is now wedded to a place: "Maggie's union with Three Loon Lake was like a happy marriage (were we married last week, or have we always lived together as one?)" (p. 84).

Vera and Hilda Severance are traditional counterparts to Maggie and Nell who have both chosen non-traditional roles. Vera makes her life a martyrdom because she does not know any better. Ambivalent about Maggie's strength and competency, she finally succumbs to her own dark night of the soul when she attempts to drown herself in the lake and fails. Like a child, she then turns to Maggie who holds her: "Maggie, bending drew Vera up and held her strong and softly in her arms until the trembling and crying went quiet" (p. 147).

Hilda rebels against her unconventional mother and chooses as conventional a life as possible for herself. Once married to Albert Cousins, she will find fulfillment as a wife and mother. Nell's true spiritual daughter is Maggie to whom she entrusts the Swamp Angel. She also gives Maggie her knowledge of a lifetime, her spiritual wisdom. In their brief visit at Kamloops, Nell finds an image for her vision:

"... I look back and round and I see the miraculous interweaving of creation ... the everlasting web ... and I see a stone and a word and this stub," and she threw down the stub of her cigarette, "and the man who made it, joined to bounds of creation ...." (p. 150)

It is up to Maggie to put the vision into practice. With her woman's knowledge and her father's training, she becomes the power centre for the group at the lodge. Haldar relies on her; Alan loves her; Vera comes to depend on her; Angus, the young Chinese boy, works well because she is there. Yet Maggie is not the "boss" in the traditional male sense. She is building a community based on work, love and trust; the Loon Lake lodge is a tangible expression of the "everlasting web".

If Maggie were ambitious, in the patriarchal sense, she would have taken up Mr. Cunningham's offer of a job. Instead, she chooses to stay where her "love service" is needed. She is a secular saint who fulfills herself through giving of her strength to others. When such a gift is placed on demand, as it was in her marriage with Eddie Vardoe, the gift itself becomes a perverted form of life. The narrator defines this perversion: ''... Maggie Lloyd, with no one to care for, had tried to save herself by an act of compassion and fatal stupidity. She had married Edward Vardoe'' (p. 16).

By freeing herself from a false relationship, Maggie is free to form true ones. The Gunnarsens become her adopted family but the lodge community also includes Angus and, implicitly, others who will come to share in the dream and the work. Beyond the nuclear family model, this community cuts across race, age, class and gender bias. The worldly world might look at them and see: a run-away wife, a crippled man, his neurotic wife, his bewildered little boy, a Chinese boy. In the context of the novel, however, we see them as: a redeeming angel, a man with a big dream, a woman and her little boy in need of love, a young man who will become a leader.

The natural setting for this community is an important aspect of its meaning. Eddie Vardoe, the fast-talking salesman, would never survive in this wilderness. He belongs where time is money and relationships are mutually predatory. By contrast, time in nature slows down, becomes a seasonal, cyclical rhythm. The novel opens with an image of migrating birds returning in the spring. This image prefigures Maggie's own flight to her true home. The novel concludes with the image of fish flickering around the Swamp Angel at the bottom of Maggie's lake. Plucked from its human symbolic context, the gun is now part of the natural order. Maggie has become the true Swamp Angel.

Nature restores, but it can also destroy. Balanced against the fawn and kitten image is that of the eagle and the osprey. Balanced against the images of water as a healing power are those of water's potential destructiveness. Maggie imagines herself as a strong swimmer but the narrator slips in a warning in brackets: ''She could never sink, she thinks (but she could)'' (p. 100). Vera tries to drown herself; Mr. Cunningham is nearly drowned.

The human relationship with the natural world is tempered by experience and caution. Ethel Wilson preserves the distinction between nature and human nature. Her view of human nature is, however, a profoundly female one.

The two poles of strength in the book are Nell and Maggie. Be-

tween them is spun the "everlasting web" of human con-
nectedness. There are sympathetic male characters (Albert
Cousins, Haldar, Henry Corder) but their roles, compared to the
women's, are minor. Power is defined in female terms: not hierar-
chically but co-operatively structured; not domination but sharing and serving; not trying to possess or exploit Nature but trying to live in harmony and balance with the natural world.

The spiritual vision is female and so is the narrator's godlike
eye which sees just how Maggie would buy a big roast so as to
leave leftovers for this husband she despises. The narrator who
sees with some compassion how Vera has been worked beyond
her strength and so welcomes Maggie's arrival:

> She was almost happy. Her load seemed for a time to
> slide away. Only a woman who pulls too heavy a load
> for her strength and skill could know Mrs. Gunnarsen's
> emotion. Not even a horse. (p. 74)

Who sees, with amusement, proud Nell Severance bowing her
head to wear a hat to her daughter's wedding. Who creates for
us the "close fabric" of these women's lives with an understanding based on experience of the traditional women's culture and
roles which have shaped these characters' lives.

Ethel Wilson is not a feminist writer in the conscious, political
sense of the term but she thoroughly explores women's experiences within the dominant male culture. Some of her women
characters transcend their roles and, in so doing, transform
themselves and make possible the transformation of others.
Wilson also understands and respects women who choose the
more traditional roles of wife/mother. She understands too the
economic and social pressures upon these women, most of whom,
like Maggie and Nell, have had little or no professional education or training. For such women, the conventional career choices
are simply non-existent. They either find a non-traditional escape
route or a man to support them. In this sense, most of the
characters in her fiction come out of a 1940's -1950's Canadian
context (with the exception of those in The Innocent Traveller) and
their lives reflect the larger social/political forces of that period
described by writers such as Betty Friedan.[4]

Yet Maggie and Nell are also avatars; they belong to and derive
from the powerful mythic structure of the female psyche, not as
described by males, but as experienced by women. Nell is the

wise Old Woman, grandmother of our soul. Maggie is the
Woman-Self who finds and heals herself. Her woman's power
allows others to heal themselves. Her element is the transfor-
mative one: water. Literally, sexually, and symbolically, the lake
belongs to her but, belonging to her, is shared with others. The
Fisher Queen restores the land, and her fish flick triumphantly
over the discarded gun.

Notes

1   Ethel Wilson, *Swamp Angel* (Toronto: New Canadian Library, 1962), p. 64.
    All further quotations will be taken from this edition.
2   "What is a rebel? A man who says no: but whose refusal does not imply
    a renunciation. He is also a man who says yes as soon as he begins to
    think for himself." Albert Camus, *The Rebel*, trans. Anthony Bowen (Lon-
    don: Peregrine Books, 1967), p. 19.
3   David Stouck, "Ethel Wilson's Novels", *Canadian Literature*, No. 74
    (Autumn, 1977), p. 85, refers to the symbol "of the grail in Maggie's
    yellow Chinese bowl."
4   Betty Friedan, *The Feminine Mystique* (New York: Norton, 1963).

INNOCENCE AND SOLITUDE: THE FICTIONS OF ETHEL WILSON

George Woodcock

Ethel Wilson always stood somewhat outside the general currents of Canadian writing in her time or any time. She was a great deal older than most of her contemporary novelists, and belonged by experience as well as birth to an earlier generation. She did not publish her first short story until she was forty-nine in 1937, when "I Just Love Dogs" appeared in the *New Statesman*, and her first novel, *Hetty Dorval*, appeared in 1947, when she was fifty-nine. Her career, after that, was remarkably short, for the last of her six books, *Mrs. Golightly and Other Stories*, appeared in 1961, and the last of her contributions to literary periodicals in 1964. Though Ethel Wilson lived long afterwards, until 1980, she withdrew in her later years into the silence of bereavement and sickness. The two items that represented the end of her career as a published writer, both appearing in the autumn of 1964, were a short story in *Tamarack Review* ("A Visit to the Frontier") and a slight autobiographical essay ("Reflections in a Pool") in *Canadian Literature*.

Thus Ethel Wilson's career as a writer lasted only twenty-seven of her ninety-two years, and her books all appeared within an even briefer period of fourteen years. In terms of publication she was the junior contemporary of much younger writers like Hugh MacLennan and Sinclair Ross, both of whom published first novels six years before *Hetty Dorval*, but in terms of age and experience she was the contemporary of writers we regard as belonging to much older generations. She was three years younger than D. H. Lawrence and six years younger than Virginia Woolf and James Joyce; she was six years older than Aldous Huxley and J. B. Priestley, and as a child she had known Arnold Bennett. When she reached Vancouver, she and the city were both in their early teens, youthful and growing, and when King Edward VII died she was a young woman in her early twenties.

I suggest that in this temporal disjunction between experience and creation lie many of the clues to the special character of Ethel Wilson's writing. For, as I remarked in an earlier and briefer essay, "She had retained, I realized, an Edwardian sensibility, but she had developed a contemporary ironic intelligence, and it was the interplay of the two that gave her books their special quality."[1]

When she began to write, Ethel Wilson carried with her — in terms of personal memories and family traditions — the rich past to which she gave fictional form in *The Innocent Traveller*, that intriguing chronicle in which the history of the young city of Vancouver is interwoven with the group biography of a transplanted Victorian family. At the same time, coming of a literary lineage (Matthew Arnold as well as Arnold Bennett haunted its past) she had remained aware of what was happening in the literary world of her time, and in her correspondence she showed a sensitive appreciation of the special qualities of novelists as varied in time and kind as Defoe and Proust.

The breadth of Ethel Wilson's literary sympathies extended to her Canadian contemporaries, and she followed with enthusiastic interest the upsurge of writing in this country during the 1950s and the early 1960s. She expressed her admiration for the achievements of Gabrielle Roy, Morley Callaghan and Robertson Davies, and recognized the originality and the lyrical power of a novel so unlike her own work as Sheila Watson's *The Double Hook*. Her very use of the adjective "dissimilar" when she talked of these writers implied that she did not need to identify herself with them. Indeed, one of the aspects of the literary calling she always emphasized was the fact that it was solitary and hence individual. In a late essay, "A Cat Among the Falcons" (*Canadian Literature* 2, 1959), she talked of her misgivings about Creative Writing courses, and went on, discussing the writers she admired:

> ... I am impelled to think that most of them — equipped with their natural and varied gifts and their early acquired processes of language — travelled their own legendary way. I cannot avoid the conviction that a writer who can already handle his tools and write, is thereafter self-taught by writing (how the view opens out), and thus a literature is made .... It is possible that a preference for early and thorough familiarity with the language, for privacy of intention, and the individual road in the matter of "creative writing" (I borrow the term, it is not mine), is a personal idiosyncrasy only; but as I look over the wide reaches of writing and at the highly personal art and act of writing, I don't think so.[2]

Clearly Ethel Wilson saw her own writing in this way — as an activity that in its creative phases was private, individual, unruled by any collective imperative. In the same essay she talked of how, in her experience, the act of creation went beyond the conscious direction even of the writer herself.

> There is a moment, I think, within a novelist of any originality, whatever his country or his scope, when some sort of synthesis takes place over which he has only partial control. There is an incandescence, and from it meaning emerges, words appear, they take shape in their order, a fusion occurs.[3]

It was this passionate sense of the personal and unconsciously motivated development of original literary works — a far cry from the doctrines of art breeding from art that Northrop Frye developed out of Oscar Wilde's *Intentions* — that made Ethel Wilson distrustful of fashions in fiction and intent on going her own way and — as she put it — "simply writing." This made her appreciate writers unfashionable among the literary intelligentsia who handled their medium lovingly and carefully. Writing to Desmond Pacey, she defended Arnold Bennett against what she regarded as Virginia Woolf's blindness to "his view of poor persons, poor houses, poor places, mean streets, and their relative beauty to those concerned — both dwellers and observers."[4] And in the *Canadian Literature* essay already cited she took up the defence of another writer often despised by academic critics and cultural snobs.

> Somerset Maugham does not pretend to sit upon Olympus, but I wonder if there is any novelist anywhere in the English-speaking world today who can write a straightforward story like *Cakes and Ale*, full of humanity and dextrous exposure.[5]

In Ethel Wilson's approach to literature there was a great deal of what she called "innocence" when she applied it to her characters — the power to look at the world with clear eyes and live with what one sees. Once she talked of the "artlessness" that is "very artful indeed," and it is this quality that is evident not only in her writing but also in her perceptions of the qualities in other people's writing that she admires. Writing about some of the writers she most admired — again to Desmond Pacey — she remarked that "my taste runs to economy in writing — with some glorious exceptions,'' and went on to say of the novelists she liked:

> I would say that the limpid style of most of them, the lack of pretentiousness, the fact that these people have something to say, with skill, with good heart, often with deep feeling yet with some cynicism, their detachment as well as their involvement, give one inexpressible pleasure. They have *style*, each his own, and without style ... how dull.[6]

Ethel Wilson did not pretend to be a critic, though at times she wrote with great insight about her craft, and for the purposes of this essay it is not important whether what she says about her favourite writers is objectively correct, though generally speaking I believe it is. The point is that in delineating the qualities of others she seems to speak of her own aims in writing, and certainly what all her works strive at — without invariably attaining — the limpid and unpretentious style, involvement distanced by detachment, irony without the loss of feeling.

Ethel Wilson was not one of those novelists who regarded critics as vermin on the body of literature. She saw the value of the critic as mediator, but she was as unhappy about fads in criticism as she was about fads in fiction, and though she herself handled symbolism sparingly but skilfully, she was especially perturbed by any broadly symbolic interpretation of her work. The critic who discusses Ethel Wilson's work should be guided by this preference on her part, for her great virtue lies in her power to record experience, not literally, but faithfully, and it is out of this recording and out of her extraordinarily clear observation of peoples and places that her symbolism and the formal structure of her novels emerge by natural extension; one never has the feeling that any symbol appearing in her books is deliberately invented, either for its own sake or to evade the difficulties of clear and direct expression.

I talked a moment ago about the clear observation of ''people and places'', and in that phrase, it seems to me, is contained the dual pattern that gives so much of its interest to Ethel Wilson's work. For she presents the unusual combination — especially in Canada — of the novelist of manners and the novelist concerned in a lyrical way with the natural world and man's place in it. She is greatly interested in the details of daily life and the modes of human behaviour and intercourse, and in representing them she has something of the wit and playfulness of a Congreve or a Peacock as well as the wry understanding of a Jane Austen. Yet she is so intensely open to the appeal of the natural setting, of the places she and her characters inhabit, that she writes of them with a shimmering intensity that reminds one — though it in no evident way imitates him — of the young D. H. Lawrence, the Lawrence of *Sons and Lovers* and *The White Peacock* celebrating the English countryside.

It is significant that what Ethel Wilson found intriguing in Proust was not so much his more obvious and celebrated preoccupation with Time, but his concern with Place, from which, as she once said, ''he took his text''. For her, Proust writing on Paris and Combray and Balbec seemed to be reaching the universal through a regional awareness, which she was careful to point out was something quite different from provincialism. She was willing to admit that there were some writers — and good writers — who were not affected by Place. But for her it was so essential that, with all her awareness of the universal implications of literature and of the intense privacy of the act of creation, her writing must be centred where her life had mainly been experienced. As she said in another late essay (''The Bridge or the Stokehold'', *Canadian Literature* 5, 1960):

> ... I am not consciously aware in my personal act of writing (how could one be?) of ''the Canadian novel'' or ''the English novel'' or ''the American novel'', as the critic or the critical reader must be aware, and as I am aware when I transfer to the position of the critical reader. When I think of the universal yet private and, I hope, critical approach of a working writer to his novel itself, the happier I am — free, and devoid of personal or national self-consciousness, which is the way I like it. Self-consciousness is a triple curse. But in retrospect I see my Canadianness, for example, in that my locale in a sustained piece of writing (that is, in a book) has to be British Columbia. There are other places that I know and love, but none that I know, and feel, and love in the same way. But I did not choose it. It chose. It is very strong.[7]

In stressing that Ethel Wilson is so intent an observer of human behaviour, and so sensitive to the setting where her novels or stories are mostly placed, I do not suggest she is ever a mere recorder, for the inventive imagination works strongly as she melds together the detail out of which her fictions are constructed. However authentic their lives may be, her characters seem rarely to be taken largely from life, and sometimes it is clear that they have sprouted and grown from a very small germ of actuality. In the essay I have just quoted, Ethel Wilson tells us:

> A novel of mine or its main character, grew directly from a few words dropped almost at random in a previous book. The words were, "... formed other connections". What connections? I had never seen and did not know the girl in question. She did not exist in my knowledge any more than a fly in the next room, but I considered certain aspects and likelihoods, and wrote a book called *Lilly's Story*. On the way, characters multiplied, their outlines at first dim, later clear. I cannot imagine willingly employing even a marginal character without knowing his outside appearance so well that he could be identified in the street by myself and for my own purposes.[8]

This imaginative construction of her characters to the point of actually visualizing them is related to the economy Ethel Wilson has been able to achieve in the text as well as in the structure of her concise yet complex novels. If she is not excessively concerned with the process of symbolization, she has always been skilful in tense, evocative writing that stimulates the mind's eye; this allows her to dispense with lengthy passages of explication and at moments to achieve the visualized shorthand of a kind of prose imagism, as in the brilliant and counterbalancing sentences that open and close *Swamp Angel*:

> Ten twenty fifty brown birds flew past the window and then a few stragglers ....[9]
> When all was still the fish, who had fled, returned, flickering, weaving curiously over the Swamp Angel. Then flickering, weaving, they resumed their way.[10]

By such simple means the whole novel is looped into its environment.

....

In the first part of this essay I have been relating what I see as
the essential qualities of Ethel Wilson's fiction to her personal attitudes towards the art of fiction, which are those of an acute,
honest and somewhat ironic self-observer. The appearance of
simplicity which her work offers demands, I suggest, this approach. We must have some idea of her general strategy to
understand how the imagination uses this limpid style, this illusion of glittering verisimilitude, this deceptively didactic manner
of narration which implies more than it ever states. Now I shall
suggest how this strategy is translated into the tactical patterns
of her various novels.

Hetty Dorval, the first of these novels, is perhaps the most striking example of the combination of a Victorian sensibility and a
modern ironic consciousness that I have noticed as especially
characteristic of Ethel Wilson. Indeed, it is the failure of these two
aspects of her literary persona to coalesce at this point that makes
it less than perfect, though an extraordinarily pleasing book. Ethel
Wilson herself described it as an "innocent novella", and indeed
it is based on the encounter of two kinds of innocence — that
which grows into experience in the sense of embracing and seeking to understand the collective life of humanity, and that which
does not.

The plot is a simple one, with strong elements of the conventional Edwardian romance. A beautiful but mysterious young
woman, Hetty Dorval, arrives to occupy a bungalow on the out-
skirts of Lytton, a small town in the British Columbian interior
at the confluence of the Fraser and the Thompson rivers. Frankie
Burnaby, the narrator, is attracted by her charm, and for a few
years Hetty weaves in a pattern of coincidences in and out of
Frankie's life, a temptress with a shadowy past of which we learn
only by vague conversational allusions. In the end, when Hetty
attracts a cousin to whom Frankie — now a young woman — is
deeply attached, there is a confrontation between them, and Hetty
leaves the field and goes off with an Austrian lover to Vienna.

> Six weeks later the German Army occupied Vienna.
> There arose a wall of silence around the city, through
> which only faint confused sounds were sometimes
> heard.[11]

Hetty Dorval is a tightly knit little book, simple in plot and written with a kind of casual candour that fits and illuminates

Frankie's character as we watch it developing. In its combination of conciseness and completeness, *Hetty Dorval* is much nearer to a French récit — by Gide or Camus, for example — than it is to the Edwardian romances usually populated by characters like Hetty. Considered in herself, Hetty Dorval seems an improbable *femme fatale*, with her strange and literally two-faced beauty.

We remained standing there and gazing at the empty sky. Then Mrs. Dorval turned her face on me and I realized all of a sudden that she had another face. This full face was different from the profile I had been studying, and was for the moment animated. Her brows, darker than her fair hair, pointed slightly upwards in the middle in moments of stress and became in appearance tragic, and her eyes which were fringed with thick, short, dark lashes opened wide and looked brilliant instead of serene. The emotion might be caused by pain, by the beauty of flighting geese, by death, or even by some very mild physical discomfort, but the impact on the beholder was the same, and arresting. Ordinarily, Mrs. Dorval's full face was calm and somewhat indolent. The purity was not there, but there was what I later came to regard as a rather pleasing yet disturbing sensual look, caused I think by the over-fullness of the curved mouth and by those same rounded high cheek-bones which in profile looked so tender. Whatever it was, it is a fact that the side face and the full face gave not the same impression, but that both had a rapt striking beauty when her eyebrows showed distress.[12]

Hetty's life is that of an adventuress who becomes involved with men not because she can love them but because they are rich and powerful; at times she turns her charm upon other people, like Frankie and her cousin Rick, and one is never certain whether she is practicing her power or acts out of an indolent unloving good nature. There are times when Hetty's life moves into melodrama, and on no occasion more strikingly than in the scene in which Mrs. Broom, her long-suffering housekeeper, shatters Hetty's illusions of being an orphan without ties of any kind by revealing that she is actually her mother. It could have been the episode that spoilt the book, but Ethel Wilson handles it with

exemplary skill and locks our attention with a final memorable
visual image.

And Hetty did exactly what Hetty would do. She did
not speak to her mother. Without a word or a look she
rose and slowly went out of the room, closing the door
behind her, and left her mother standing there, looking
after her with a ravaged face.

Mrs. Broom had forgotten me. She now looked down
at her hands, and so did I. Her hands, with the
pressure upon the table, were red and looked swollen
and congested. She held up her hands and regarded
them strangely, turning their roughness this way and
that to the light. What she thought as she regarded her
worn hands so strangely I could only guess.[13]

If one makes the leap of credulity and accepts Hetty as
something near to an allegorical figure, then the novel takes on
two aspects. It is first, as I have suggested, a study in two kinds
of innocence, and secondly a fascinating study of the process of
growing up, in which flesh-and-blood Frankie becomes the central figure and Hetty becomes a foil to Frankie's changing attitudes
to existence.

Hetty's innocence is the negative kind that manifests itself in
a failure to feel for or with other people, and, more than that,
a dominant desire to remain untouched by them. Hetty is not
wholly insensitive; she responds with deep feeling to the wild
geese in whom she sees made manifest her own desire to fly for
ever free. But she is incapable of developing loves or loyalties.
"People only existed when they came within her vision. Beyond
that she had neither care nor interest."[14] She has no malice, as
Frankie observes, but she resents attachments that limit her
freedom or interfere with her "self-indulgence and idleness." "It
is preposterous, the way other people clutter up and complicate
one's life," she says. "It is my own phobia ...."[15]

Thus Hetty's innocence takes the form of an inability to proceed beyond the self-bound world of the infant, an inability to
acknowledge herself "a piece of the Continent, a part of the maine
...." Frankie, on the other hand, has been taught by her mother
the truth of John Donne's statement (which is the epigraph to
the novel) that "No man is an Island, intire of it selfe ..." and
so she shows the natural growth from innocence into experience.

John Donne was to Ethel Wilson much more than a convenient source of epigraphs. "My own discovery of John Donne, almost before he has again entered the Re-Establishment, dazzled me,"[16] she remarked in "A Cat Among the Falcons", and there is no doubt that Donne's central statement about the unity of all mankind continued to be an inspiration throughout her writing life, so that her characters can be divided between those who through love move into the world of experience and realize that they are irrevocably "involved in Mankinde."

It was less the spiritual content of Donne that Ethel Wilson absorbed than his abounding sense of the reality of existence and the unity of all beings. She pays tribute to the pious, like the mystical and saintly Annie Hastings in *The Innocent Traveller*, but it is the people who belong to the visible rather than the invisible world that she portrays with the greatest understanding and involvement. Life as she projects it in *Hetty Dorval* no less than in her other novels is the whole world in which we live, including the human communities to which we belong, as Frankie belongs to Lytton and the country around it with its mixed population of whites and Indians and Chinese, but also the whole environment, for everything that happens in the human heart finds its echoes and correspondences in the natural world.

This is why Ethel Wilson's precise and lyrical description of the country of sagebrush hills and great rivers in which so much of *Hetty Dorval* takes place is so important. We read it not merely for its evocative representation of the natural setting but also because we are aware of being offered a kind of mirror in which the human condition is illuminated, just as Frankie's room in Vancouver contains a mirror in which she sees the mountains framed into forms whose power she had never realized before. Frankie herself recognizes the importance of the "genius of place", and remarks:

> My genius of place is a god of water. I have lived where two rivers run together, and beside the brattling noise of China Creek which tumbles past our ranch house and turns our water wheel, and on the shore of the Pacific Ocean too — my home is there, and I shall go back.[17]

And water does indeed play a constant and varying role in Frankie's existence. A sea voyage to England marks the beginning of her growth into maturity; she leaves Canada a girl and quickly in Europe becomes a sophisticated and responsible young woman. And perhaps the most potent image in *Hetty Dorval* — an image generating a vast symbolic power — is that of the confluence of the two rivers, the Fraser and the Thompson, and the Bridge from which one sees them; it is an image to be repeated in Ethel Wilson's best novel, *Swamp Angel*, which shares so greatly the terrain of *Hetty Dorval*. She describes it thus in her first novel:

At the point where the Thompson, flowing rapidly westwards from Kamloops, pours itself into the Fraser, flowing widely and sullenly southwards from the Lillooet country, is the Bridge. The Bridge springs with a single strong gesture across the confluence of the rivers and feeds the roads and trails that lead into the northern hills which are covered with sage, and are dotted here and there with extravagantly noble pine trees. The way to my own home lay across the Bridge.

Ever since I could remember, it was my joy and the joy of all of us to stand on this strong iron bridge and look down at the line where the expanse of emerald and sapphire dancing water joins and is quite lost in the sullen Fraser. It is a marriage, where, as often in marriage, one overcomes the other, and one is lost in the other. The Fraser receives all the startling colour of the Thompson River and overcomes it, and flows on unchanged to look upon but greater in size and quantity than before. Ernestine and I used to say, "Let's go down to the Bridge," and there we would stand and lean on the railing and look down ... at the bright water being lost in the brown, and as we walked and laid our own little plans of vast importance for that day and the next, the sight of the cleaving joining waters and the sound of their never-ending roar and the feel of the frequent Lytton wind that blew down the channels of both the rivers were part and parcel of us, and conditioned, as they say, our feeling.[18]

The image — like all potent images — can be read in several ways. It can stand in potent isolation, like the image in a haiku, suggesting everything, stating nothing. It can be read as a rendering of direct experience, and, given the plot of the book, as a portent of what follows, for soon Ernestine will be destroyed by the "sullen Fraser" when she plunges in to try and save a dog (thus providing the extreme contrast to Hetty's persistent non-involvement with other beings). It can be read symbolically. Rivers run together and all rivers run into the sea, which means much the same as Donne's imagery of islands and continents. Lives run together, as rivers do, so, irrevocably, something from Hetty's life (the brown of the Fraser or the blue of the Thompson?) has flowed into Frankie's life. Or, finally, we can return to our concepts of innocence and experience, and learn that no life continues forever in the innocent blueness of origins; experience muddies and hides it, just as Hetty's sparkling and careless beauty in fact flows into a river of murky consequences.

The Innocent Traveller is a more complex and also a more ponderous book than *Hetty Dorval*, mainly because it attempts to be two things, the life-story of an eccentric personality and the history of a family. In both respects it is highly readable and conducted with wit and wisdom, but the fusion is incomplete.

The novel begins in Staffordshire, Ethel Wilson's ancestral county, and there is no doubt that family traditions and her own memories have contributed to its content, just as one of the younger members of the fictional family, Rose, shares much of Ethel Wilson's youthful experience and perhaps also her point of view.

The innocent traveller is Topaz, at the beginning of the novel a small child, "innocent as a poached egg," telling Matthew Arnold with embarrassing enthusiasm about the newly installed water closet in the Edgeworth house that goes "Whoosh! Whoosh!" She ends far away in space and time from that Staffordshire home, for she has passed a hundred when, in Vancouver, she finally dies, as self-centred, as avid, as innocent, as she had always been.

> Topaz is dying, there is no doubt of that. She — gay, volatile, one hundred years old, the last of her generation, long delayed — is uneasy. She is very restless. She shows no fear and yet she seems to be in some kind of anguish. Plainly she is awaiting something, an affirmation or release. What is that she is saying? She wants to go, she says. She is being prevented. The poor volatile bird.

"Let me go immediately ... immediately ..." she mur-
murs in her imperious way. "A hundred years ... I
shall be late ... me, the youngest." Then the small face
lightens. "Quick, get me some fresh lace for my head,
someone! I'm going to die, I do declare!" Evidently she
is pleased and confident. What an adventure, to be
sure!

Away she went. Now she is a memory, a gossamer.[19]

Topaz becomes "a memory, a gossamer" because she had no
love and no true attachment. Yet, thanks to circumstances and
especially to the love of others, she has been able to live out her
life with happiness and zest and to retain to the end the special
kind of innocence that enables her to survive in emotional insulari-
ty until death gathers her in to the continent of the one experience
that, after birth, all mankind must share.

In this way, of course, though it reads as a very different kind
of book, much busier and more crowded, *The Innocent Traveller*
is an extension of *Hetty Dorval*, presenting the comic rather than
the tragic face of innocence. If Topaz is incapable of love, she has
an extraordinary zest for living, yet in her own strange way she
remains immune from the effects of experience, which leaves her
unchanged while it moulds and modifies the other major
characters in the novel. The very innocence that keeps her from
forming deep personal attachments also enables her to confront
each encounter in life with an open kind of enthusiasm. It also
makes her tolerant, so that she suffers neither from snobbery nor
from any other prejudice and is willing to accept people as she
sees they are. Conventions and conventional distinctions mean
nothing to her, and she is as devoid of prejudice as she is — like
Hetty — lacking in malice.

One of the crucial scenes in the book concerns the black man,
Joe Fortes, an actual figure in Vancouver's history who used to
teach the children to swim at English Bay and who rescued many
from drowning. A woman taught by Joe is presented for membership of the Minerva Club, and a "pudding-faced lady" asserts
she has been "seen more than once in a public place, bathing
in the arms of a black man."[20] Topaz valiantly defends both Joe
Fortes and the maligned woman, who is elected to the club with
acclamation, and when she gets home tells her saintly sister Annie and her niece Rachel. And Rachel, who has often been an-
noyed with Topaz, listens to the tale, and then remarks: "I have

never heard you say an unkind thing about anyone. I have never heard you cast an aspersion on anyone. I really believe that you are one of the few people who think no evil."[21]

What Rachel says takes on its full meaning only if we think of it in relation not only to Topaz, but also to Hetty, that other innocent incapable of self-denying love. For Topaz is able to retain and nurture the honesty and fairness that represent the positive side of her innocence only because she has been brought up and protected to the end of her days in the warm nest of the family. Hetty seems less kind and more devious because she has never lived in the emotional shelter a family like the Edgeworths provides. The only relative she knew — and she did not know until the end that this was a real relative — had been Mrs. Broom, the mother masquerading as a servant, and all her years since girlhood had been a long campaign to gain the life of ease she desired without sacrificing the freedom that made the wild geese almost her totem birds. In one poignant scene on an Atlantic liner, Hetty approaches Frankie and her mother, and begs them not to reveal what they know about her, because she hopes to achieve a marriage that will bring her the security she had never known. Topaz's innocence has always flourished in security, and so it has manifested itself in genial eccentricities and a fearless acceptance of life.

Topaz could never have survived as she did, mentally and physically, without the support of that family, some of whose members understood better than she the reality of love. But the family could have survived without Topaz, and in the reader's eye it takes on a life of its own, as a kind of collective character that provides the other stream of interest in the novel.

We encounter the Edgeworths in the first chapter as a solid Staffordshire pottery family which has made money on teapots admired by Queen Victoria at the Great Exhibition and on chamber pots which an African tribe ordered in large numbers, reportedly for use as headgear. The Edgeworths are cultured enough to be the guests and associates of local politicians, though they have remained chapel folk, true to the Methodism that was the militant cult during the industrial revolution.

The Victorian patriarchs die, the children spread over the Empire, to die in India, to prosper in Australia and South Africa and Canada, and finally the remaining nucleus of the family — the saintly Annie, her daughter Rachel and the feckless Topaz,

emigrate to Canada. Once again, a sea voyage brings a change
of perspectives, and the Edgeworth women find in the new land
a place where their natures can expand into a new fulfilment.

> Topaz had at last reached open country. British Col-
> umbia stretched before her, exciting her with its moun-
> tains, its forests, the Pacific Ocean, the new little fron-
> tier town, and all the new people. Here was no time
> limit, no fortnight's holiday. Here she had come to live;
> and, drawing long breaths of the opulent air, she began
> to run about, and dance for joy, exclaiming, all through
> the open country.[22]

Vancouver, when the family arrives, is still little more than the
rough settlement that sprang so quickly into existence when the
C.P.R. reached over the mountains.

> Modest one- or two-storied buildings rose, to everyone's
> admiration, where the nobler forest had lately been. The
> forest still was, and winding trails through the woods
> ended at small hidden shacks, almost within the town
> itself. Vancouver was only a little town, but propheticall-
> ly it called itself a city.[23]

Vancouver's growth into a real city is one of the themes of *The
Innocent Traveller*, but it is so woven into the experience of the
novel's main characters that one perceives it rather as one
perceives Balzac's projections of Louis Phillippe's France; as a
living fictional entity, with Joe Fortes who was a historical individual and Yow the Chinese cook who was a historical type
at home within the half-imaginary, half-documentary but wholly self-consistent world of Topaz and her relatives and their
middle-class friends of British origin.

It is not the relative authenticity of the imaginative vision that
troubles one in *The Innocent Traveller*. It is rather the awkwardness of the structure. The novel is highly episodic in form. Three
chapters, "Down at English Bay" (about Joe Fortes), "The In-
numerable Laughter" (about Topaz scaring herself by sleeping
out one night in the Gulf Islands), and "I have a Father in the
Promised Land" (an ironic and amusing account of a revivalist
meeting) were all published separately in periodicals, where they
stood happily on their own, as self-contained as short stories. This
autonomy of the chapters gives the book as a whole a somewhat
jerky motion. It is no great improvement that the cracks which

result are often papered over by passages of authorial comment, sometimes too ponderous and sometimes too arch. Occasionally such comment actually serves as a flashforward, telling the reader with clumsy confidentiality the future consequences of acts committed in the present.

Ethel Wilson never again attempted a novel as large or as complicated in structure as *The Innocent Traveller*. She returned to shorter fiction with relatively simple structure and a single dominant line of development. Her next two novels, *Tuesday and Wednesday* and *Lilly's Story*, were in fact so short that they were published in a single volume, *The Equations of Love*, which altogether — with its 90,000 to 100,000 words — is no longer than an average novel.

At first sight, except that each of them is concerned with the varieties of emotion and relationship we bring together under the name of love, these two novels — or novellas — seem very different. *Tuesday and Wednesday* is entirely urban, set in a later Vancouver than the little town where Topaz and her sister first arrived. Its action, leading through comedy into tragedy, is completed in the two days of the title. Its characters have no time to change and grow; they merely reveal their true natures through the harrowing of stress and calamity. *Lilly's Story* encompasses the greater part of its heroine's life. It begins in the city and takes refuge in the country. And its very core is the changing and maturing of a personality. Lilly Waller, the pale girl with taffy-coloured hair who works in Lam Sing's restaurant and arouses the passions of Yow (the Edgeworths' cook) is in the beginning an innocent very much like Hetty Dorval, but she is born into life on a lower level, so that her struggle to survive is necessarily more ruthless and predatory. Experience changes her when she devotes her life to providing the best possible future for the child, Eleanor, whom she has by a passing liaison.

It is curious that no previous critic has linked these two novellas with Ethel Wilson's admiration for Arnold Bennett. For in fact they present just what she thought to be good in Bennett — "view of poor persons, poor houses, poor places, mean streets, and their relative beauty to those concerned ...." They are, apart from a few stories, the only writings in which Ethel Wilson left the middle class to which she belonged and imaginatively entered the minds and lives of people who lived outside the sophisticated world that was her own.

There is no suggestion in these novels that Ethel Wilson had been led to write about the poor by any political imperative. In her inclinations she was indeed liberal, and she had read widely in political polemics ever since she was introduced to the *New Statesman* in the 1920s, but, though politicians appear as characters in at least two of her novels, and she would have agreed that the novelist cannot ignore the political any more than other dimensions of life, the idea of writing to make propaganda for any partisan viewpoint was remote from her view of the role of literature. But to show through the glass of the imagination the true lives of poor people — to show them with compassion and understanding — was to her, as much as it had been to Dostoevsky, a part of the novelist's function, provided it were done in a work of literary art, true to and within itself.

Tuesday and Wednesday carries an epigraph from *Bleak House* — Mr. Chadband asking, "Now, my young friends, what is this Terewth ... firstly (in a spirit of love) what is the common sort of Terewth ..." And, somewhat like Jesting Pilate, the novella proceeds to consider how we can judge of human actions, and how the same actions, seen by different people, can seem heroic or despicable, without either viewpoint being objectively correct. Mortimer and Myrtle Johnson (Mort and Myrt) are a feckless working class couple living in an untidy room off Powell Street near the docks in Vancouver. Mort is good-natured, lazy, a born fantasist who turns every gardener's job he loses from idleness into a big landscaping contract. Myrt, who goes out cleaning, is less given to dreaming of this kind, for her small, acrid personality is self-contained and self-fuelling. Losing one job during the days of the novel, Mort almost gets another, and is walking home in a self-congratulatory glow when he encounters his dearest friend, the high-rigger Eddie Hansen, who is — according to his wont — roaring drunk on Powell Street. Eddie forces Mort to accompany him down to the docks on a futile search for a lost suitcase. Eddie staggers over the end of the wharf, and Mort either falls or dives after him — it is never quite clear which — and is dragged to his death by the panic-stricken logger, who cannot swim.

Later, in the Johnsons' flat, various versions of the truth are brought in confrontation with each other. Myrt believes the policemen who tell her of Mort's death. According to them the two men were seen staggering together down the street, and therefore they were presumably both drunk. Myrt thinks only

of herself and bitterly laments what Mort has done to her by getting drunk again with the detested Eddie. But shortly afterwards
her timid cousin, Victoria May Tritt, makes an appearance. On
her way to church Vicky has seen Mort walking soberly along
the street and being accosted by drunken Eddie. On her way back
from church, she has heard Mort's name mentioned by a group
of men talking in the street about the tragedy. On the spur of
the moment, it occurs to her to vindicate Mort's memory by in-
vention, and, reproaching Myrtle with uncharacteristic vigour,
she declares that Mort acted heroically, deliberately diving in to
rescue his drunken friend. Neither version is the whole truth,
but Victoria speaks with the passion of conviction, and Myrtle
in astonishment accepts her story.

> Something grew warm within Myrtle and she saw the
> simple picture of Morty putting his hands together and
> diving in to rescue Eddie Hansen and she became, as
> Victoria May had said, the widow of a hero, and she
> became proud of Morty, but prouder of herself for be-
> ing the widow of a hero. Vicky, seeing what she had
> achieved, expelled a long breath, and relaxed. How sim-
> ple it had been![24]

It is a world of simple, ill-educated people with primitive reactions among whom Ethel Wilson moves, a dripping Vancouver
world where minds are inclined to be as foggy as the skies, and
one wonders, when the equation of Mort's and Myrt's love is
worked out, just how the sum comes out. For underneath the
comic, almost Dickensian masks worn by Myrt and Mort and
Vicky and the self-indulgent Mrs. Emblem, Myrtle's aunt, one
senses emotions of compassion and loyalty and love that are unar-
ticulated or at best articulated in the debased language of the
cinema and the radio. (Television had yet to come.)

Lilly's Story begins in the same depressed area of Vancouver
as *Tuesday and Wednesday,* for the gambling houses where Yow
spends his nights and the café where he meets and becomes
obsessively enamoured of Lilly, a runaway girl working as a
waitress, are not far from the Powell Street areas where the
Johnsons lived.

Yow had already appeared in *The Innocent Traveller,* as lacking
in innocence as Aunt Topaz was full of it, yet capable of love.
He boasted, and probably truthfully, of having killed two men

in China, one quickly and one slowly, but he was devoted to the saintly Annie, Topaz's sister, and he loved Lilly with a ferocity that led to his ruin, for he stole on a large scale from the Edgeworths to win her heart. When Yow was arrested, Lilly — who had never loved in her life — thought only of saving herself from the police, and became a "pale slut who is running through the dark lanes, stopping, crouching in the shadows, listening, hardly daring to look behind her."[25]

If Aunt Topaz stands on one side of Hetty Dorval as the innocent who was sheltered and so saved from having to live in the appalling amorality of endangered innocence, Lilly stands on the other side — the child who never knew even the strange love with which Mrs. Broom had protected Hetty, her unproclaimed daughter. When she flees from the police and disappears to surface again on Vancouver Island, Lilly knows the meaning of love even less than Hetty or Topaz.

> No one had loved her, and she did not even know that she had missed love. She was not bitter, nor cruel, nor was she very bad. She was like the little yellow cat, no worse and no better. She expected nothing. She took things as they came, living where she could, on whom she could, and with whom she could, working only when she had to, protecting herself by lies or by truth, and always keeping on the weather side of the police.[26]

In Nanaimo Lilly goes to live with a Welsh miner, but there is no love. Lilly is still as innocent and uncaring as an animal, as Ethel Wilson suggests in the strangely harsh way in which she describes the relationship.

> Ranny was only a kennel into which a homeless worthless bitch crawls away from the rain, and out of which she will crawl, and from which she will go away leaving the kennel empty and forgotten.[27]

The rest of the novel tells of Lilly's transformation from "a homeless worthless bitch" into a loving and responsible human being, her difficult passage from innocence into experience. With one of those haunting resonances that in Ethel Wilson's work pass on from novel to novel, there is a second echo here of *Hetty Dorval*. The young Lilly, the taffy-haired girl for whom Yow lusted, may have been a debased counterpart of Hetty, but her later life uncannily resembles that of Hetty's mother, Mrs. Broom. Pregnant by Ranny the miner, she leaves him to have her child, and then assumes another self. She is no longer Lilly Waller, the slut who has an illegitimate child. She gives herself a new name, and with the new name a different history, so that she is now Mrs. Walter Hughes, the widow of a prairie farmer, better bred than herself, who was killed by a horse before their daughter was born. In this guise she sets about finding the circumstances in which she can best bring up her daughter and give her the kind of life she has missed.

To begin she becomes housekeeper to a British ex-officer and his wife at Comox, and there are some idyllic years until Lilly realizes that in the village Eleanor is know as "the maid's daughter". She departs and becomes housekeeper at a hospital in the Fraser valley; here she ages as her daughter grows up, and lets her looks fade, and resists the approaches of men, for all she can feel is the possessive love that binds her to her daughter.

The final opening out of that love comes when Eleanor has gone to Vancouver for training as a nurse, has married and herself had children. Lilly, in her hospital, seems to be withering into a loveless existence, when fate and coincidence thrust her back into the stream of life. One day, looking out of the window of her cottage at the hospital, she sees a figure of dread walking in from her past. It is Yow, come to work at the hospital as cook.

> Year after year now she had lived in an obscurity that was so planned and safe that there were times when it seemed that the years of vagrancy had never been. They had become a dream and hardly a dream, yet a recurring dream. Her faked past had almost become her reality. She had forgotten the associates of her vagrant years, and here was Yow, the most dangerous, the most violent of them all.[28]

Reappearing with such melodramatic suddenness, Yow paradoxically liberates Lilly from the life of fear and concealment into which her care for Eleanor has involved her. She flees once again, this time to Toronto, where she works as chambermaid in a hotel. There she meets widowed Mr. Sprockett, and Mr. Sprockett falls in discreet love with her, and Lilly, for the first time since Ranny, accepts a relationship with a man. But this time it is different. Ranny was the unloved provider in whom she found refuge as a fugitive. But Sprockett talks of love, and asks her for love, and Lilly begins to see love as a mutual caring:

> If loving Mr. Sprockett meant looking after him and
> thinking for him and caring for him and guarding him
> from harm and keeping things nice like she'd always
> done for Eleanor and for Matron, then she could love
> him, and she was his, and he was hers.[29]

She senses, in this relationship where she would give as much
as she would be given, "She would be without fear; nothing,
surely, could touch her now." And so, after the long years of
love as sacrifice, Lilly comes to the realization of love as mutual
caring, love as union.

Just as in some ways *Lilly's Story*, that modest and moving
novella, develops elements that had their origin in *Hetty Dorval*,
in other ways it anticipates *Swamp Angel*; perhaps most notably
in the way it develops the correspondences between human life
and the natural world. Its most dramatic scene is one of conflict
between wild creatures, when Lilly and Eleanor, still a child, are
on a little promontory at Comox, with the child's kitten. They
see a robin attacking a tiny snake; the kitten stalks the robin until the shadow of an eagle falls upon it, but before the eagle can
swoop down he in turn is attacked and driven away by a crow
and a seagull. The scene makes Lilly uneasy; she relates it to her
own life, and to her it "seems like everything's cruel, hunting
something." It is beyond Lilly to see — though her daughter
Eleanor may — what Ethel Wilson describes on the next page in
one of her authorial asides as

> The incorporeal presence in air, and light, and dark,
> and earth, and sea, and sky, and in herself, of
> something unexpressed and inexpressible, that
> transcends and heightens ordinary life, and is its
> complement.[30]

Nowhere in Ethel Wilson's work is this sense of a spiritual force
imminent in the natural world more powerfully expressed than
in *Swamp Angel*, the best of her novels. Maggie Vardoe, the
leading character, runs away from her present, as Lilly Waller
had done. She too changes her name to indicate her change of
living, though in her case she takes back an old name, Maggie
Lloyd, which means that she is rejecting the interlude in which
she sought to live according to bourgeois conventions with the
pathetic materialist Edward Vardoe.

Maggie Lloyd is a much more complex figure than the earlier characters with whom one naturally compares her, Hetty and Lilly. She has always known and understood the reality of love, in her relations with her father and later with her first husband, killed during the war. Her love for that dead husband does not vanish, but she married Edward Vardoe for compassion, and only when she realizes that this vain, coarse man is unchangeable does she decide to leave him. Having made her decision, she plans her departure carefully, earning money secretly, arranging her flight with care, and leaving no clues that will enable Vardoe to track her down. In this respect she resembles Lilly saving and planning before she leaves Ranny the miner to have her child.

But Maggie is not really choosing a new way of life. She had been brought up at a fishing lodge beside a lake in New Brunswick, where she helped her father and learnt from him the skill of fly-tying which she uses to finance her flight. It was in that past that she developed the self-reliance, manifesting itself in both resourcefullness and secretiveness, to which she now turns.

> Maggie, brought up from childhood by a man, with men, had never learned the peculiarly but not wholly feminine joys of communication, the déshabille of conversation, of the midnight confidence, the revelation. And now, serenely and alone, she had acted with her own resources ....[31]

There is something uncanny, even slightly repellent about the serenity with which Maggie makes her plans and acts and deals with people. For cruelty is never far from compassion, not only in her view of nature, but also in her own actions. Perhaps compassion has failed with Edward Vardoe, but the way Maggie leaves him, slipping out in the middle of dinner, seems calculated to create the greatest bewilderment and pain, and the same duality exists in her attitude to nature. She loves the wild and the creatures of the wild, yet fishing and all that goes with it are at the heart of her life, and — not being callous — she is aware of the cruelty. After she leaves Vardoe on her flight into the hinterland, Maggie stops for a couple of days beside the Smilikameen River, and fishes there.

> In the pleasure of casting over this lively stream she forgot — as always when she was fishing — her own

existence. Suddenly came a strike, and the line ran out, there was a quick radiance and splashing above the water downstream. At the moment of the strike, Maggie became a co-ordinating creature of wrists and fingers and reel and rod and line and tension and the small trout, leaping, darting, leaping. She landed the fish, took out the hook, slipped in her thumb, broke back the small neck, and the leaping rainbow thing was dead. A thought as thin and cruel as a pipe fish cut through her mind. The pipe fish slid through and away. It would return.[32]

At the moment of landing the fish, Maggie is as totally and naturally absorbed in her task and unconscious of its implication as the osprey she will later watch with such admiration, until the thought like a pipe fish slips through her mind and separates her from the world of nature.

Maggie goes on, through Lytton, where the meeting of the waters is again splendidly described, and on to Kamloops, where, up in the hills, she gets a job as cook at the lodge run by the Gunnarsons at Three Loon Lake. From now on this is her world and her life, and she cannot even envisage returning to the city. The lake, like her, is both cruel and kind. It gives Maggie physical and mental vigour, but two people are almost killed by it, and brought back to life by Maggie's care. A strength emerges in her. She is no longer the discontented powerless wife of Edward Vardoe. She moved to create a life in which her self-reliance can flourish, a life without attachments, though not without the desire to help others as she helps the Gunnarsons. But as she helps she shapes, dealing as capably with Vera Gunnarson's jealousy as she deals with the practical problems of running and expanding the lodge. She uses her very decency to impose her will on others, manipulating them even if it is for their own good, so that in the end one has a sympathy for poor weak Vera's obsessive feeling that Maggie is running the Gunnarson's lives. There are times when her very helpfulness robs other people of their personal sense of dignity.

In this way the main plot and the sub-plot of *Swamp Angel* come together and the title is explained. Leaving Vancouver, Maggie has left not only Edward but also her real friends, Hilda Severance and her old mother Nell. Hilda's unlikely marriage comes about and flourishes as Maggie's own marriage with Vardoe ends, and in the background the eccentric Nell Severance plays with her souvenir of a lost life, the pistol known as the Swamp Angel. For Nell has been a professional juggler in her day and remained romantically attached to the circus world of illusion, yet curiously practical as she now juggles with other people's lives, turning Vardoe aside from his murderous anger towards Maggie, and pushing Hilda into making up her mind to marry Albert Cousins. It is appropriate that when Nell feels the Swamp Angel is a dangerous toy to keep, she sends it to the other juggler, Maggie, and when Nell dies it is Maggie who takes the pistol and throws it into the lake as if it were Excalibur.

> She stood in the boat, and with her strong arm she threw the Angel up into the air, higher than ever Nell Bigley of the Juggling Bigleys had ever tossed it. It made a shining parabola in the air, turning downwards — turning, turning, catching the sunlight, hitting the surface of the lake, sparkling down into the clear water, vanishing amidst breaking bubbles in the water, sinking down among the affrighted fish, settling in the ooze. When all was still the fish who had fled, returned, flickering, weaving curiously over the Swamp Angel. Then flickering, weaving, they resumed their way.[33]

The Swamp Angel, which "in its eighty years or so has caused death and astonishment and jealousy and affection," nevertheless belongs to the temporal world of human artifice, and when it is gone, it will soon be "not even a memory, for there will be no one to remember it." The lake into which it falls represents the timeless world of nature where the fishes flicker and weave a dance that never ends. And so another duality of the novel is projected; we live in time but belong to the timeless, just as the land in which we live is rocks and trees and water but also in other ways a map of the human heart.

Swamp Angel offers Ethel Wilson's most successful structure as a novel, every part tuning with the other, just as Maggie Lloyd is her most developed and most convincing character. Perhaps there is a shade too much of the melodramatic in Nell Severance; perhaps Edward Vardoe is too absurdly contemptible, but otherwise the characters and their relationships exist entirely convincingly in their autonomous world.

Ethel Wilson's last novel, *Love and Salt Water*, was also her least successful. It is a neatly written and well enough constructed book about the growing-up of a middle class girl and her difficulties — which finally end — in achieving the kind of marriage that satisfied her. But the urgency of feeling that burns through the other books is no longer present. The essential plot is perhaps no more unpretentious than that of *Hetty Dorval*, but Ellen Cuppy does not develop through the same sensitively evoked opening of the perceptions as Frankie Burnaby, and there is no enigma in the book as interesting as Hetty. Even the minor characters are less tellingly portrayed as those that crowd *The Innocent Traveller*, and the wit has somehow faded from the narrator's tongue as the irony has from her eye. There is only one point in the whole book at which the reader becomes urgently involved. That is when Ellen takes her little nephew Johnny out in a dinghy in Active Pass to look for seals and they are nearly drowned when the riptide overturns the boat. The feeling of the British Columbia coast and its waters is at times pleasantly recalled, but rarely does it become the commanding environment of *Hetty Dorval* and *Swamp Angel*.

It is perhaps significant that this was the time when Ethel Wilson began to think consciously about her art as a writer, and to write about it almost as a critical outsider. For what is lacking in *Love and Salt Water* is precisely the sense that here is a writer led on half-consciously and only half-willingly by her own creation, which was so strongly present in her earlier books. *Love and Salt Water* is a well-made novel of manners, but the clear flame of feeling and insight one remembers from her earlier books does not shine through the translucency of its prose.

Thus Ethel Wilson's significant novels embrace an even shorter period than the full list of her books suggests. They were published in a mere seven years, from *Hetty Dorval* in 1947 to *Swamp Angel* in 1954, and the period over which they were written was doubtless no longer. But these few short books have an unchallengeable place in the record of Canadian fiction, not only for their own qualities and their influence on younger writers, but also because they were the first successful attempt to bring the physical setting of western Canada convincingly into fiction, so that their comedies of manners and their dramas of feeling were played out against superbly described backdrops of landscape, for Ethel Wilson was unrivalled in her time as a novelist of Place.

Notes

1   George Woodcock, "On Ethel Wilson", in his *The World of Canadian Writing: Critiques and Recollections* (Seattle: University of Washington Press; Vancouver: Douglas and McIntyre Ltd., 1980), p. 122.
2   Ethel Wilson, "A Cat Among the Falcons", *Canadian Literature*, No. 2 (Autumn 1959), pp. 13-4.
3   *Ibid.*, p. 16.
4   Desmond Pacey, *Ethel Wilson* (New York: Twayne Pub., 1967), p. 21.
5   Wilson, "A Cat Among the Falcons", p. 15.
6   Pacey, p. 18.
7   Ethel Wilson, "The Bridge or the Stokehold: Views of the Novelist's Art", *Canadian Literature*, No. 5 (Summer 1960), pp. 43-4.
8   *Ibid.*, p. 46.
9   Ethel Wilson, *Swamp Angel* (Toronto: Macmillan, 1954; rpt. McClelland and Stewart, 1962), pp. 13.
10   *Ibid.*, p. 157.
11   Ethel Wilson, *Hetty Dorval* (Toronto: Macmillan, 1947; rpt. Toronto: Macmillan, 1967), p. 92.
12   *Ibid.*, p. 15.
13   *Ibid.*, pp. 83-4.
14   *Ibid.*, p. 25.
16   Wilson, "A Cat Among the Falcons", p. 14.
17   Wilson, *Hetty Dorval*, p. 57.
18   *Ibid.*, pp. 6-7.
19   Ethel Wilson, *The Innocent Traveller* (London: Macmillan, 1949), p. 275.
20   *Ibid.*, p. 154.
21   *Ibid.*, p. 157.
22   *Ibid.*, p. 122.
23   *Ibid.*, p. 123.
24   Ethel Wilson, *Tuesday and Wednesday* in her *Equations of Love* (London: Macmillan, 1952), p. 123.
25   Ethel Wilson, *Lilly's Story* in her *Equations of Love* (London: Macmillan, 1952), p. 145.
26   *Ibid.*, p. 156.
27   *Ibid.*, p. 164.
28   *Ibid.*, p. 243.
29   *Ibid.*, p. 276.
30   *Ibid.*, p. 194.
31   Ethel Wilson, *Swamp Angel*, p. 20.
32   *Ibid.*, p. 38.
33   *Ibid.*, p. 157.

ERNEST BUCKLER

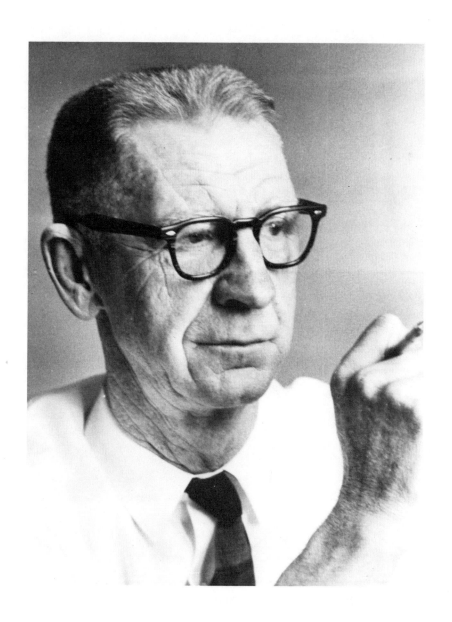

THE GENESIS OF ERNEST BUCKLER'S
THE MOUNTAIN AND THE VALLEY

Alan R. Young

A year after Ernest Buckler had published *The Mountain and the Valley* (1952), he gave a radio talk in which he mentioned that the novel had taken him six years to write.[1] However, Buckler's correspondence and manuscripts, now deposited in the Thomas Fisher Rare Book Library at the University of Toronto, reveal that the gestation period for this now acknowledged classic of Canadian literature was much longer.[2] My intention here is to trace the course of that gestation and to show how Buckler's comments on the novel, taken in consideration with his early short stories that were reworked into its fabric, collectively provide a unique glimpse of the processes of his creative imagination and at the same time suggest that certain aspects of the novel may hitherto have been overlooked by its interpreters.

The first hint of Buckler's desire to become a novelist occurs in a letter to *Esquire* in 1937 in which he quotes from the novel he himself is supposedly writing:

> ... When David closed his eyes at night, all the strange horde of imagination swarmed, seething, into his brain — the bewildering multiplicity of memory, the teeming variety of perception, the infinite permutations of speech ... the ephemeral, cloud patterns of ideas, constantly recast into a new galaxy, never still enough to have form or meaning or to crystallize and outline themselves in the mold of words; shimmering and wandering, through each other, insubstantial and bodiless, like the interstitial weavings of a puff of smoke.[3]

Here, complete with typical Bucklerian simile, is an intriguing but unconscious anticipation of the inner turmoil of David Canaan which is to become the central concern of the completed novel some fifteen years later. A few months later, in response to another letter to *Esquire* in which Buckler had pretended that his own fiction was superior to that of the magazine's contributors (among whom were Hemingway and Fitzgerald), Burton Rasco, the influential *New Yorker* critic, sent Buckler a telegram praising his "excellent sense and command of vigorous and effective English prose" and expressing his willingness as advisor to a publishing company to see whatever Buckler considered his "best unpublished work."[4] Buckler's bluff had been called for he had little to send, least of all a novel. Nevertheless, in 1939 in a letter to Rasco he mentioned that he was thinking of writing a "farm" novel.[5]

No further references to his plans for a novel occur until 1946. Meanwhile Buckler had been writing plays for the CBC, had managed to move from the correspondence to the fiction columns of *Esquire*, and had begun what was to be a fruitful relationship with *Saturday Night* by publishing a number of poems, articles and stories. However, in 1946, encouraged by these successes, Buckler seems to have returned to the idea of a novel, and he wrote to Edward Aswell of Harper and Brothers (the publishers) asking whether it was "too late for a book which has anything to do with the war."[6] Buckler mentions that "the short stories I did about the war, the ones I wrote from the truest compulsion, got editorial praise but no print." What troubles him is that these stories "are still gnawing at me inside my head, the way only stories you really believed in, but which were still-born, can." Out of this frustration, however, emerged the plan for a novel, for, enclosed with the letter to Aswell, are three stories which, Buckler claims, are "connected, my best, and have in them the foetus of a novel."[7]

Today the three stories are immediately recognizable as the barely-formed "foetus" of *The Mountain and the Valley*. In the letter Buckler explains that his "main theme is embodied in the one, 'The Trains Go By', the frustration of a young man who has to see it all happen to someone else," and his theme is "suggested also in 'Thanks for Listening'." A glance at "The Trains Go By" quickly reveals that the story was later modified and reshaped to form the bulk of Part Six "The Train" in the novel. The story concentrates upon Peter's isolation and frustration and the effects on him of the visit of his sister Martha and her sailor husband David. Whole passages and stretches of dialogue recur in the novel where, of course, the characters' names are changed to David, Anna and Toby respectively.[8] The pattern of the plot is also retained. Peter, who lives alone on the farm, is visited by his sister and brother-in-law prior to this latter's departure for the war. A remarkable understanding develops between the two men, but this is shattered at the end when Peter observes David's departure in the train and realizes the *"It was always someone else,* that was the panic of it. There had been these things while he was alive and young but they had all been for other men. The trains had all gone by and the grey smoke settled on the fields and he was standing there alone, with a hoe."[9]

A sequence of Peter's subsequent bitter reflections follows which reaches a climax when he slashes at his turnips with his hoe. The only basic difference between the novel and the story is that in the latter the two men are meeting each other for the first time and, rather than going hunting in the old orchards (see Chapter XXXVI) as they do in the novel, they walk to the top of the mountain. Presumably Buckler later made these adjustments so that the contrasts between the two men, who know each other from childhood on, could be sustained throughout the book and expanded to symbolize the pervasive dilemma facing David who is torn between his love for the land and his desire to move beyond the limitations of his rural culture. Given the symbolic importance in the novel of David's final climb up the mountain, which suggests his ultimate transcendence over his dilemma, it is also clear why Buckler should transform the mountain climb of the story into the hunting sequence.

"Thanks for Listening", the second of the stories sent to Aswell, reappears in the novel as the story which David sets down in his scribbler in Part Six while Toby and Anna go into town.[10] In the short story, so Buckler admits in his letter to Aswell, "the writing is a little overblown and doesn't quite come off even if the intention is honest." In fact the story is sentimental and self-pitying in its portrayal of the point of view of the one who did not go to the war. However, Buckler transforms this defect into a virtue in the novel since this key sample of the way David does write, as opposed to the way he thinks he writes, then becomes part of a planned pattern of irony that will be commented upon again in a moment. As he writes, David is excited by his own creative processes: "He said the phrase out loud. It was true. It was his. He felt like crying. Oh, it was wonderful, to be able to do a thing like this ...."[11] The reader, however, is meant to take a more objective view and be unimpressed by what David actually writes.[12]

The third of the stories sent to Aswell is entitled "Indian Summer", its subject, according to the letter, being "the relation of the man and the woman who are really *in* the war (Anna, here,

being the Martha of 'The Trains Go By')." The story later became
Chapter XXXVIII in Part Six of the novel, the section in which
Toby and Anna climb to the top of the mountain alone and share
one moment of consummate perfection which for Anna is described as "the peak of her whole life." In the novel the function of
this section is to underline ironically the fact that David has never
achieved a fulfilled relationship with anyone and that, in spite
of his desire to climb the mountain throughout the novel, the symbolic implications of which have already been mentioned, he has
yet to achieve that goal.

In both novel and story, it is Indian Summer, and the treachery
of the season is revealed when all turns cold as both characters
descend the mountain and the wife intuitively perceives that this
will be their last day together and that her husband will be lost
at sea. The novel provides a more concise version than the
story,[14] though Buckler adds a reference to Toby's and Anna's having "sloughed off the city way" during their visit, a passage comparing their silence to that of children in a place of enchantment,
a description of Anna's smile, Anna's memories of Christmas
with her twin brother when they were children, and an important paragraph in which the fact that Anna is wearing the clothes
of both her husband and brother serves to enforce Buckler's
deliberate fusing of the identities of the two men elsewhere,[15]
and to reveal the impending near-tragic situation of Anna ("...
now these clothes gave their definition to her. She looked small
inside them. As a child looks small who has no *other* clothes but
the discards, always cruelly too large, of someone else." p. 270).

The three stories sent to Aswell were politely returned by
Elizabeth Lawrence in Aswell's absence with the accompanying
suggestion that, since war themes are "desperately unpopular
with the public at this time," Buckler should broaden the base
of his idea "and make the war only an incident in the story of
a young man forced to watch life from the sidelines."[16] Whether
directly as a result of this suggestion or not, this in effect is what
Buckler went on to do. David Canaan is unable to participate in
the world into which he has been born on account of his physical
incapacities and the alienation he suffers because of his education and highly developed sensibility. At the same time the opportunities of city-life are rejected since they appear to deny this
innate love and attachment to the land. His inability through
physical disability to get enlisted for war service in Part Six is thus

merely a minor addition to an already established broader pattern of frustrated alienation.

Part of Buckler's reason for writing to Aswell was to seek some objective judgement as to whether he should risk the financial sacrifice involved in devoting his available writing time to a novel:

It's something I would like very much to do, but naturally if the idea has all the strikes against it at the start, there would not be much point in attempting it. Particularly when bread and health are such a problem with me that I literally couldn't abdicate the short story market unless there was something definite to hope for in the long run gamble. One must write to sell to live, even if it's only so that one may live to write.

We must be thankful that, in spite of Elizabeth Lawrence's somewhat lukewarm encouragement, Buckler decided to take on the gamble. In the process of broadening the base of his original plan for a war novel, Buckler went back to several of his other stories. One of the most interesting of these is an unpublished work called "The Locket".[17] This portrays the feelings of its narrator (David) who, torn between loyalty to family and desire to experience the world beyond the limited horizons of his rural situation, steals away early one morning to go to sea. His blind grandmother, with whom he has always had a special relationship, hears him and calls him to her. She tells of her hiding of a sailor on the run when she was young and gives David a locket. He recognizes the face in the locket as a kin to his own and realizes that the call to the sea in his blood and his grandmother's sympathetic attitude are due to this concealed part of his family history. Here evidently is an early version of David Canaan's relationship with his grandmother Ellen in *The Mountain and the Valley* and in particular the story of her relationship with a sailor about which she tells Anna in Chapter III. Significantly in the novel the call of the sea and the sound of a train are equated by Ellen,[18] thereby anticipating the climax of David's situation in Part Six when the train passes by bearing Toby to the sea. Similarly, in the novel Anna's future relationship with Toby is also anticipated when she says "I think I'll marry a sailor."[19] The gift of the locket to David occurs much later in the novel, but the crucial self-identification with the sailor is there, as is Ellen's empathy with David, who has just previously attempted to leave home:

> This locket had something to do with what had happen-
> ed today. She'd sensed somehow what had happened.
> She'd sensed it because she too knew what it was like
> when the moonlight was on the fields when the hay
> was first cut and you stepped outside and it was lovely,
> but like a mocking ... like everything was somewhere
> else.[20]

Another unpublished story exists in three different versions entitled "Children", "Hares and Hounds" and "The Day Before
Never" respectively.[21] It depicts two country children who are
isolated from their peers, the boy because of his cleverness at
school, and the girl because of society's unspoken attitudes
towards her mother who is widely suspected of being sexually
promiscuous. The story develops a theme which Buckler once
described as always being "an insistent one" for him: "The theme
of lonely people who, because their true inner warmth and vitality
is never suspected, come to be cruelly labelled by others as of
one negligible 'type' or another."[22] The cruelty of the girl's situation is revealed in a powerful schoolroom scene in which she is
made victim of ribald smirks when she has to read from the Bible the story of "The Woman Taken in Adultery". The boy's isolation develops into an acute frustration which causes him to smash
his favourite kite. The two children understandably find relief for
their isolation in their friendship.

Clearly these stories anticipate the David/Effie relationship in
the novel though the two incidents mentioned above do not, of
course, occur there. However, the fact that Buckler did conceive
of David and Effie in much the same way as the protagonists of
these earlier stories is clear from some "Notes on David and Effie" which he sent to Doris Mosdell of the CBC in November 1964
in which he states that Effie is " 'set apart' by her consciousness,
no whit less acute because it is not altogether explicit, that her
mother is subtly shunned. And David is somewhat of a stranger
to the others because of his precocity."[23]

The enormity of David's betrayal of Effie in the novel would
have been much greater had Buckler initially made more of the
parallel situations of the two characters. By pruning some of the
material in the stories, he seems, in this instance, to have inadver-
tantly fallen short of his intentions, for the parallels that he
assumes in his "Notes" are in fact hardly apparent.

In another of the early stories, "One Quiet Afternoon", Buckler explored the situation of the prototype for Effie's mother, Bell Delahunt.[24] The story is portrayed through the eyes of a motherless boy (David) who feels a special attachment to the woman (Martha Legros). The insinuations of society cruelly isolate her, and, when her husband begins to accept society's view of her and calls her "a whore", she commits suicide by drowning, a tragic climax parallel to that of her counterpart in *The Mountain and the Valley*.[25] In a letter to Desmond Pacey, Buckler admitted that "One Quiet Afternoon" had been reworked into the novel, and in the same letter a similar admission is made concerning "The First Born Son",[26] which provides an anticipation of the important rock-clearing scene in Chapter XXIV and the ensuing rift between David and his father.[27]

Clearly, as Buckler set out to transform himself from short story writer to novelist, the material of his stories (both published and unpublished) was the first thing he turned to. Already he had the makings of an imaginative world where characters, themes and plot-motifs overlapped from one narrative to another. The choice of a semi-autobiographical protagonist must have followed naturally, for the sensitive, intelligent, isolated country boy, separated from his peers by his precocious learning and desire for something beyond that which rural culture appeared to offer, had already appeared many times in his fiction, sometimes even with the name "David". Equally natural, perhaps, was the decision to make the central focus of the novel the complex development of this protagonist as he passes from childhood to adulthood and gradually emerges as an artist. Two early unpublished sketches among Buckler's manuscripts suggest the growth of this concept. One sketch is entitled "Would you know if you fell over it?" which is a portrait of Karl who, like Buckler, is from the country, is clever and goes to college. Like Buckler and the later David Canaan, he suffers from headaches: "Never resilient physically, the striving to do everything perfectly put a strain on his health he could not stand."[28]

Discovering that he cannot make money, Karl takes up writing as a substitute for competing. Like Buckler he is nearly thirty at the time, and he too returns to the country where he discovers that "Happiness (sic) was where he had left it, snug, unasking, in the country village."[29] Like David Canaan, who never in fact leaves the country at all, he suffers nonetheless from the knowledge that his rural neighbours are "empty, uninhabited by any of the feelings that their secretive masks suggested." More recognizable as an early draft for the novel is a much longer manuscript entitled "Excerpts from a Life" in which the central character is David Redmond (the latter being Buckler's second name). The father is called Martin (the same as David's father in "The First Born Son") and the mother Anna.[30] The prototype for Bess Delahunt is called Ada Legros. Her daughter's name is Effie, and, as in the novel also, the name of the protagonist's grandmother is Ellen.

The two sketches mark successive shifts away from the purely autobiographical towards the fictional world of Entremont and the Canaan family, though, as Buckler later admitted, the principal characters in the book still owe much to his family.[31] In the years following the letter to Aswell there is little in Buckler's correspondence about the novel, but he must have been encouraged following his winning the Maclean's Fiction Prize in 1948 when a number of publishers, including Macmillan and McClelland and Stewart, made enquiries about its progress. In 1950, four years after the Aswell letter, in a letter to Naomi Burton of Curtis-Brown, the publishing agents, Buckler remarks that the structure of the novel is all blocked out and a good bit of the first draft is complete.[32]

More details do not emerge until a year later when Buckler wrote to Dudley H. Cloud of Atlantic Monthly Press who held an option on the novel. The original desire to depict "the frustration of a young man who has to see it all happen to someone else" against a war background has expanded into the complex psychological portrait of the "recurrent dichotomy in David's nature (Country boy or city boy? Naive or sophisticated? Harsh or tender? Over-child or over-adult? Serious or comic? Homebody or alien?).[33] Furthermore, the all-important delineation of the passing of a whole way of life that is so much a feature of the novel and those works that are to follow is now very much to the forefront of Buckler's thoughts as he talks of his concern with "the gradual dispersal of family oneness and (in parallel) in the village itself, as progress(?) laps closer and closer." Of significance also is his comment on Ellen's rug, which, as many critics have remarked, is a major unifying symbol in the novel. According to Buckler this was how the rug was intended for it exists "to show

how the apparently blind and capricious turns of their [the characters'] fortune are the inevitable outcome of circumstance and inheritance."

More is revealed about the composition of the novel in a second letter to Cloud which Buckler wrote after Atlantic Monthly Press had rejected the book.[34] Rather surprisingly, in view of what has here been said, Buckler claims that David's death was "the very first thing I wrote; the foundation for the whole thesis." Originally, he explains, he had planned to begin with David's death, but later he "split the opening chapter and shifted that part to the epilogue." In retrospect we can see that the structural unity resulting from the subsequent "framing" effect of Prologue and Epilogue was a happy stroke in the novel's composition. Not only does it make clear that David's final situation is the sum and substance of his entire past, but, by delaying David's death, Buckler reserves a dramatic climax for the novel that would have been hard to match had we known of David's fate in advance.

What Buckler then says in this letter about his intentions regarding David's death is of such interest that I think it is worth quoting in full:

> It was to be the crowning point of the whole dramatic irony (and, of course, the most overt piece of symbolism in the book), that he should finally exhaust himself climbing the mountain, and, beset by the ultimate clamor of impressions created by his physical condition and his whole history of divided sensitivities, come, at the moment of his death (prepared for, not only by long accounts of the result of his fall, but by the medical officer's advice to him at the time of his enlistment examination; and, more immediately, by the excitement, the panic, the climbing), achieve one final transport of self-deception: that he would be the greatest writer in the whole world.[35]

The objectivity displayed here by Buckler towards his semi-autobiographical protagonist confirms a point Warren Tallman touched upon but never fully developed in his perceptive article on *The Mountain and the Valley*,[36] in which he mentions David's uncritical and over-idealized view of his father. The ironic use of "Thanks for Listening" discussed above suggests that in *The Mountain and the Valley* Buckler indeed intended that the reader share a measure of detachment and perceive that there is a strong vein of irony involved in the portrait of David, an irony, which, as the letter to Cloud shows, is designed to reach a "crowning point" in the final pages. No critic who has discussed the novel has ever suggested an interpretation of the book that matches Buckler's apparent intentions.

This is no place to digress into a consideration of the "Intentional Fallacy" whereby a writer's intentions are mistaken by the critic for the actuality of the finished work of art. Nevertheless, as I hope I have shown, there may well be cause to re-read *The Mountain and the Valley* with some care in the light of Buckler's various statements about the novel. In addition, as I have also tried to show, our understanding of the material he incorporated into it from earlier published and unpublished stories may give one further insight preparatory to a re-reading of the book. If nothing else, the material described here provides an intriguing view of a major Canadian artist at work.

Notes

1   "My First Novel", CBC Radio, Toronto, 2 Dec. 1953. The talk has been published in *Ernest Buckler*, ed. Gregory M. Cook (Toronto: McGraw-Hill Ryerson Ltd.), pp. 22-27.
2   Grateful acknowledgement is given to Ernest Buckler and to the Thomas Fisher Rare Book Library, University of Toronto, for permission to quote from the material in the Ernest Buckler Manuscript Collection, hereafter referred to as "BColl".
3   *Esquire*, Nov. 1937, p. 10.
4   The telegram is quoted by Gregory M. Cook in "Ernest Buckler: His Creed and Craft", M.A. thesis, Acadia University 1967.
5   Letter to Rasco, 1 Dec. 1939. BColl. Box 4.
6   Letter to Edward Aswell, 10 Sept. 1946. BColl. Box 4.
7   The three stories ("Indian Summer", "Thanks for Listening", "The Trains Go By") were never published. They are now in BColl. Box 3.
8   The appropriate sections occur in *The Mountain and the Valley*, New Canadian Library Edition (Toronto: McClelland and Stewart, 1961), Part Six, Chapters XXXV, XXXVI, XXXIX, pp. 245-59, 272-74, 276-78. All subsequent quotations will be from this edition.
9   Cf. *The Mountain and the Valley*, pp. 274 and 276.
10 *Ibid*, pp. 260-63.
11 *Ibid*, p. 261.
12 To his credit David is more clear-sighted in his self-evaluation when Toby later confronts him with the manuscript: "David grabbed the sheet from his hand almost savagely. If Toby read what he'd written, he thought he'd die. The whole thing seemed unutterably shameful. How could he have put down anything so damned sickly and foolish? War was about as much like that as .... He opened the stove and thrust the

papers into the flames" (*The Mountain and the Valley*, pp. 263-64).

13 *Ibid*, p. 269.
14 The most significant cut is the wife's description of a dream she has had. Like many of the dreams later used in the novel, it is foreboding in its implications. It concerns her playing hide and seek with her husband. Whenever he is out of sight, she feels "lost and really like a child" and the dream turns "dark and frightening", the same feelings as she then experiences when they descend the mountain.
15 Cf. *The Mountain and the Valley*, pp. 135, 180, 226, 252, 253.
16 Letter from Elizabeth Lawrence, 1 Oct. 1946. BColl. Box 4.
17 BColl. Box 2.
18 *The Mountain and the Valley*, p. 34.
19 *Ibid*, p. 35. Cf. her anticipation of his early death, p. 52.
20 *Ibid*, p. 172. The importance of David's relationship to Ellen is defined in a note Buckler prepared for the projected T.V. dramatisation of *The Mountain and the Valley* in which Ellen is described as the "source of David's imaginative streak: the one grown-up to whom he can talk and confide in" (BColl. Box 2).
21 BColl. Box 3.
22 Biographical note for *Chatelaine*. Copy in BColl. Box 11.
23 BColl. Box 2.
24 *Esquire*, April 1940, pp. 70, 199-201.
25 *The Mountain and the Valley*, p. 295.
26 *Esquire*, July 1941, pp. 54-55, 114.
27 Letter to Desmond Pacey, 7 June 1961. BColl. Box 6.
28 BColl. Box 2.
29 After completing his B.A. at Dalhousie University and his M.A. at Toronto, Buckler worked for some years in Toronto for the Manufacturers Life Insurance Co. before returning permanently to his Nova Scotia home in the Annapolis Valley in 1936 at the age of 28.
30 BColl. Box 2.
31 "Mona is my youngest sister. (I think I'm giving no secrets away if I say that she is kind of roughly the Anna of the book.) Bob is Robert Simpson, her [navy?] husband. (Not totally unlike Toby and Rex)." Unaddressed fragment of letter from Buckler, 11 Dec. 1969. BColl. Box 11. Buckler also says in this letter that his mother was related to the "Jonathan Swift bunch" (cf. Ch. XII, p. 92, in the novel). His father was the "son of Joseph Buckler and Ellen (Kenny) Buckler. Ellen is, roughly, the Grandmother in the book." The circumstances of her marriage are much as those described in Ch. III of the novel (p. 31).
32 Letter to Naomi Burton, 25 Feb. 1950. BColl. Box 5. He also mentions that the novel is "psychological".
33 Letter to Dudley H. Cloud, 24 Mar. 1951. BColl. Box 15.
34 Letter to Buckler from Atlantic Monthly Press, 4 May 1951. BColl. Box 15. Letter to Dudley H. Cloud, 15 May 1951. BColl. Box 15.
35 This last point ends David's succession of desires to be the greatest general in the world (p. 41), the greatest actor (p. 82), the best doctor (p. 178), the most famous mathematician (p. 209), and the most wonderful dancer (p. 291).
36 "Wolf in the Snow" in *Contexts of Canadian Criticism*, ed. Eli Mandel (Chicago Univ. press, 1971), p. 238.

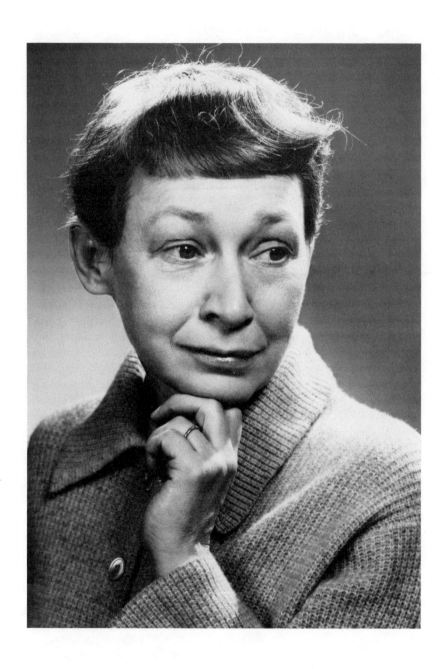

SHEILA WATSON, TRICKSTER

George Bowering

The prepared reader

In the fall of 1973, Sheila Watson gave her first public reading from *The Double Hook* at Grant MacEwan Community College in Edmonton. She prefaced her reading with a few minutes of talk about the writing and publication of the book that was to become the watershed of contemporary Canadian fiction. Here are the last three sentences of that preface:

> I don't know now, if I rewrote it, whether I would use the Coyote figure. It's a question. However, it begins with a dramatis personae, I suppose, and that is in the mouth of this figure who keeps making utterances all through the course of the novel.[1]

Sheila Watson then uttered the novel's famous first words: "In the folds of the hills under Coyote's eye ...."

Since then, people have been wondering why she might drop Coyote (though they should keep in mind the unlikelihood of a rewriting). On being asked the obvious question, Mrs. Watson said simply that she was responding obliquely to the extensive critical speculations on the function of the Coyote figure.

But Mrs. Watson, as those who have listened to her know, is a wily conversationalist. Return to that oral preface and notice that she said that the dramatis personae is in the mouth of Coyote. It is manifest to the reading eye that the roster is surrounded by white space, indented like verse, and thus that it resembles the poems of Coyote found throughout the text, as on page 115:

> Happy are the dead
> for their eyes see no more.[2]

But the dramatis personae is a different matter, isn't it? It does not sound oracular as the other verses do. It is an enumeration, an introduction of the inhabitants of the creek land. It is, though, because it does not appear the way an unobtrusive realist novel first appears, clearly a voice. It brings attention to its source. And its source is the author. Perhaps when Sheila Watson said "in the mouth of this figure," we should hear a syntactical rime with the reporter's "in the view of this correspondent ...."

As everyone now knows, Mrs. Watson went through a few

years of botheration in trying to see her eccentric book published; and even when McClelland & Stewart published it in 1959,
the publisher presented a text whose introductory design and
punctuation had been tidied by the British printer. Still, the book
appeared as a delicious oddity, a self-conscious departure from
the Canadian norm of eastern realism and western naturalism.
People found it hard to read and delightful to attempt. One reason
for this stir was the syntax and the lyricism: "A stone breathed
in her hand. Then life drained to its centre" (p. 35). Another
reason was Coyote.

Some people thought that *The Double Hook* was an electrifying
or charming oddity, a magic pool beside the Canadian
mainstream. Others, casting an eye less than a year later on the
similarly-designed *Mad Shadows* by Marie-Claire Blais, thought
they sighted a literary revolution. Here were two books that did
not provide windows on the harsh Canadian landscape, but
rather directed the eye and ear to their own pages, their language.
Mrs. Watson was not much interested in a revolution in the Canadian tradition. She has always felt her tradition to be defined by
what she read, and she has always thought of art as opaque, of
writing as writing, not social studies:

> There was nothing particularly revolutionary in Ger-
> trude Stein's theory. At the end of the nineteenth cen-
> tury Konrad Fiedler, one of the German fathers of
> stylistic history, had maintained that "each art expresses
> only itself and the value of its work cannot depend
> upon what an extra-artistic interest reads into it," in
> fact that "the various forms used to express human in-
> tellectual activity express only themselves." Each art
> moreover utters itself in its own form-language ....[3]

Figures in a ground

A typical early response to the book was Elliot Gose's review in
the first number of *Canadian Literature*.[4] He liked the mythical and
symbolic elements, critically assimilable material ever since the
creation of the Romantic novel of the nineteenth century, and seen
in a few Canadian fictions such as *Tay John* (1939), and *Wacousta*
(1832). But, says Gose, the reader will have to decide whether
to approve of "the short bits of poetry Mrs. Watson occasionally
includes in connection with the coyote."

Poetry, or that   poetry   is the ceremony of the word, don't we agree? It is not the signal, but the bringing of transformation. It is creation itself and logos itself. It is, as the first poetry was, naming and counting. (A piece of archness, if I may: if Coyote were Hesiod, Kip would be his wandering and blind Homer.) If poetry appears in a novel especially, it is language drawing attention to its physicality, and hence to the author as invisibly present, just like Coyote.

The Canadian literature of 1959 was presented with these pages given to an unsual amount of whiteness. The action was seen to be, then, within the shape of the page, indicating that the book is a spatial art, unlike film or music with their passive audiences, more like sculpture or architecture. So the reader stays aware of his own movement, aware that he is not at the end of the line, that he is continually looking at the material from his point of view. Mrs. Watson disrupted the 1959 reader's reading habits, so that he was made aware almost of a kind of threat, of at least a laughter beyond the reach of the reading lamp. Many of us are still 1959 readers, at least vestigially. We notice the white space and the short paragraphs, the refusal to describe, the scarcity of furniture, the closure of any distance in narration. The one-to-one relationship of word to world, found in the usual Canadian prose (Rule, Munro), does not hold here. We do not see characters in a setting, but rather what the artist calls "figures in a ground."[5]

"Figure" is a nice word, because it is used in all the arts. It means something fashioned, shaped, and always implies the activity of the author, composer, painter or dancer. In poetry it is another word for the stuff of metaphor. The concept of "character" suggests realist fiction, in which the author tends to convince us that she is less actual than Hagar Shipley. *The Double Hook* resembles *The Waste Land* more than it does *The Grapes of Wrath*.

Margaret Morriss has noticed that "Mrs. Potter is more of a force than a character in the novel."[6] But is she really more so than the rest of her family and her neighbours? A fictional character is someone you are convinced you have seen, though she is not there. In that sense the posthumous Ma Potter is more real for Felix and Ara than they are for us. In truth they are all equally figures, made of words. If they live, it is under Coyote's eye. Our reward for reading the book is language, not character development, not edification, not diversion, but language. This language, as anyone exposed to the first page will know, is not at rest and not seeking rest, but challenging us to form a logos out of our own unknowing. Robert Kroetsch sees "the text not as artifact but as enabling act. Not *meaning* but the possibility of meanings." He then goes on to say of

the artist him/her self:

in the long run, given the choice of being God or Coyote, will, most mornings, choose to be Coyote:

He lets in the irrational along with the rational, the pre-moral along with the moral. He is a shape-shifter, at least in the limited way of old lady Potter. He is the charlatan-healer, like Felix Prosper, the low-down Buddha-bellied fiddler midwife (him/her) rather than Joyce's high priest of art. Sometimes he is hogging the show instead of paring his fingernails. Like all tricksters, like Kip, like Traff, he runs the risk of being himself tricked.[7]

Under the eye of the critic

Then who or what is Coyote? The critics of *The Double Hook*, like those figures living in the folds of the hills, have numerous notions. Beverly Mitchell, in a Christian reading, sees Mrs. Watson referring to the Biblical myths and then "displacing" them. Coyote's remarks often resemble those of the fierce God in the Old Testament, and his deeds are equally fierce. He is perhaps the hound of heaven. The people of the creek respond to him with fear, and even create him as an objectification of fear. Beverly Mitchell argues that the various responses of the people demonstrate "the fact that their concept of God is frequently the result of psychological projection."[8] So with their concepts of Coyote, a kind of reversal of the usual process of characterization performed by an author. In this scheme, the birth of baby Felix imitates and introduces the New Testament, in which redemption is offered to the community. Mitchell's allegorical reading, especially in light of her interiorizing of the landscape that seems to her at first damned, a Biblical and otherwise mythical familiarity, would seem one way of finding accord with Mrs. Waton's statement against regionalism.[9]

Margaret Morriss, too, sees Coyote as a symbolic projection, and the fear of him as "the fear of vision, knowledge, and immortality."[10] When he speaks he does so with metaphorical or more properly allegorical language. John Grube says that *The Dou-ble Hook* is a symbolic novel, in the mode of *The Old Man and the Sea*. One suspects, especially as Grube's essay is the introduc-tion to the college edition of the novel, that he is trying to find familiar ground for students (he also calls it a parody of Faulkner). So the coyote is something like a marlin or a bear — Grube sees the animal as "fear" turned by Indians into a god, as is death, and describes that fear as "the nameless fear of the unknown." But the Indians, and the figures in the text, seem awfully familiar at least with Coyote's presence.

Nancy Corbett reads Coyote as "detached from the communi-ty, uninvolved and therefore merciless as he laughs at what he observes."[11] That would make a fine description of the author of a naturalist comedy; but in this case, I think we have a more coy author, a trickster. J. W. Lennox calls Coyote "the clairvoyant overseer"[12] which would be a pretty good description of an ironic Victorian author. Coyote, he says, comments on what he sees, rather than initiating events. With Ma and Kip he forms a ghost-ly trinity that keeps appearing as meaning that the rest of the figures would like to do without.

Most critics of the book make only passing mention of Coyote as trickster in the native stories of the Salishan people of the west, and especially here in the British Columbia Interior. Some point out, correctly I think, that Mrs. Watson layers the Coyote story with others, such as the Hebrew and Mediterranean ones, to achieve a universality beyond regionalism. Barbara Godard, for instance, notes that Coyote echoes Jeremiah, and that we get only "fragments" of each story, a hint at the deracination that bedevils the isolated community.[13] Not only does the layering of myths and sources suggest universality, but it also turns attention back upon the people doing the layering — reader and author. I agree that Mrs. Watson rangles Coyote with figures from other myths, that she even invokes the Greek Euros:

> In my mouth is the east wind. Those who cling to the rocks I will bring down I will set my paw on the eagle's nest. (p. 24)

Later we observe Ara's observation of the smoking doorsill of the destroyed Potter house. "The door of the house," she remarks, "had opened to the east wind. Into drought" (p. 114).

But the most interesting aspect of Coyote is his function as trickster, and I think that Mrs. Watson layers him with two other tricksters (three, if you count the author) in the scene wherein James blinds the servant of clairvoyant Coyote. Says James, daring the tricksters of America, Africa and Eurasia: "If you were God Almighty, if you'd as many eyes as a spider I'd get them all." (p. 67)

Leslie Monkman takes more notice of the Indian Coyote than do the other critics, noting especially the contraries in the figure's nature, his aspects of giver and negator, creator and destroyer, duper and duped. He points out that Coyote possesses no moral values, but that he challenges and creates them by his actions. Thus again Coyote, who is invisible though "the whole landscape is presented as embodying his immediacy,"[14] is a projection of various fears and guilts. Over that bridge Monkman also carries the Coyote story into an allegory of Old Testament dialectic. He suggests Coyote as Satan to Nod's Jehovah, and posits a drama occurring under "God's eye vs. Coyote's eye." So his interpretation of Indian myth employs Biblical ideas, seeing "Indian myths which relate that the world was originally created as an Eden until Coyote released from a sack the spirits of fatigue, hunger and disease."

All the readings of Mrs. Watson's Coyote suggest that she has taken the figure from Indian myth in her own mouth and dropped him into her text, where he will always be a reminder of artifice. However I am still unsatisfied. The emphasis on Coyote as projection employs Freudian notions peculiar to Romantic and realist fiction, in which revelation of character is a premier aim. The allegorical readings acknowledge the pleasure and aptness of the literal, but in their next decisions depart from the image of the trickster. Though one must admit that Mrs. Watson connects Coyote more with fear than with fun, one also would like to point out that most of the critics have concentrated almost exclusively on the experiences of the creek people, and hardly at all on the experience of the reader — this despite the constant signals made on the surface of the text. So it was with great pleasure that I found Robert Kroetsch identifying Coyote with a sly author.

The Indians' Coyote

Then who was the Coyote of the Indian people west of the Rockies?

John Berger has pointed out that "what distinguished man from animals was the human capacity for symbolic thought .... Yet the first symbols were animals."[15] In western Indian stories the animals are people, with speech and human foibles. Or put another way: when narrative enters, so does the singular and the humanoid, so that there are coyotes, part of the surround, and there is Coyote, a personality.

There is no scarcity of white men's scholarly treatments of the Coyote stories, but the one I like best is an address by Gary Snyder, who is, happily, both a trained ethnologist and a poet. It is called "The Incredible Survival of Coyote" and accounts for the passage of the Coyote figure into the literature of the white culture that has settled in the North American northwest. The figure he describes seems marvelously apt to *The Double Hook* — both to its narrative and to its composition.

People with European and literary backgrounds are used to gods or spooks with ultimate power over the elements and human lives. Even though the Greek gods symbolized qualities seen in the human psyche, they did not have human personality. It is Coyote's failure, his idiocy, that make him a puzzle to white folk. He has power, but he does not have ultimate power. He is a kind of person, but not one who can be assimilable to the conscious and rational mind. That is why critics can so readily treat him as a projection upon the landscape of the human subconscious. He says, perhaps, you are on your own, but I am always here, watching, and when I get an urge, meddling. That statement might as well be attributed to an author as to a subconscious. An author may meddle whenever she wants to, but in a fiction she does have to deal with materials that readers are accustomed to — such as "dramatis personae".

Gary Snyder points out that Coyote is stupid, bad, indecent, and tricky.[16] He did not make the physical or social world — Earthmaker did. Coyote is Shapeshifter, a meddlesome goof. It is interesting, given the plot of *The Double Hook*, that Coyote taught people how to fish, and that he showed them how to make fire; also that he got them interested in the possibility of death, though that was more from thoughtlessness than from malice. (Comparative mythologists might see him as a foolish rime, then, of Christ, Prometheus and Satan.)

As to Coyote's daily life: he is tricked as often as he tricks (p. 61). He is the funster who is always forgetfully tripping his own booby-traps. He is always travelling, though often wherever you are. Over and over he dies a stupid death and comes back. He can not leave well enough alone, so is always introducing a wonderful new idea into the world (as an author does into a setting). Other animals and people are always trying to deflate his eager busybodiness. Lily Harry, who lives at Dog Creek, where Sheila Watson did, says that Coyote got his yellow colour when Skunk turned around and expressed a popular impatience.[17]

The comic elements of Coyote might seem inappropriate to those readers who see him always associated with fear in *The Double Hook*. But really, isn't that a pretty funny book? Aren't there a lot of fools along the creek and down in the town? Don't we hear at least an echo of Rachel Cameron's escape from "that fool of a fear" as she removes herself from the thralldom of her own Ma and the latter's doctor, whose name was Raven?

Coyote does not represent a clear psychological dualism, then. He is a powerful fool, a smart goof who copes, an anti-hero of his own story, and for the writer who did not want to write a Western,[18] a nice change from the Western's silent hero and rescuer. Remember, though, that Sheila Watson can present not Lily Harry's Coyote, but only her own, only the white person's, only the writer's Coyote. Only, literally, the writing.

Under Coyote's mouth

The word "myth" gets tossed around a lot, by people who may have forgotten for a while that it comes to us from Greek *muthos*, meaning mouth and speech, and is related to Old Slavic *mudh*, meaning to think imaginatively, and even Lithuanian *mausti*, to yearn for, to desire. Myth is not a story about desire (for salvation), but is the expression, the body of desire itself. The desire of the author is in the text itself, and if it is to mean anything, the reader too must experience his own. Roland Barthes has written: "in the text, in a way, I *desire* the author: I need his figure (which is neither his representation nor his projection), as he needs mine ...."[19] (Note that Barthes' translator, Richard Miller, has used some words particular to our concern here.)

As heard in the Edmonton reading, *The Double Hook* emanates from the mouth of "this figure" Sheila Watson; and the desire for more (more novels, please) has been perhaps the most often spoken in the past two decades of Canadian reading. I believe that there is a peculiar reason why our readership has yearned for more of her voice, that it has to do with the revolutionary announcement her novel made. As Gertrude Stein once said, we do not need any more stories about our lives, but we need writing. Of the revolutionary discontinuity in Flaubert's work, Barthes wrote: "there is no longer a language *on the other side* of these figures (which means, in another sense: there is no longer anything but language)."[20]

The figure of Coyote is never "seen" by readers of *The Double Hook*, though his footprints are. Although the novel is structured by the occurrence of seeing, and eyes are the organs by which we know most of its figures, after the first sentence we know Coyote mostly by what our ears hear of his mouth.

From his mouth he breathes cactus into the grassland (p. 22). He boasts that the drought-bringing east wind is in his mouth (p. 24). He announces several times that if one will enter his mouth one will enter darkness and rest.[21] Perhaps somehow by his agency, Ma Potter goes into the darkness when James (whose name means "usurper") speaks from his own mouth. She goes "into the shadow of death. Pushed by James's will. By James's hand. By James's words" (p. 19). Whether that is a sequential order or a climactic one, it is a suggestive one.

When Coyote opens his mouth and uses thunder to call his servant Kip, Ara hears it and loses for the moment her life-giving grace (p. 36). The thunder means nothing to Felix (p. 38), who considers ceremonial words to be God's servants (p. 51). But at one point even he dreams *a* coyote like a eucharist in his mouth (p. 68). Kip reports that he has seen Coyote carrying Ma in his mouth, as if she like Kip were his pup (p. 57). The voice out of Coyote's mouth is heard when the human component is shifting, at Greta's death and at young Felix's birth. In town, where James first questions his matricidal motivation as if he were a character in a realist text, Coyote's mouth tells him that he was really trying to punish and end himself. It is interesting and appropriate that when the novel goes to town and plays with referential regionalism for a while, Coyote becomes a Freudian fool.

And ambiguous Coyote has the last word ('world'). If one speaks (or cries, as he does) his final lines, one will begin once with high short vowels and end with low long ones, then do it again, with the latter more drawn out this time. Coyotes sounded like that in the hills of my childhood. When we tried to chase one he would easily dash away, then sit and grin at us. But if it was also dark and we could hear one, it was not clear how much of the delicious feeling was neighbourly comfort and how much fear.

The writer writing

There is one critic who has taken wise note of the comic *Double Hook*. Eli Mandel, in *Another Time*, says: "A rough and wicked humour, not unlike that in a mediaeval morality play, cuts deliberately across the high poetic lines, the buzzing energy of the novel."[22] If there is one thing that characterizes Modernist realism, and especially Canadian western naturalism, it is the lack of humour, except for the high-toned cosmic irony. Most fiction in the post-modernist, anti-realist mode is comic (Kroetsch, Hawkes, Calvino) for that reason and others. The "intrusion" of the author is generally, in our time, a matter of wit. In this case, it is the laughter of a coyote.

"Coyote made the land his pastime" (p. 22), we are told, and I cannot think of a quicker way to describe the relationship between author and setting. The realist (regional and otherwise) pretends that he just observes, but that can only happen in books, as they say. Or really, out of them. In a book, which is made of language, one does not have to pretend that some things are real and some illusions. Everything is equally real. A reading from a realist viewpoint says that the people along the creek would only think that there was a creature Coyote, that he is a figment rather than a figure. But realism says that there is no author, too, though there are people inside the book. The opposite, of course, is true.

Everyone notices that the main difficulty in reading *The Double Hook* for the first time is in following the narration, so trained are we to look beyond the sentence toward its referent. The narration is here obtruded upon; or at least we are made to see the foregrounding of syntax, rime and image. So, as Jan Marta has said, "the reader experiences the book as a process, not simply as a product,"[23] and especially not product somehow of environment and character. That is, we observe the writer writing, and we are aware of the reader reading. When John Moss says of the story that "over the whole is an unobtrusive God,"[24] we have to rejoin that in a novel, God is another created figure, equal, nominatively, to all the others.

The calmly presented Coyote was a means by which Sheila Watson could make a non-realist yet non-Romantic text in the 1950s. We needed, perhaps, a reference to "exotic" though indigenous myth in order to swallow the antinomian, the antinominalist. Mrs. Watson's remark that she might not use Coyote in an unlikely rewriting might mean that one does not now need him to declare one's freedom from the orthodoxy of cause-and-effect.

Cause-and-effect is another way of seeing time and motivation, whether the plot is straight or curled with flashbacks. In *The Double Hook*, as in a poem, such as *Four Quartets*, we are led from image to image, back and forth, listening for full truth at all times, not just at the end. If we did the latter we would hear only a coyote's laughing cry.

Downhill to realism

Mandel and Grube have both called *The Double Hook* a parody. I think that Part Four, the account of James's visit to town, is perhaps a parodic departure in mode from the rest of the book, that it trifles with conventional regional mimesis, and that it is then left, rejected by the author in favour of the syncretic writing in the other four parts of the book.

Part Four is characterized by unusual attention to conventional setting, plot, character and theme (what John Hawkes has called the main enemies of fiction), to dialogue that reveals character, to local colour. (I also know that Act IV in a Shakespearian play is crammed with action.) Myth fades in favour of cause-and-effect, and the duality of good and evil. Sex and money, the materials of nineteenth-century realism, are foregrounded. The language becomes less the author's and more an extension of place and character. The book becomes for a while the Western abjured by Watson in her Edmonton talk. Landscape becomes something against which the people are clearly marked. And the "wicked humour" of the earlier writing is replaced by comic visitors from another more common kind of book or movie — a conniving whore, a notorious parrot (ironist instead of trickster), a town schemer whose name is fart sounded backwards.

Yet this is a necessary scene in narrative terms. Not only does the scabrous town full of minor opportunists contrast unfavourably to the *communitas* seen in Part Five; its presentation contrasts to the language of that last part in such a way as to ensure that we see the last part as authentic. What happens at the end is not totally good, just as what happens in the New Testament is not all flowers, but is true.

The last part is not, however, totally like the first three parts. In the last part, while the figures converge toward community, they seem to decide the course of the narrative a little more, as the author backs away slightly and permits them to handle the language. It is as if they have taken as much mimesis as is proper from the intervening Part Four. It is as if they have joined to take responsibility for their own lives once the book is finished, as if their creator has set their feet on soft ground.

Though the ground is not firm, then, it is not stony either. All readers of the text agree that we have a more-or-less happy ending, a kind of transformation, or resurrection, a new testament. A revelation (I, Coyote, saw this) under the seer's eye. Some readers have gone a little too far in their view of James as redeemer and renewer. He did, after all, murder his mother and blind a young man before returning to the pregnant lass he had abandoned.

But a Modernist, realist book would probably have had James dead in a ditch in the town, his pockets turned out; and a Canadian naturalist novel would have had the weather and objects in nature doing something nasty though unemotional to his corpse. The despair of the Modernists is understandable, given the shocking obliteration of the individual in the twentieth century. But the post-modernists live in a second stage of twentieth-century irony, and they are interested in some kind of reconstruction beyond despair — that is why their fictions are characterized by both laughter and non-realistic treatment. One cannot deny contemporary plagues of war and starvation, but one knows that a further documentation of them is a dead-end street with another blighted youth at the end of it.

Hence the qualified or sometimes demented joy at the end of our contemporary comedies, the unprovable transformations and transcendence of social angsts, the obviously constructed endings of our fictions, the prospects we are left with: not Lieutenant Henry plodding away in the rain, not Duddy Kravitz begging for bus fare. See the fantastic communal uplift at the end of a Jack Hodgins book, or one by Robert Kroetsch, Roch Carrier, or *The Double Hook*.

When James Potter is "freed ... from freedom" (p. 121), so that he must return to the hills, he is freed from the world of the realists. The realist writer says: I put my character into the world

and then he takes on a life of his own, and all I can do is observe
and record. That is why James' return is so important: he has
rather a part to play in the author's writing. He cannot pass into
the world any more than his author can create anything other
than a design of language.

The language makes allusions, of course; or rather the reader
makes associations between words and things. In *The Double Hook*
the associations with the dry Interior of British Columbia and with
literature are equal — neither has precedence. Coyote is a denizen
of both. The author writing was living in both. Her setting was
where she was sitting. We do not see the author "in" the book,
but the other figures of language there catch glimpses of her, as
do the figures of other fictions catch glimpses of "Nabokov",
"Joyce", "Vonnegut" and "Calvino". I suppose that we readers
catch glimpses of those figures catching glimpses of those figures
that we all associate with the authors of the books. In this way
we also come under Coyote's eye for a while, and we hear his/her
voice. In this situation it is hard to remain or become "objective",
isn't it? One is not on this side of this text, receiving meaning.
One is in the realm of meaning just as the story is. We cannot
"bolt ... out of the present" (p. 91) any more than James could
when he tried to escape into plot and setting, to the town where
he and we spent most of our time trying to keep track of time
and money, till he ran out of both.

The prepared text

The questions remains: why might Sheila Watson not use the
Coyote figure if she were to rewrite the novel?

There are many possible answers. As Sheila Watson has said,
she is not patient with all the interpretations of Coyote that have
been offered over the past two decades, and it is more than likely that the one above will not make her happier. Perhaps she
simply feels that the Indian myth figure was a structural imposition on the story of those other figures, something a little too wily, too tricky. Maybe she felt that those human figures are on one
hook and the readers on another, and so Coyote incorrectly let
off the hook. It might be, too, that the book does not need both
Coyote and Watson. If Ma Potter is more a presence, a force, than
a "character" and if her disappearance leads to the birth of young
Felix and hope for *communitas*, maybe she might represent the
controlling author as well as Coyote does. Coyote does appear

once as the ghost of the old woman (p. 35). Sheila Watson might even be saying that she has second thoughts about using Coyote because in person and as an author she was a visitor to the land, an outsider from a canned-food environment. She can create only a white Coast author's Coyote.

I lean toward the answer that by 1973 our literature had evolved to such a condition that one could simply write a fiction that was not naturalistic, not regional, not "about" the west or Indians, not thematic; and that one did not any longer have to prepare the audience by suggesting a structure based on indigenous myth instead of sociology.

In any case, Sheila Watson will not rewrite the book, of course. It could not be done, anyway. So the question remains. And why not? The reader who does not in his heart want to bolt out of the present does not so much desire to know what Coyote is but rather what she says.

Notes

1   Sheila Watson, "What I'm Going to Do", *Sheila Watson: A Collection, Open Letter,* Third Series, No. 1 (Winter 1974-75),p. 183.
2   Sheila Watson, *The Double Hook* (Toronto: McClelland and Stewart, 1958; rpt. Toronto: McClelland and Stewart, 1966, introduction by Malcolm Ross). Further page references will appear within parentheses in the text.
3   Sheila Watson, "Gertrude Stein: The Style is the Machine", *Sheila Watson: A Collection,* p. 170.
4   Elliot Gose, "Coyote and Stag", *Canadian Literature,* No. 1 (Summer 1959), p. 80.
5   Sheila Watson, "What I'm Going to Do", p. 183.
6   Margaret Morriss, "The Elements Transcended", *Canadian Literature,* No. 42 (Autumn 1969), p. 63.
7   Robert Kroetsch, "Death is a Happy Ending: A dialogue in thirteen parts", (with Diane Bessai), *Figures in a Ground,* eds. Diane Bessai and David Jackel (Saskatoon: Western Producer Prairie Books, 1978), pp. 208-9.
8   Beverly Mitchell, "Association and Allusion in *The Double Hook," Journal of Canadian Fiction,* II, No. 1 (Winter 1973), 68
9   Sheila Watson, "What I'm Going to Do", p. 182
10 Morriss, *op. cit.,* p. 57.
11 Nancy Corbett, "Closed Circle", *Canadian Literature,* No. 61 (Summer 1974), p. 48.
12 John W. Lennox, "The Past: Themes and Symbols of Confrontation in *The Double Hook* and 'Le Torrent' ", *Journal of Canadian Fiction,* II, No. 1 (Winter 1973), p. 70.
13 Barbara Godard, "Between One Cliche and Another", *Studies in Canadian Literature,* III, No. 2 (Summer 1978), pp. 154-5.
14 Leslie Monkman, "Coyote as Trickster in *The Double Hook", Canadian Literature,* No. 52 (Spring 1972), p. 72.

15   John Berger, "Why Look at Animals" in his *About Looking* (New York: Pantheon, 1980), p. 7.
16   Gary Snyder, "The Incredible Survival of the Coyote" in his *The Old Ways* (San Francisco: City Lights, 1977).
17   Lily Harry is the informant for linguist Dwight Gardiner who has been researching the Shuswap language and stories.
18   Sheila Watson, "What I'm Going to Do", p. 182.
19   Roland Barthes, *The Pleasure of the Text*, trans. Richard Miller (New York: Hill and Wang, 1975), p. 27.
20   Barthes, *op. cit.*, p. 9.
21   The tricksters, Coyote, Raven, Spider, are not food.
22   Eli Mandel, *Another Time* (Erin, Ont.: Press Porcepic, 1977), p. 60.
23   Jan Marta, "Poetic Structures in the Prose Fiction of Sheila Watson", *Essays in Canadian Writing*, 17 (Spring 1980), p. 46.
24   John Moss, *Patterns of Isolation* (Toronto: McClelland and Stewart, 1974), p. 166.

W.O. MITCHELL

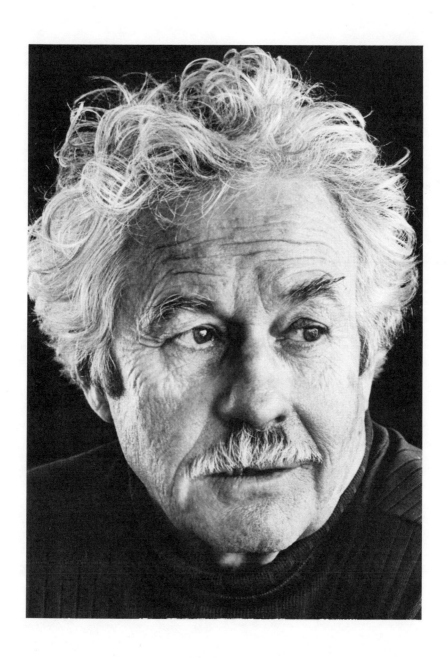

THE UNIVERSALITY OF W.O. MITCHELL'S
WHO HAS SEEN THE WIND

Ken Mitchell

When W. O. Mitchell's novel *Who Has Seen The Wind* was published in 1947, and for some years after, it was generally relegated
to the limbo of "regional" writing, with the limitations that label
implies. In recent years, the novel has been more carefully re-
examined with respect to the use that Mitchell makes of his
geographic setting, Southern Saskatchewan, but it seems to me
that even those views still treat the setting as incidental when
in fact, it is profoundly basic to the rather sophisticated theme
developed in *Who Has Seen The Wind*. Such simplistic readings
overlook the carefully controlled structure, the subtlety and
strength with which the author fuses prairie symbolism with a
theme much broader and more significant than a mere account
of a boy "growing up" in a small town. For what Mitchell has
attempted, in his portrayal of young Brian O'Connal's maturation, is to reconcile the conflict between good and evil in the
universe, to discover an equation of life and death, creation and
destruction. It is only through finding balance for these elements,
Mitchell implies, that any human being such as Brian O'Connal
can understand the dilemma of human existence.

In this apparently rustic setting of a small Saskatchewan town,
clinging to the very edge of the bountiful yet threatening environment of the prairie, the author establishes a microcosm of the
universe. It would be far too easy to assume that the prairie, as
beautiful and idyllic as it seems from Mitchell's description, is
equated with good or righteousness. Nor is the unnamed town
which borders on the prairie neatly symbolic of evil, despite the
corruption and mendacity which often seem to pervade it. And
it is to Brian O'Connal's credit that he avoids such over-simple
observations himself as he comes to sense the presence of conflicts in his world.

It is certainly true that most of Brian's primary observations are
made in the "natural" world of the prairie. His most important
friendship is with the Young Ben, who personifies the wildness
and freedom of habitat; he is always present when Brian makes
the discoveries which lead him to later wisdom. He is deliberately portrayed as animal-like, silent and wild as the coyotes that

228   W.O. MITCHELL

drift across the plains, and the perfect antithesis to the complicated social framework that holds him captive in school. In fact, the Young Ben has withdrawn from human society before it can cast him out. He becomes a spiritual guide to Brian in his search for a divine plan, a combination of priest and disciple. There is "a strengthening bond between them, an extrasensory brothership."[1] Any verbal, or intellectual, communication between them is unnecessary, perhaps even impossible. Yet it is from this vagabond that Brian discovers the essential quality of the prairie.

But Brian learns from the town, too. The other main teacher in his life — more literally — is the school principal, James Digby. He is the Young Ben's thematic opposite, but is at the same time one of the few citizens who show sympathy for the Young Ben. *He* personifies intelligence and rationality (including its weaknesses: consider his failure with Miss Thompson). Unlike his counterpart, Digby depends on thought and formal communication. He likes nothing better than arguing with the minister Hislop and Milt Palmer, the town philosopher. His teaching is as crucial to Brian's development as the Young Ben's is. It is he who articulates — as much as is ever possible — Brian's relationship with God and the universe.

In acquiring his wisdom, his sense of *place* in this puzzling existence, Brian must as Mitchell says, see "the realities of birth, hunger, satiety, eternity, death. They are moments when an inquiring heart seeks finality, and the chain of darkness is broken."[2]

The novel is divided into four major sections, each of which is roughly two years apart and represents a different plateau in Brian's development. One of the motifs that show this development is death, a phenomenon naturally disturbing to a young boy curious about life. It is, after all, that part of the cycle of life which is most difficult to equate with a smiling, bountiful Deity. I think too, that with this motif, Mitchell shows himself in most complete control of his imagery and his theme.

In the first section of the novel, Brian is four years old and ignorant about the forces controlling his life. He is not the lisping innocent that sentimental readers might prefer. His baby brother, Bobby, is ill with fever and in danger of dying, but Brian only resents the attention Bobby is given by the family. In his ignorance, he wishes a cruel and violent death on his grandmother.

He hoped Jake would bring his policeman's knife and

chop her into little pieces and cut her head off, for making him go outside to play. (p. 5)

Brian's first direct involvement with death comes after he fails to get an interview with God at the Presbyterian Church. He discovers a caterpillar inching across the sidewalk.

> He squashed it with his foot. Further on he paused at a spider that carried its bead of a body between hurrying thread-legs. Death came for the spider too. (p. 11)

Brian is represented as a careless "killer", who has no more regard for life than the most primitive animal. It is from this level that he progresses. Later in the first section, when Brian's pet pup is taken away, he adopts a baby pigeon as a companion. Through his ignorance and boyish carelessness, he inadvertently causes its death, too. Brian is shocked to tears as a result of his first obvious encounter with a lifeless being, a creature once warm and now gone cold in his hands. Because it touches him personally, he begins to understand the fact of death. He has reached the first plateau of wisdom, and decides to bury the dead pigeon on the open prairie.

> "Where the Young Ben is," said Brian. "There is where — not with houses." He was aware of a sudden relief; the sadness over the death of the baby pigeon lifted from him. (pp. 58-9)

As it turns out, Brian has accurately anticipated the Young Ben's presence. He "attends" the burial, crouched behind some bushes, a priest of the prairie ensuring that life returns to the earth to give life.

The first section of the novel ends with Brian's pup returned to him. He is now prepared for its companionship, having learned something of responsibility for life in the incident of the pigeon.

> Within himself, Brian felt a soft explosion of feeling. It was one of completion and culmination. (p. 60)

This is the first of many times the "feeling" will come to Brian O'Connal. These experiences seem to be part of what Mitchell calls the "moments of fleeting vision" that come to the boy in his search for the meaning and balance of life.

The second section of Who Has Seen The Wind is an extrapolation of Brian's initial awareness. He learns that death comes to all things, including people, even to those things on which love is focused, like his pet dog. He learns, too, something of the paradox of death, its occasional rightness, its justice, and its inevitability.

We see this most clearly when Brian takes part in a gopher-drowning expedition with his pals. With discomfort, he watches Artie Shaw ripping the gopher's tail off, an act of gratuitous cruelty. Suddenly the Young Ben appears, almost literally rising out of the earth to enforce the natural law of life and death. With "one merciful squeeze" he kills the gopher; in the same movement he attacks and punishes the ignorant Artie Shaw.

> And Brian, quite without any desire to alleviate Art's suffering, shaken by his discovery that the Young Ben was linked in some indefinable way with the magic that visited him often now, was filled with a sense of the justness, the rightness, the completeness of what the Young Ben had done — what he himself would like to have done. (pp. 127-8)

> He senses, without understanding, that the gopher's death is necessary, not merely to "put it out of its misery", but because somehow that is part of the divine plan in nature. Months later, he and Bobby find the corpse on the prairie, "strangely still with the black bits of ants active over it. A cloud of flies lifted from it, dispersed, then came together again ...." (p. 128)

There is an echo in this of Steinbeck's novel *The Red Pony*, in which Jody Tiflin, a boy slightly older than Brian, also learns that life thrives on death. Mitchell's task in handling this theme is much more difficult than Steinbeck's, however, for he must by his own definition account for a Divine Being behind all this. Here is Brian's observation:

> Prairie's awful, thought Brian, and in his mind there loomed vaguely fearful images of a still and brooding spirit, a quiescent power unsmiling from everlasting to everlasting to which the coming and passing of the prairie's creatures was but incidental. He looked out over the spreading land under intensely blue sky. The Young Ben was part of all this. (pp. 128-9)

Not long after, Milt Palmer the shoemaker explains the process to Brian, in his own special idiom:

> "Somebody dies, they're right handy with the Heavenly

Land on High an' a shiny box an' flowers an' a lotta
things ain't got nothin' whatsoever to do with bein'
dead. You know what death is? Rotting — stink — dust
— an' you're back to the prairie again. Take birth —
what's that? Sprinkling with water? Announcement
cards? Seegars? Hospital ward? Hell no! Blood an' water
an' somethin' new for a while — mebbe a shoemaker
that wishes he was a tree." (p. 139)

Brian discovers too that birth and death are never far apart — are,
indeed, inter-related. Forbsie Hoffman's pet rabbits spawn litter
after litter of young; Brian is quite naturally fascinated by the process. But the increase grows alarming as none of the rabbits seems
"to have heard of the Malthusian theory." Food grows short
despite their sheltered, domesticated environment. The natural
elements of population control are missing, and one night Forbsie's desperate father exterminates the lot. Brian is shocked, but
he feels an "uneasiness that recalled to him ... the day on the
prairie when Art had torn the tail from the gopher" (p. 169).

In this section of the novel occurs the first human death, that
of old Wong, owner of the Bluebird Restaurant. The town's
Establishment has callously taken Wong's children away from
him to place them in foster homes, after subjecting the family to
a long history of prejudice and neglect. "Two weeks after his son
and daughter had left, Wong was discovered, still with his red
toque on, swinging from a rafter in the dark kitchen ..." (p. 172).
Wong's suicide springs from the same almost inadvertent
carelessness which resulted in the death of the baby pigeon. This
is not observed by Brian, apparently; but for the reader, the conclusion is inescapable.

The plateau Brian reaches by the end of Part Two is the grievous
loss he feels when his dog Jappy is killed by a passing dray. This
is the first death that strikes right into his heart, and he is not
yet mature or wise enough to accommodate it. He cannot explain
the death to Bobby — just as his father could not earlier explain
the pigeon's death to *him*. Perhaps Mitchell is saying that this
understanding can come only through non-rational, non-verbal
learning, which cannot be communicated to others. All Brian does
know is that "a lifeless thing was under the earth. His dog was
dead" (p. 181).

Once again, the Young Ben materializes for the burial on the
open prairie. He helps Brian cover the grave with rocks, but his

presence does little — this time — to alleviate Brian's loss.

> Somewhere within Brian something was gone; ever
> since the accident it had been leaving him as the sand
> of an hourglass threads away grain by tiny grain. Now
> there was an emptiness that wasn't to be believed. (p.
> 181)

It is his blind self-pity that creates this emptiness.

The third section emphasizes the inevitability of death. Brian's father falls ill, and the boy is sent to his Uncle Sean's farm, where he protests the killing of a runt pig. He seems to ignore the lesson of the gopher, shrieking profanities and refusing to listen to his uncle. "Killing a thing's no favour!" he shouts. What Brian may be lacking is the rational maturity that would enable him to connect the gopher and the pig — a quality he later learns through Digby. At least this is what Ab, the outraged hired man, defines as Brian's problem: "You don't think," he says (p. 233).

The third level of awareness is reached after the death of his father, which creates in Brian an unsettling flux of emotions. Standing once again on the prairie, he "did not feel like crying. He did not feel happy, but he did not feel like crying" (p. 238). This is not intended to show the developing "manhood" of a boy who refuses to be reduced to tears. It is the growing recognition that his father's death is part of the vital process — inevitable and even necessary to the ultimate survival of life. He thinks:

> People were forever born; people forever died, and
> never were again. Fathers died and sons were born; the
> prairie was forever, with its wind whispering through
> the long, dead grasses, through the long and endless
> silence. Winter came and spring and fall, then summer
> and winter again; the sun rose and set again, and
> everything that was once — was again — forever and
> forever. (pp. 246-7)

Suddenly, inexplicably, Brian does begin to cry — as he goes outside himself and realizes the loneliness his mother must feel. "His mother! The thought of her filled him with tenderness and yearning. She needed him now. He could feel them sliding slowly down his cheek; he could taste the salt of them at the corners of his mouth" (p. 247). His tears are for his mother, a display of selfless compassion which takes him away from grief and mourning to a new consideration for life and the living. And Mitchell employs a perfect touch to reinforce the theme of the all-pervading unity of life:

> A meadow lark splintered the stillness.
> The startling notes stayed on in the boy's mind.
> It sang again.
> A sudden breathlessness possessed him; fierce excitement rose in him.
> The meadow lark sang again.
> He turned and started for home, where his mother was.
> (p. 247)

In Part Four, Brian reaches physical maturity and the highest level in his quest. He is twelve, on the brink of puberty, and during this last summer of the novel, from spring to fall, he makes the greatest progress in his spiritual development.

He visits Milt Palmer's shop and overhears an argument between Digby and Palmer about the nature of existence. "Who the hell's me?" asks the shoemaker.

> "Shoes, folks, churches, stores, grain elevators, farms, horses, dogs — all insidea me. You — the kids — this shop, insidea me — me insidea my shop; so that means I got me insidea me. Who the hell's me?"
> Fascinated, Brian stared at the shoemaker; he thought of Saint Sammy; he thought of the feeling. "You got a feeling?" (pp. 291-2)

But Palmer, an adult and an agnostic, does not get "feelings".

> "— I guess that ain't there no-more." He said it, thought Brian, sadly. The shoemaker turned to Digby. "I still don't know who 'me' is." (p. 292)

A little later, Digby ventures an explanation: "You're inside Him, Milt. When I get outside that door, I'm out of you, but I'm still inside Him."

Out of this oblique, Berkleyan discussion, Brian learns enough to decide he's "on the right track" (p. 294). He proves it in the incident of his grandmother's death. In the intervening years since babyhood, Brian has grown much closer to Mrs. MacMurray, listening to her tales of early pioneering days on the prairies. Now as she nears the end of her life, the two have grown particularly close and they spend a great deal of time together. She is bothered by the clock in her room, a "crazy, quivering, enamel box trying to tell all the time in all the world. It had measured out little of her past life, and now it thought it was going to dole out what was left" (p. 289).

Brian senses her hatred for the clock and halts the symbolic progress of time. He "killed it for her; he pulled its plug and turned it around on the dresser" (p. 289). As she increasingly senses the closeness of death, she seems to feel a corresponding need for the presence of the natural world, the prairie. She asks Brian to open the window, that is, to remove the barrier between herself and the outdoors — the wind and the presence of her God. Earlier, she has valued the open window to her room, "teasing her old nostrils with the softness of spring, the richness of summer, or the wild wine of fall" (p. 277). At one point, during a storm, she has kept the window open and "seemed to have drawn new life from the storm" (p. 274). Now, Brian opens it again, against his mother's instructions.

> It slid the full length of his arms, and the warm room was suddenly filled with the mint freshness of the outside. Stray flakes of the winter's first snow floated out of the afternoon and into the room, to melt in mid-air. (p. 290)

(This symbolic association of snow and death is interestingly developed. The slow passage of the old woman's time is described this way: "The eighty-two years of her life had imperceptibly fallen, moment by moment piling upon her their careless weight ....") (p. 277). But Brian's apparently sympathetic gesture has an unexpected effect, because the combination of the open window and her weakened condition causes Mrs. MacMurray's death.

> Feathering lazily, crazily down, loosed from the hazed softness of the sky, the snow came to rest in startling white bulbs on the dead leaves of the poplars, webbing in between the branches. Just outside the grandmother's room, where she lay quite still in her bed, the snow fell soundlessly, flake by flake piling up its careless weight. Now and again a twig would break off suddenly, relieve itself of a white burden of snow, and drop to earth. (p. 294)

The only possible conclusion is that Brian *kills* his grandmother, perhaps sensing her need and desire to return again to the prairie.

Mitchell does not force that conclusion, but intentionally or not, Brian is the agent of his grandmother's death. This would make no sense if it were simply another example of death caused by human neglect and carelessness (even if it is not malicious). The only explanation, in view of Brian's cumulative wisdom, is that he takes an active part in ensuring that the process of creation and destruction goes on — although it is probably an unconscious decision that he makes. At any rate, this atavistic impulse represents his supreme awareness of the function of death

If all of this seems to indicate some macabre predilection of W. O. Mitchell's, it should not. What Brian is faced with learning is an understanding of the universe, the meaning and existence of God. This is the central theme of the novel, and the motif of death makes an especially illuminating contribution. It is a part of nature, and nature — Mitchell asserts — is God. The concept of God is another puzzling subject for Brian's tenacious mind, and here again he proceeds gradually and haltingly to awareness, moving from his naive conception of the Deity as a little elf — ''R. W. God'' — to something very close to Digby's belief in a universal Presence.

It is here that Mitchell uses his most effective symbol: the wind. The ingenious use of this device unifies the novel and illuminates Brian's search. "Who has seen the wind?" he asks (or states) rhetorically — rhetorically, because of course no one has seen the wind, just as no one (with the possible exception of saints and lunatics) has ever seen God Himself. Despite his innocent childhood pilgrimage to the Presbyterian church, or his vision of God stirring the prairie like a bowl of porridge, Brian can no more visualize God than he can the wind that passes by.

The wind is a common literary device for symbolizing God's presence, but it is especially effective in *Who Has Seen the Wind*. In this prairie setting, it is — like nature (or God) — hostile and benign, creative and destructive. At the outset, even before Brian is introduced, Mitchell outlines this paradox. The prairie lies,

> ... waiting for the unfailing visitation of the wind, gentle at first, barely stroking the long grasses and giving them life; later, a long hot gusting that would lift the black topsoil and pile it in barrow pits along the roads, or in deep banks against the fences. (p. 3)

"Symbolic of Godhood" as Mitchell suggests, the wind brings

both rain and drought to the prairie — holding the power of life and death over the settlers.

On his initial quest to look for God in the church, Brian feels "the wind ruffling his hair" as he knocks on the door. As he awaits an answer, "a fervent whirlwind ... rose suddenly, setting every leaf in violent motion, as though an invisible hand had gripped the trunks and shaken them" (p. 8). The minister's wife gives Brian his first vital information about the God he seeks: " 'It's someone — something you can't hear — or see, or touch' " (p. 9).

With this beginning, it isn't surprising to discover the wind's presence at certain critical points in the novel, those instances when Brian makes a crucial discovery or experiences his "feeling". In the first section, for example, as Bobby lies near death, "the night wind, stirring through the leaves of the poplar just outside [Brian's] room on the third floor, strengthened until it was wild at his screen. He thought again of the strange boy on the prairie and felt, as he did, a stirring of excitement within himself, a feeling of intimacy" (p. 20).

Yet when the incompetent school-teacher, Miss MacDonald, threatens Brian with Divine punishment for a lie in school, the wind turns threatening and harsh, reflecting Brian's perception of the Deity. Vengefully, the wind sweeps "down upon the town ... lifting the loose snow and driving it into the children's faces, stinging their eyes and noses above the scarves tied around their mouths" (p. 94). Terrified of the impending punishment, Brian lies awake, feeling the "gathering Presence in his room as the wind lifted high, and higher still, keening and keening again, to die away and be born once more .... Fearful — avenging — was the gathering wrath about to strike down Brian Sean MacMurray O'Connal ..." (pp. 94-5).

More often, however, the wind blows gently in Brian's presence, usually co-incident with some manifestation of God, or Brian's "feeling". One Sunday, there is a "turning point in Brian O'Connal's spiritual life" (p. 106). At the age of six, he experiences what can only be called a transcendental vision while staring at a few drops of dew nestled among new spirea leaves in the spring.

> As he bent more closely over one, he saw the veins of
> the leaf magnified under the perfect crystal curve of the

drop. The barest breath of a wind stirred at his face,
and its caress was part of the strange enchantment too.
Within him something was opening, releasing shyly
as the petals of a flower open, with such gradualness
that he was hardly aware of it. But it was happening:
an alchemy imperceptible as the morning wind .... (p.
107)

This is really the first time Brian clearly feels and recognizes the
depth of emotion that occurs with his discovery of God in his
world. "He was filled with breathlessness and expectancy, as
though he were going to be given something, as though he were
about to find something" (p. 108). And yet he never does, in an
intellectual sense; he feels vaguely incomplete and unsatisfied.
Moreover, he finds that

... many simple and unrelated things could cause the
same feeling to lift up and up within him till he was
sure that he could not contain it. The wind could do
this to him, when it washed through poplar leaves,
when it set telephone wires humming and twanging ....
Always, he noted, the feeling was most exquisite upon
the prairie or when the wind blew. (pp. 122-3)

The care and precision with which Mitchell develops this symbolic motif is worth examining. It ranges from the look on Art's
face when he is attacked by the Young Ben like that of "a man
whose home has just been levelled by a prairie tornado" (p. 127)
to the "dead and yellowed leaves" Brian sees sliding along the
walk ahead of him "at the bidding of the wind" when his dog
is struck down. As the dog dies, "the wind carried the settling
dust of the street sideways" (p. 179). The darker element of nature
and God is suggested by the "feverish little dust devils" which
whirl through town at certain times, such as when Brian's father
is ill and nearing death.

Mr. O'Connal dies far away, in Rochester, but at the moment
of his death Brian experiences a new intensification of his feeling. Having run away from his Uncle Sean's farm, he is physically
isolated, alone on the prairie during the night.

The night wind had two voices; one that keened along
the pulsing wires, the prairie one that throated long and
deep. Brian could feel its chill reaching for the very centre of him, and he hunched his shoulders as he felt the

wincing of his very core against it. (p. 235)

I take this passage to indicate not only that he is naked and vulnerable to the action of God (as well as to the elements), but also that he experiences the sudden solitude of independence, that cold chill brought on by the loss of a child's dependence on his father.

> As the wind mounted in intensity, so too the feeling of defenselessness rose in him. It was as though he listened to the drearing wind and in the spread darkness of the prairie night was being drained of his very self. He was trying to hold together something within himself, that the wind demanded and was relentlessly leaching from him. (p. 236)

The next day, just before he learns of his father's death, he has "an experience of apartness much more vivid than that of the afternoon before — a singing return of the feeling that had possessed him so many times in the past" (p. 237).

The wind also brings awareness to Brian when he goes out onto the prairie after the funeral to reconcile himself to the loss of his father.

> All around him the wind was in the grass with a million timeless whisperings.
>   A forever-and-forever sound it had . ... Forever and forever the prairie had been, before there was a town, before he had been, or *his* father, or *his* father. ... Fathers died and sons were born; the prairie was forever, with its wind whispering through the long, dead grasses, through the long and endless silence. (p. 246)

With this vision of the cyclical pattern of the birth and death of seasons, days, and people — its inevitability and its beauty — he reaches the third plateau. The meadow larks shrill but natural melody expresses his new positive belief: a "fierce excitement rose in him" (p. 247).

The enigmatic quality of the wind is presented most effectively in Mitchell's portrayal of Saint Sammy, "Jehovah's Hired Man", who lives in an abandoned piano box on Magnus Petersen's south eighty. Although this character is often praised — and dismissed — as a colourful portrait done in brilliantly humorous idiom, Sammy's stature in the novel assumes a great deal more than that of a comic lunatic. In fact, he is the archetypal figure of the visionary madman. The Lord speaks to Saint Sammy, beginning at the time of his canonization in "the bad hail year, when Sammy had stood on the edge of his ruined crop, looking at the countless broken wheat heads lying down their stalks."

> As he stared, the wind, turning upon itself, had built up a black body from the topsoil, had come whirling toward him in a smoking funnel that snatched up tumbleweeds, lifting them and rolling them over in its heart. The voice of the Lord had spoken to him.
> 'Sammy, Sammy, ontuh your fifty-bushel crop have I sent hailstones the sizea baseballs. The year before did I send the cutworm which creepeth an' before that the rust which rusteth.
> 'Be you not downcast, fer I have prepared a place fer you. Take with you Miriam an' Immaculate Holstein an' also them Clydes. Go you to Magnus Petersen, who is even now pumping full his stock trought. He will give ontuh you his south eighty fer pasture, an' there you will live to the end of your days when I shall take you up in the twinkling of an eye.
> 'But I say ontuh you, Sammy, I say this — don't ever sell them Clydes, fer without them ye shall not enter
> ....
> 'Hail, Saint Sammy!' the Lord had said. 'Hail, Jehovah's Hired Man!' (pp. 264-5)

But the materialistic, machinery-oriented farmer Bent Candy is coveting Sammy's Clydesdale horses and is threatening Sammy with eviction unless he sells them. This sacrilege, in Sammy's mind, both guarantees and justifies the violent vengeance the Lord will undoubtedly wreak on Bent Candy.

Brian has earlier been fascinated by Sammy's peculiar relationship with God, and at this point goes out to see the recluse. Together they wait in the strengthening wind for the storm to strike.

> As far as the two could see, the grasses lay flat to the prairie earth, like ears laid along a jack rabbit's back. They could feel the wind solid against their chests, solid as the push of a hand. (p. 270)

As the Lord speaks to Sammy, His voice "scarcely distinguishable from the throating wind," Brian is "filled again with that ringing awareness of himself."

> "Sammy, Sammy, this is her, and I say ontuh you she is a dandy! ... "In two hours did I cook her up; in two hours will I cook her down! An' when she hath died down, go you ontuh Bent Candy's where he languishes an' you shall hear the gnashing of teeth which are Bent Candy's an' he shall be confounded!" (p. 270)

True to His word and to Sammy's vision, the Lord destroys Candy's new barn as though it had "been put through a threshing machine and exhaled through the blower" (p. 272).

The point of this little parable (which at first reading seems to be a humourously sentimental digression) is not only to reveal to Brian God's capacity for destruction. This is already evident in the ravaging drought of the 1930's, and in the frequency with which he encounters death. The incident suggests that a man like Saint Sammy, mad hermit and an outcast from society, living on the open prairie like one of his own Clydes unbroken and gone wild, is a man much closer to God than, for example, Bent Candy, a deacon of the Baptist Church. And despite his somewhat Old Testament viewpoint, he is much more a Christian man than the Reverend Mr. Powelly, the Presbyterian minister who *seems* to profess Christian virtues but who is a man guided by social, not spiritual laws. Indeed, there are many characters in the novel who claim to be pious, but who are completely ignorant of the natural forces that reveal a Divine Presence. Saint Sammy is a man who *has* seen the wind, and who has come to his vision through suffering and humility.

This contrast between Saint Sammy and Reverend Powelly is a neat example of the central conflict in *Who Has Seen the Wind*. As I said before, one must avoid the tendency to see the conflict as one of rural innocence versus urban corruption. There is corruption on the open range, too. The Old Ben, despite an appealing frankness, is a callously insensitive man. He has all his son's irresponsibility with none of his innocence (and from this, perhaps we can deduce that the Young Ben will become an Old Ben). Bent Candy, too, is anything but a dedicated son of the soil, although he is the most successful farmer in the district. In fact, there seems to be more destruction and desolation in "God's country'' than there is on the streets of the little town. Instead of a contrast between town and country, I believe Mitchell intends a parallel.

The comparison is simply this: that there is a balance maintained between positive and negative (good and evil; creation and destruction) both in the social community and in the natural one. The positive influences on Brian do not come only from the pastoral environment; Digby and Miss Thompson, for example, also have an important effect on Brian's development. There are others, like Hislop, the banished minister, and Milt Palmer, not to mention Brian's parents. The negative element in the community is obviously (one might say, *too* obviously) represented by Reverend Powelly and Mrs. Abercrombie. It is the cruel and meddlesome interference of these two which causes the destruction of Wong's family. Their unswerving dedication to the breaking of the Bens is both impressive and revealing. Through these acts, Brian sees that havoc occurs in the town as well as in the country, possibly for the same reasons, and is therefore inevitable — given the formula of human nature.

Brian, by the end of the novel, is able to fuse his experience of both environments as a result of his special capacity and his insights. It is important to realize that, despite his admiration for the Young Ben, Brian is not at all inclined to run wild on the prairie (or like Huckleberry Finn, to flee from ''sivilization''). What he learns in school and from Digby is ultimately as valuable as what he learns on the prairie from the Young Ben. In his decision to become a ''dirt-doctor'', we see that he is determined to apply the formal ''intellectual'' education he acquires through Digby to the love of land he associates with his Uncle Sean, Saint Sammy and the Young Ben.

This decision of Brian's is one expression of the balance he finally achieves in his new view of the universe, a view that incorporates reason and emotion, hatred and love, creation and destruction — then makes them all one in himself, through an almost mystical process.

Near the end of the novel, he is puzzled by an emotion he recognizes as being long familiar to him. ''It was as though he were recognizing again an experience that his memory had stored for him, but not too well.''

It had something to do with dying; it had something

to do with being born. Loving something and being
hungry were with it too. He knew that much now.
There was the prairie; there was a meadow lark, a baby
pigeon, and a calf with two heads. In some haunting
way the Ben was part of it. So was Mr. Digby. (p. 299)

But he cannot intellectually comprehend this experience,
although he some day hopes to be satisfied. "The thing could
not hide from him forever," he thinks. But Brian is mistaken here.
He can never understand what happens in a rational sense — just
as he will never see God, or the wind. Only madmen like Saint
Sammy can do that. The wind goes on, Mitchell observes in the
final paragraph, oblivious of all, turning "in silent frenzy upon
itself, whirling into a smoking funnel, breathing up topsoil and
tumbleweed skeletons to carry them on its spinning way over the
prairie, out and out to the far line of the sky" (p. 300). Brian's
accomplishment has been to *feel* the wind, to sense the presence
of God in nature. That, Mitchell implies, is all that he or any man
can do — and all that is necessary to advance into maturity.

Notes

1 W. O. Mitchell, *Who Has Seen the Wind*, Macmillan of Canada, (Toronto,
   1947), p. 89. Page references are hereafter given in the text.
2 Author's epigraph.

THE VANISHING POINT: FROM ALIENATION TO FAITH

Catherine McLay

In his third novel *The Vanishing Point* published in 1973, W. O. Mitchell explores a central truth of modern existence, man's sense of alienation and his need for community to give purpose and meaning to life. In an interview with Donald Cameron, Mitchell comments on the role of fiction:

> To me the only justification for art is that this particular narrative, these particular people, shall articulate some transcending truth .... It's not a new truth or a fresh truth, but it's the first time this truth has been filtered through this particular artist, in this particular part of the world, at this particular point in time. It isn't the truth that's important so much as the illusory journey to that truth, through the artist's illusion bubble.[1]

Mitchell's previous novels *Who has Seen the Wind* (1947) and *The Kite* (1962) have examined the relationship of man both to death and to life, and *The Kite* celebrates the triumph of life in the person of Daddy Sherry, the magnificent old patriarch of one hundred and eleven. In *The Vanishing Point*, the quest for truth is both broader and deeper. For the central character, Carlyle Sinclair, must not only come to terms with death and life; he must also accept man as a social being and attempt to reconcile the division between the individual and his society, the Indian world and the white. Like Thomas Carlyle whose name he bears, he must pass through the "Everlasting No" to come to the "Everlasting Yea". His journey from alienation and doubt to faith in himself, in the Stony peoples, and in society as a whole, is the central theme of the novel. *The Vanishing Point* is Mitchell's most mature work, the clearest statement of his essential humanism, his faith in the human race.

Man's sense of alienation, of separateness and isolation, is one of the central themes of the twentieth century. Like Matthew Arnold, Mitchell sees men as islands, forever yearning yet forever unable to bridge the division between self and self. In a mood of despair, Carlyle Sinclair asks:

> ... wasn't all communication between all humans

> hopeless? Out of my skin and into yours I cannot get —
> however hard I try — however much I want to! ....
> What a weak bridge emotion was for people to walk
> across to each other — emotion swinging, unable to
> hold the heavy weight of communication .... Just illu-
> sion after all, for once the passage was made, the door
> was always closed. You stopped at the eyes, and you
> had never left the home envelope of self anyway (216).[2]

The roots of *The Vanishing Point* lie in this concept of alienation. In 1953, Mitchell's novel *The Alien* won the MacLeans' Fiction Award and excerpts appeared in *MacLean's Magazine* from
September to January 1953-4. But the novel as a whole was never
published; Mitchell withdrew it and it remained in the back of
his mind for some twelve or thirteen years. Like *The Vanishing
Point*, *The Alien* was based on Mitchell's own experience as a
teacher for some months on the Eden Valley Reserve west of High
River, Alberta. Both novels concern the life of Carlyle Sinclair,
teacher on the Paradise Valley Reserve, and his search to bridge
the gap between Indian and White, man and man. In each, Victoria Rider is central. A student of Carlyle's who has completed
her Senior Matriculation and entered nursing in a city hospital,
she is, as her name suggests, a symbol of Carlyle's success or
failure in adapting the world of the Indians to modern urban
society.

It is largely in the ending that *The Vanishing Point* differs. For
"the alien" in the earlier version is, in a very literal sense, Carlyle
himself; half Indian and half white, he is alienated from both
cultures. Overwhelmed by Victoria's pregnancy and his consequent failure, he refuses to accept less than perfection and, in
one version, commits suicide. *The Vanishing Point* is the work of
an older and more mature writer. Mitchell remarks to Donald
Cameron:

> ... about fourteen years ago I worked on a novel, very
> close to when I thought it was finished, and then I was
> unhappy with it. I returned to it several times over a
> period of about five years or more — it became a King
> Charles' head with me — and then about four years ago
> suddenly I realized that what had grown, indeed, said
> No. It ended with despair, and while the piece of work
> had grown to say No, I myself hadn't; and this is what

had crippled it so terribly for me.[3]

In the middle sixties, Mitchell was attracted to Steinbeck's philosophy, in particular *The Grapes of Wrath*. For Mitchell, the giant turtle, sliding back two steps for every three ahead, becomes a symbol of mankind which not only survives but slowly and surely, despite pain and suffering, progresses towards its destination.[4] The artist, Mitchell claims, "either says Yes to man or he says No to man." *The Alien* said No but in *The Vanishing Point* Mitchell now says Yes.[5]

Carlyle's movement in the novel from death to life, from despair to commitment, is framed by his initial journey into the city, and his final return two weeks later to Paradise. Part One relates the present situation of Carlyle and of Paradise Valley Reserve, and introduces the two complications of the action, the search for the lost Victoria Rider and the approaching death of her grandfather, old Esau.

Part Two regresses to 1950 and traces Carlyle's eight years in Paradise from the beginning to the present. Part Three picks up the thread of events from Part One and moves toward the conclusion, Esau's death and the marriage of Carlyle and Victoria, interweaving events in the present with flashbacks into Carlyle's distant past. Interrelated with these events and memories are the wind-up of Heally Richards' Rally for Jesus, Archie Nicotine's appeal to Heally to save old Esau, and the activities of Norman and Gloria Catface. The tone alternates between comedy, tragedy and black humour, with tragedy predominating until the final pages. Despite certain structural weaknesses and the blurring of view-point at times, the events and characters of the novel are all integrally related to the central theme, Carlyle's search for understanding between man and man, race and race.

In this search all the relationships of Carlyle's past become central and take their place in shaping his thought and character: relationships with his father and Aunt Pearl, with his dead wife and daughter, with his teacher Old Kacky, with Archie Nicotine and the Riders, Powerfaces, Wildmans, Left-hands, and Baseballs of his Reserve days. Gradually he comes to realize the Victoria is not the cause of his search but merely the precipitant:

> The loss of Victoria had shattered something inside him. He knew that now. He knew he was not simply trying to find her. He knew that he must put back together

something he had been trying all his life to keep from being splintered — broken beyond repair. It was something mortally important to him, and it had never — ever — been whole for him really; Aunt Pearl and Old Kacky had seen to that. And his father.

Victoria Rider had grown essential; he must find her and he must do it to save himself as well. (p. 323)

The ending of the novel, the marriage of Carlyle and Victoria, is not merely a romantic cliché but a comic resolution, a logical outcome of the events and problems of the novel. Carlyle must ultimately choose between life and death. In existential terms, the rejection of suicide is itself an affirmation, an embracing of life over death. In one sense the "vanishing point" of the title is the point of decision, the point of choice between being and not-being. But in another sense, it is the point of understanding, the point at which man imposes meaning and perspective upon the chaos of life, order and form on events and characters seemingly disparate and unrelated. Carlyle's acceptance of this order and meaning is his acceptance of life as symbolized by his marriage and Victoria's coming child.

Carlyle Sinclair's journey in *The Vanishing Point* from death to life is paralleled in the movement of the novel from winter to spring. The opening passages prepare for this movement:

Spring — actual spring by God! ... Mountain spring exploded in his face. Fifteen years and he still wasn't emotionally ready for the chinook stirring over his cheek and breathing compassion through the inner self that had flinched and winced for months from the alienating stun of winter. Full reprieve! (pp. 3-4)

But Carlyle is still dominated by winter and death. Spring is his "cup of water on the desert." It accentuates his isolation, his aloneness: he is "starved for the thrust from self to the centre of a loved one" (p. 4). He identifies with the male grouse "drumming life inside, membrane throatbag flushed with blood." But the image of potency is transposed into an image of death in the balloon of dead little Willis which the child Carlyle blew up and released in the play-room: "It died without warning in mid-air, dropped to the floor — a stilled and shrunken scrotum" (p. 5).

The predominance of death and isolation in these early pages symbolizes Carlyle's past. His mother died when he was seven and Aunt Pearl was no substitute, for her life was shaped by her dead husband and her dead son Willis. The death of his father was only the final stage in an already existing estrangement and Carlyle sees their relationship reflected in the hymn "You in your small corner and I in mine" (p. 336). His friend Mate died from diphtheria, contracted from Carlyle. Before coming to Paradise, he lost his wife and unborn daughter.

On the Reserve, the years have been marked by deaths from pneumonia, appendicitis, diabetes, eclampsia, fire: "Each spring death seemed to play a counterpoint to bud and sprout and rising sap and river flow" (p. 224). As he looks back from the vantage point of his ninth year, Carlyle meditates: "All the deaths he died in nine years: Each one leaving him older — sadder — more helpless" (p. 20). The figure of the dying Esau Rider, an almost fleshless skeleton, symbolizes this dominance of death over life. Even the wick of the lamp in Esau's room is described in terms of disease as a "pale, giant tapeworm preserved and floating within the lamp's clear belly' (p. 8). But although the events of the novel move toward the climax of Heally's restoration of Esau and his subsequent death, Carlyle is moving in the opposite direction, towards life as indicated by his recognition: "his own life was just as urgent as poor Esau's death" (p. 9).

The two settings of the novel represent the two worlds in which Carlyle exists and between which he is divided. The city, not specifically identified but recognizably Calgary, is an alienated world from which Carlyle has been absent for many years but from which he is not totally free. Unreal and even, to Carlyle, fantastic, it represents the confused values, the isolation and lack of commitment of modern man. Paradise Valley, the world of the Stonys, is also remote to Carlyle despite eight and a half years there. Between the two lies a suspension bridge which cannot be crossed by cars and which symbolizes the separation of Paradise from the modern world, Indian from white.

Carlyle's journey into the city in Part One is a journey from the past into the present. On the borders live the "periphery people" who "resisted anonymity, clung still to first-name informality" (p. 32), and who raise budgies or operate cottage enterprises. The city proper is impersonal and faceless. Its buildings could be anywhere: the Devonian Tower, the Empress Hotel and Beer Parlour, the Liberty Cafe and in the alley behind, the lair of Norman and Gloria Catface sheltered by orange parachutes, the Bonneydoon jail where the Stonys spend much of their city time, the Foothills Carleton Hotel, the Super-Arcade. Carlyle sees these as unreal, a pantomime or movie set: "when he left this evening they would all be taken down" (p. 58). His fantasy of the life of mannekins in department stores is a reflection not only of his own isolation but also of the emptiness and superficiality of modern city life. The flow of traffic becomes for him a ritual dance of negation, a sterile counterpart to the vital Prairie Chicken Dance: the cars "meet opposite partners; swing and pass each other in opposite direction." And the pedestrians are weighed down with humanity:

> ... almost all of them carried something. Those who did not seemed to; the white-egg burden of their own lives perhaps .... all were engaged in a communal pantomimist illusion of walking up an invisible slope. (pp. 57-8)

Anonymous and impersonal, the city is typified by the bus station. It is "not a place where people met people" but an unloading place where the passengers "looking slightly dazed, as though they had just stepped bewildered from a car wrecked in a highway accident" (p. 301). Everywhere Carlyle meets the "lonely accosters" who fix him with an unflinching gaze and spill "precious intimacy" (p. 63). The old man in the bus station attempts to relive his whole past; the pathetic man in hospital is convinced his heart-pacer is linked up backwards; the man in the drug store faces life alone after the death of his wife; and the man in the Super-Arcade, when Carlyle turns away from him, reacts sadly "as though he had just confirmed something again for himself" (p. 97). All these are represented by Luton. As he leans on the car window, pouring out his whole life with his rancid breath, Carlyle fantasizes about the "moat which has separated him from all human contacts" and sees the whole proliferation of plaster garden ornaments as Luton's reaction to isolation, his choice of a company which will not show revulsion. While the surface in all these cases is comic, the comedy is undercut by tragic recognition of man's separateness within the bonds of his own skin.

The city's crowning symbol is the Devonian Tower, a "concrete erection" with a "May basket balanced on its tip ... [and] a red oil derrick to spear the last fifty feet" (p. 42). The explicitly sexual symbolism underlines its negation of sex. In its shadow Gloria and Norman Catface live off the proceeds of prostitution. From it as centre the city reaches out menacingly, threatening to submerge the surrounding countryside with its commericialism and industry. The oil derricks in the outlying areas are "great metal birds tipping and sipping from deep in the earth, releasing the stink of hydrogen sulphide" (p. 28). The city encroaches upon Paradise Reserve where coloured ribbons mark the sites of future wells and its seismic drillings have reduced Beulah Creek far up in Storm and Misty Canyon to a feeble trickle. It even endangers the Arctic, building pipelines across the tundra to transport oil and gas to the urban world and disturbing the ecological balance of caribou and Eskimo.

Its entertainment is cheap. The Shelby rodeo with its parade of chuckwagons, decorated tractors and floats, its merry-go-round, its wheel of fortune and kewpie dolls, is shallow and gaudy. In this setting the Indians become farcical, a travesty of their forebears in buffalo horn headgear, paint, war bonnets, and breechcloths over dyed pink underwear. Its art too is machine-made. Luton's brother and his wife do a vast trade in plastic flowers all over the West while Luton mass-produces sleazy plaster ornaments, rows and rows of identical does and Bambis, bear cubs, geese and flamingoes which represent the true antithesis of art. Carlyle fantasizes that Luton may renounce his ornaments for a Kentucky Fried franchise or a Kiddyland near Banff. But the flamingoes and bambis and bear cubs will not be renounced. Fornicating among themselves, they take control of Luton and in a final nightmare vision Carlyle sees the whole world "up to its arse in fluorescent flamingoes" (p. 41).[6]

In the city the Indians are doomed to fail, unless like Jake Rider they conform fully to white life. Jake's grey business suit, white shirt, Stetson and hand-tooled kangaroo hide boots cost more, Carlyle speculates, than his half-brother's funeral. It is the realization of Victoria's inevitable fate in the city which motivates Carlyle to make such a desperate search for her. And her experience confirms this fear. Her job as waitress in the Liberty Cafe is short-lived when she discovers that "extra services" are required in the evenings. She is "rescued" by Norman and Gloria Catface who live on the proceeds of prostitution and sell her to meet their expenses. Other members of the band too are out of place here. Carlyle habitually visits the city to bail out various members on charges of "drunk and disorderly." For years Archie has dropped by the Express Bar and drunk up the funds he intends to buy rings and a rebuilt carburetor for his car. And he is bailed out by Heally Richards when he is arrested for relieving himself in an alley behind the hotel.

Paradise Valley Reserve is in direct contrast to the city. Although the Stonys may be alienated from modern urban society, they are part of a great oneness, what Mitchell terms the "living whole". But Paradise Valley lies between two modes of life, the city and the present, and the past as represented now only by Storm and Misty Canyon. Carved by the "millennia of wind and frost and water" (p. 109), Storm and Misty is a place of refuge for youth, the hunting-ground for the whole band, and the source of water and food for the Reserve. In it no whites can survive for long. Here Caryle loses his way although even the smallest of his Indian children is at home. And here Archie finds the white hunter, who betrayed the rule of the wilderness, frozen in the snow. Storm and Misty is the centre of old Esau's vision; it is a "shaman place" where he could "purify and prepare, and be absolved from self" (p. 108). But Esau's dream of leading his band back here into the past dies with him. For Stormy and Misty represents what the Stonys have left behind:

> Before white people come to this country Indian had a good livin' — never hungry for himself — for his horse .... We lost all that now; we lost the Indian good life. Those days we had buffalo-hide wigwam that was wind-proof — cold-proof. Now we haven't. The Indian child get sick out of it. There is why my people suffer in their heart. (p. 378)

The new way of life is imposed upon them in part by the church and the government and in part by their own desire to share elements of white society as represented by cars and liquor. In his unconventional but vivid prayer, Ezra Powderface expresses their dilemma:

> We want to live the white way now and put the suf-fering out of our souls. I know the old people cannot do this .... [But] Thou take the young ones, Heavenly Father — the kids and the like of that .... These are the ones will live the white way and there is why we thank Thee for sendin' us Mr. Sinclair to teach them (p. 126)

But their success in adapting is very partial. They continue to live in summer in airless tents and in winter in cabins which are unrepaired and draughty. Carlyle persuades a few to grow hay for their numerous horses but the day it is ready for cutting they have departed for Shelby's annual rodeo. A few grow gardens but the vegetable diet cramps the bowels used to moose and bannock. Despite the protests of the Reverend G. Bob Dingle and Ezra Powderface, the young couples continue to be united by "blanket marriages", unblessed by the church. Spring is "grabbin'-hold-of-time" in Paradise and the fulfilling of natural urges is immediate and unselfconscious. Both children and adults are embarrassingly uninhibited; not only the boys but also the girls relieve themselves in the open, and Archie is naively innocent of wrong when he urinates in the alley behind the Empress Hotel.

The Stonys are vulnerable to disease and Archie does not speak in jest when he claims that hospitals are places where Indians die. They insist on minor medications such as liniment and castor oil, epsom salts and aspirin, and refuse treatment for tuberculosis, diabetes and pneumonia. As Dr. Sanders remarks bitterly to Carlyle "Your dispensary takes cares of them — when they want me they're moribund" (p. 127).

Their closeness to nature influences their culture. In contrast to the sterile art of the city, Indian art is individual, free and spontaneous. The children draw in coloured chalks on the blackboard: buttercups and tigerlilies, galloping horses, moose and elk. The women embroider on doeskin or bead moccassins. Their dances are ritual and follow the rhythms of animal life, the Rabbit Dance, the Owl Dance or the most popular Prairie Chicken Dance. But this closeness to nature has its negative side, and the beat of the drums, Carlyle feels, is "lobotomy", linking them to animal nature rather than thinking mankind: "right from birth they've got that drum ... with their mother's milk — every week — every month — every year .... It's what we're up against" (p. 204).

A recognition of white attitudes to the Indians is an essential part of Carlyle's education. Much of the white world is hostile, like the Greek owner of the Liberty Cafe who propositions Victoria but later tells Carlyle: "I do draw the line — somewhere — at smoked meat" (p. 280) or the prison officials who express their contempt of Archie in crude humour, or the taxi-driver who patronizingly calls Archie "chief" when he fails to tip him. Even Officer Dan who refers to the lost Victoria on T.V. as "one of our fine young Indian friends" (p. 269) reveals himself when he apprehends Gloria Catface supposedly for soliciting Heally Richards: "You got no licence to sell your Girl Guide Cookies between here and the Devonian Tower" (p. 283). And the Indians retaliate. When Carlyle looks for Victoria at the Indian Friendship Centre, they threaten and punch him, first high on the cheekbone, then in the groin (p. 299).

The dedicated whites, the government officials, teachers and preachers who attempt to bridge the gap between white and Indian, are themselves often patronizing and, even at their most sincere, often as little aware of real Indian needs and desires. Perhaps the most idealistic of these is the Reverend G. Bob Dingle with his blatant health posters and his simplistic religious verses. Dingle sees the Indians as "good people — gentle — happy — just children" (p. 151), and he has a blind faith in their, and man's, perfectability. He lives by illusion, as Carlyle discovers when Dingle insists that the children eat greedily the Minimal Subsistence Biscuit. And the Stony phrase he proudly quotes "No-watch-es-nichuh" means, not "You please very much" as he supposes, but "bull-shit" (pp. 174-5).

Less naive but even less effectual is Sheridan, the agent in charge of Hanley and Paradise Valley. Sheridan shows little interest in Reserve affairs and has little time for Carlyle's plans to upgrade the stock, raise oats, grow vegetables and keep cows and chickens. His life lies in the past and his only real achievement in a lifetime of service has been his development of a baseball team on the Reserve. Dr. Sanders remarks:

> After thirty-five years it doesn't matter whether you lived or died — or retired — all comes to nothing. You could have been added — subtracted — divided — multiplied, and the result would have been exactly the same — except for one thing — those champion Hanley Wolverines. (p. 182)

Another idealist is Fyfe, agent of the federal government and living in Calgary. Even he questions his success. On the verge of retiring he remarks: "Can't help wondering what you've actually accomplished in forty-five years" and admits he only "held the fort" (p. 88). Fyfe is cautious and non-commital. His favourite policy is "wait to see what transpires" and his favourite advice, "don't let yourself get personally involved" (p. 87). His main achievement has been the Fyfe Minimal Subsistence Cookie, an indigestible oatmeal biscuit which the children scatter in parts and wholes over the classroom floor. Responsible, honourable, practical, dedicated, he nevertheless fails to bridge the gap between white and Indian for his whole philosophy has been wrong. He sees the Indians as "terminal cases to be made as comfortable as possible within the terms of the reserve system — the budget and the Indian Act" (p. 91).

The wisest of the whites associated with the Stonys, Dr. Sanders functions in the novel as Carlyle's mentor and guide. Sanders is clear-sighted and sympathetic to the Indian problems:

> They are children, but with adult drives — grown-up hungers — mature weaknesses — envy — love of power — of their own children; they have vanity and — what's very — the key — terrible feeling of inferiority. If you know that — and that they are child-like ... then you won't rant at them because they failed to carry what you piled on them. Don't expect too much of them — don't let them get you angry .... Be a good guardian. (pp. 130-1)

And he sees in the paternalism of the Reserve System a slough which has weakened their resistance: "the more you do for them the more you sap their strength" (p. 183). Despite his insight and understanding, however, Sanders is unable to bridge the gap between races, and in Carlyle's eight year he is forced to retire from the scene to win a personal battle against tuberculosis and death.

It is left to Carlyle, then, to act as intermediary between the Indians and modern urban society. He sees the old suspension bridge across the Spray River as a symbol of communicaton between race and race, human and human, to "carry hearts and minds across and into other hearts and minds" (pp. 12-3). But to this point he has failed. He asks himself:

> Had he ever made it across to any of these people? ... How the hell could he ever know! How could he hope to understand what any of them sheltered secret inside themselves. (p. 13-4)

Verbal communication is ineffective. His talk with Esau Rider indicates the circumlocution: "they could go on all morning, circling nose to tail" (p. 8). Conversation with any of them but Archie is almost impossible, "like trying to play catch with someone who wouldn't throw back the ball" (p. 16). And communication without language is even more difficult. They withdraw: "He could not know what went on inside their heads — behind the eyes that refused to hold his" (p. 203). While Carlyle is not a Bob Dingle who teaches Stony children to sing "Bringing in the Sheaves" in Cree or murmers "bull-shit" when he means "You please me very much," he is little more successful than Dingle in bridging the gap, and his insistence on using English indicates the core of the problem: it is Indians who must conform to white standards.

Victoria then becomes central to Carlyle's purpose of communicating with the Stonys. She has been the first and only one to respond to him since the day when at twelve she held his hand on the way to the dentist: "two worlds had merged .... He and she were no longer so vulnerable on this concrete and asphalt planet" (p. 216). But in seeing her as a symbol of his success, he has sacrificed her as an individual, with individual needs and wants. Her growth and maturation have threated his own purposes so that he has chosen to ignore them. He has been in part aware of her sexuality and has seen the budding of her breasts as "poignant as young ferns' tight thrust through earth" (p. 225). But he has disregarded Sanders' warning that at sixteen she is a year older than Martha Bear who disappears up Storm and Misty with Wilfrid Tailfeather. And he has insisted, "She can make it to matriculation. I can get her through" (p. 233).

Victoria completes her Grade Twelve and enters nursing in the city. But it is not in her nature to accept Carlyle's plans for her, and her answer to him, her pregnancy, is the only answer that he will accept. As she says to him: "you are — asking me to turn the mountains upside down ... Stop the spring run-off" (p. 374). Her predominant emotion is not the loss of her career but shame at disappointing him. As Archie remarks, "With white people it's easy for us people to be ashamed in front of them .... You know, Victoria — I come to a conclusion — they want it that way" (p. 296).

Carlyle begins to recognize his blindness as early as the day he learns of her disappearance although he is unable to grasp the significance of his discovery until later. In admiring Fyfe's prize orchids, he favours one with handsome lavender flowers which Fyfe labels a failure. Carlyle objects:

> ... has the orchid been disappointed? Does it consider itself a complete miss? .... You're trying to — for

something that hasn't anything to do with what the orchid wants ... the orchid's concept — destiny — it takes
a little longer than the few years you — what it has
wanted for millions .... (pp. 85-6)

He rejects the scientific breeding which reduces beauty to a
mathematical formula. But he asks himself if he could be equally
"dispassionate about his misses" (p.86). And he comes gradually to realize that he too has interfered with natural growth. He
has tried to impose his standards and his classifications upon Victoria and indeed upon all the Stonys with due consideration for
their inborn needs and desires.

It is only in Part Three that Carlyle is prepared to achieve his
quest. The combined perspectives of the loss of Victoria, the
recognition of the roles of Aunt Pearl and Old Kacky in his past,
and his identification with Heally Richards lead him to see his
own limitations. The memory of Aunt Pearl is significant. The
child Carlyle opposes her desire for ritual and order through
deliberately rearranging the objects on her dressing-table. But her
love of order becomes more, a denial of the natural and spontaneous elements of life, even of the physical body itself, as
Carlyle discovers when Aunt Pearl comes upon him with the
magic lantern, projecting onto the wall the image of his penis,
magnified many times. In his weeks with Aunt Pearl, she imposes
upon him the personality of little dead Willis and his defiance
of her is his reaction to her unnatural rigidity, her life-denying
force.

His memory of Old Kacky too leads to this recognition. Old
Kacky, like Aunt Pearl, imposes order and ritual upon the chaos
of life. And in so doing, he rules out all the natural and
unregenerate areas as represented by Billy Blake's nosebleeds or
Maitland Dean's repertoire of wind-chords (p. 317). Language
becomes grammar; history becomes an account of systematiza-
tion, of governments, laws and constitutions. The parts of the
body are abstracted under scientific Latin names. And art becomes
not an exercise in creativity but a rigid adherence to a set of rules.

The child Carlyle admits that the illusion of perspective works.
But the illusion which he himself has created takes on a power
of its own which to the child is terrifying:

... his eyes travelled straight and unerring down the
great prairie harp of telephone wires ... down the

> barbed-wire fence lines on the other side of the
> highway. And as the posts and poles marched to the
> horizon, they shrank and crowded up to each other,
> closer and closer together till they all were finally suck-
> ed down into the vanishing point. (p. 318)

Carlyle, in adding a pine-tree and a poplar, is asserting the
freedom of art and the imagination to defy rules and logic and
for this Old Kacky straps him. Carlyle's reaction is not repentance
but fear. This moment marks the beginning of the alienation
which is to possess him for more than twenty years:

> Here he stood by himself, and outside the office walls
> were all the others properly together and busy all
> around his own empty desk. He had vanished from
> them. Old Kacky had vanished him from them to
> vanishment. And then the really crazy though happen-
> ed. He was being vanished from himself ... stepping
> outside and getting smaller and smaller and smaller ...
> dwindling right down to a point. (p. 322)

His immediate physical reaction, the cramping of the bowels and
their release in Old Kacky's drawer, is more than Mitchell's attempt to shock or titillate. It is, like Victoria's pregnancy, the
response of the physical body to an order which refuses to take
account of it. The pervasive imagery of elimination throughout
the novel serves the same purpose; it counters the idealistic and
spiritual in man with a recognition of the primary needs and basic
requirements which make him truly human.

Carlyle's friend Mate insists that the vanishing point is only
an illusion: "the rails don't meet .... C.P.R. couldn't run their
engines if they did" (p. 325). But Carlyle does not wholly escape
from this illusion until he is able to recognize how he himself,
in rejecting Old Kacky and Aunt Pearl, has become another Kacky
himself, another Aunt Pearl. He is not only divided from others,
alienated; he is also separated from himself, schizophrenic. Body
and mind have become rivals; instincts and reason are not part
of a greater whole but distinct. From this point on he is moving
towards the vanishing point of his own life, towards the moment
of choice between being or non-being.

It is Heally Richards and his Rally for Jesus which ultimately
prepares Carlyle to choose between life and death, society and
isolation. The ground has been laid in Part One for Heally

Richards' role in Part Three. Although there is perhaps an overemphasis on Richards and a consequent diversion of interest from Carlyle, the Heally Richards' section is integral to Carlyle's search. Certain elements of Heally's past parallel those of Carlyle and Heally's failure leads to Carlyle's recognition of his own parallel failure.[7]

Unlike Aunt Pearl and Old Kacky, Heally cultivates the dramatic in human life and his religious ritual satisfies the human craving for meaning and significance. He succeeds essentially by what Carlyle calls "primitive oversimplification" (p. 17). His appearance is striking. The pure lard-white of his shoes, socks, suits, tie, hair and eyebrows, contrasted with his tanned face, suggests to Archie the magic of the "backward people" and to the more sophisticated Carlyle a photograph negative. In the Rally he plays on the dramatic elements of redemption and his deployment of Norman and Gloria Catface is brilliant, Gloria in the white doeskin costume of Miss North-West Fish and Game, Norman with the sinister scar cutting across his right cheek, both fresh from their solicitings in the neighbourhood of the Empress hotel. His oratory too is brilliant in subject, rhythm and style.[8] His final address seizes upon a simple incident, the pitch stains on the green wood of the altar steps, and turns it into a striking sermon on man's need for redemption.

The source of Heally's power lies in the needs of his audience. To Archie and the Paradise people he offers something they yearn for, a replacement perhaps for their lost religion, for the tales and legends of Bony spectre and Weesackashack. His appeal is simple and direct and their confidence in his healing powers is absolute. As Archie says "They wouldn't let him onto the radio if he couldn't do it" (p. 18). But he satisfies an even more basic need. Carlyle comes to realize: "he promised to shrive them of their mortality, to lift from them the terrible burden of their humanity, the load of their separateness" (p. 358).

Carlyle comes to realize too the flaw in Heally Richards. His apparent faith, his search for God, is in fact a search for power. Our glimpse into Richards' mind confirms this. The miraculous cures are essential to him for they salvage his flagging self-esteem, assuage the life-long feelings of rejection and inferiority. They cause him to seek for larger and larger audiences, for more and still more conversions and healings. He imagines to himself the building-up of glory through a series of healings to the dramatic resurrection of Esau Rider before the audience and the cameras of CSFA-TV:

> Oh, God, please — please choose — through Heally
> Richards — to lift up that old Indian from that stretcher
> before the Mercy Seat! Raise up that feathered buckskin
> Lazarus with Your revivin' pahr! "Esau — Esau — take
> up thy stretcher and walk!" ... Rise up, Esau! And
> Heally Richards too! Right up out of the evangelic bush-
> league — clear to Billy and Gipsy and Aimee and Oral!
> Hallelujah! (p. 348-9)

Esau's sudden restoration and as sudden death in front of the vast audience and the T.V. cameras is Heally's answer from above. It is not for man to interfere with life and death, to play with these for his own selfish ends. So different from Aunt Pearl in all ways but one, he is yet alike. For, concludes Carlyle, he is "ordering them into a moral box to suit himself only — not them" (p. 354).

But Carlyle is not able so easily to see his own failure with Victoria and the Stonys. It is only in the dark hours following his meeting with Victoria and his discovery of her pregnancy that he comes to see that he too has placed them in a moral box. He has fulfilled his own cravings for self-importance at the expense of theirs. In these hours he descends into the "Everlasting No". He has tried to be a mirror to Victoria and the Stonys, to show them to themselves. But they have responded with tricks; for him they have "capered and postured and made faces" (p. 367). The mirror tells them they are separate, ashamed. He has failed. And all have failed with him: Victoria, Fyfe with his Minimal Sub-sistence Cookie, Heally Richards with his laying-on of hands, even Esau Rider whose faith has died with him. He becomes nihilistic: "He hadn't known that it was no use at all — that nothing could be done at all" (p. 366). And ultimately he despairs not only of the Stonys but of humanity as a whole: "Victoria is one knocked-up mess! I am! The Stonys are! Right from the begin-ning the whole human race has been one God-damned mess!" (p. 374).

At this point, he must choose between life and death. It is the beat of the drums in the ritual Prairie Chicken Dance which recalls him to life. For the pounding rhythms annihilate past and future, anesthetize from pain and suffering, illness, loss, injustice. They give the sense of oneness which man has sought in love, in sacrifice, in religious faith, the breaking of the bonds of the self:

> Only the now remained to them — the now so great that only death or love could greaten it. Greater than pain, stronger than hunger or their images paled with future — dimmed with past. Only the now — pulsing and placeless now? Song and dancer and watching band were one, under the bruising drum that shattered time and self and all other things that bound them. (p. 385)

The revelation is sudden. While man is part of nature, of the "living whole", he is also alien to it. And only man can share this sense of alienation; in accepting responsibility for others he enters a new social unity, becomes committed to life: "Man lifted bridges between himself and other men so that he could walk from his own heart and into other hearts" (p. 385). In leaving Victoria on that city street he has destroyed a bridge between himself and the Stonys. His return of faith is essential: he might "try again — for them — for himself — for her!" (p. 385).

The consummation and marriage which ends the novel in the traditional manner of comedy thus becomes an important statement of faith in humanity as a whole. For only through love can man heal the separation between mind and body, between man and man, between race and race. Carlyle's acceptance of Victoria marks his acceptance of his physical self, of the life force. The child to be born of Victoria will share his life, and their future children will help to heal the division between Indian and white. his dedication as a teacher must also be reaffirmed. The little Powderface boy experimenting in the dust before his cabin with a system of ditches and canals will be his next challenge. But this time will be different. He will be aware of the child's needs and desires, of his individuality and his significance as a person, not merely of him as a symbol of his race. For they need each other, he and his pupils; only in working together can they be truly successful and truly human.

The novel closes in the fullness of spring and morning. The trees are in full leaf, the grouse is drumming triumphantly and the pulsing rhythms of the Prairie Chicken Dance are still in the air. Carlyle's revelation, his moment of perfect faith, is marked by two important events on the Reserve: the renascence of Beulah

Creek and the flowing once more of the live-giving waters, and the resurrection of Archie's car signifying the ultimate success of the Indian in adapting to the best elements of white society. Life has triumphed over death, society over alienation. Mitchell has said "Yes" to man.

Notes

1 Donald Cameron, *Conversations with Canadian Novelists* (Toronto: Macmillan, 1973), pp. 51-2.
2 W. O. Mitchell, *The Vanishing Point* (Toronto: Macmillan, 1973). All quotations are from this edition.
3 Cameron, *op. cit.*, pp. 61-2.
4 W. O. Mitchell in discussion with students at the University of Calgary, March 1971.
5 Cameron, *op. cit.*, p. 61.
6 The working title of the novel in 1970 was "The Fluorescent Flamingoes".
7 Mitchell's discussion with students at the University of Calgary.
8 In an interview with William French, Mitchell remarked that he attended many sessions of the Emmanuel Chapel of the Free Assembly of God to capture the rhythm and style of Heally's speeches. See *The Globe and Mail*, Saturday, July 7, 1973.

ABOUT THE CONTRIBUTORS

David Arnason teaches Canadian literature at St. John's College, University of Manitoba. He is a former editor of the *Journal of Canadian Fiction* and is now an editor for Turnstone Press. He has published a number of short stories and a book of poetry, *Marsh Burning*.

Stanley S. Atherton is Professor of English at St. Thomas University, Fredericton. He has contributed articles to scholarly journals and is the author of *Alan Sillitoe: A Critical Assessment*, and co-editor (with Satendra Nandan) of *Creative Writing from Fiji*.

George Bowering's criticism includes books on Al Purdy and *Three Vancouver Writers*, as well as articles on James Reaney, David McFadden, Fred Wah and Margaret Atwood. A collection of essays on Canadian poets is imminent. He also writes poetry and fiction.

Elspeth Cameron is coordinator of the Canadian Literature and Language Programme at New College, University of Toronto. She has published articles on Margaret Atwood, Scott Symons, Marian Engel and others, and books on Robertson Davies and Hugh MacLennan, including the recent critical biography, *Hugh MacLennan: a Writer's Life*.

Wilfred Cude is author of *A Due Sense of Differences*, an evaluative study of four classic Canadian novels. A free-lance writer living in Cape Breton, he is currently working on a critical appraisal of the North American doctorate, and a novel on William Henry Jackson, Ontario secretary to Louis Riel.

John Goddard is a reporter from Peterborough, Ontario, who recently opened a northern bureau of The Canadian Press in Yellowknife. He has worked for C.P. in Toronto, Ottawa and Montreal, and has travelled widely to cover news events abroad, including the release of American hostages from Tehran in 1981.

Henry Makow's Ph.D. dissertation at the University of Toronto was on Frederick Philip Grove's theory of art. His articles on Grove have appeared in *Canadian Literature, Dalhousie Review* and the *University of Toronto Quarterly*.

Catherine Mclay teaches Canadian literature at the University of

Calgary. She has edited *Canadian Literature: The Beginnings to 1910*, and has published articles on Shakespeare, Willa Cather, Margaret Atwood, Margaret Laurence and W. O. Mitchell. She is currently working on a critical biography of Mitchell and an anthology of fiction by Canadian women.

Lorraine McMullen teaches Canadian literature at the University of Ottawa. She has published articles on Malcolm Lowry, Leo Kennedy, Frederick Philip Grove, Leo Simpson, Frances Brooke and others; and is the author of *Introduction to the Aesthetic Movement in English Literature* and *Sinclair Ross*.

Ken Mitchell teaches literature at the University of Regina. He has written for radio, television and cinema, and has published novels, poetry and plays. His published works include *Wandering Rafferty*, *The Meadowlark Connection* and the folk-opera *Cruel Tears*.

Donna E. Smyth teaches literature at Acadia University. She has published two plays, *Giant Anna* and *Susanna Moodie*, and a novel, *Quilt*. She has also published short fiction and was a founding editor of *Atlantis: A Women's Studies Journal*. She is currently working on a project on feminist aesthetics.

Lee Briscoe Thompson teaches Canadian literature in the Canadian Studies Programme at the University of Vermont. She has presented and published papers in Canada, the United States and overseas on a variety of Commonwealth and Canadian topics.

George Woodcock was the editor of *Canadian Literature* for almost two decades. His many books include works of philosophy, history, biography and literary criticism: included among them are *Odysseus Ever Returning*, *Canada and the Canadians*, *Rejection of Politics* and *The Crystal Spirit*, for which he won the Governor General's Award.

Alan R. Young is Professor of English at Acadia University. His scholarly interests are divided between Renaissance literature and Canadian literature. His books include *Henry Peacham*, *The English Prodigal Son Plays* and *Ernest Buckler*. He has recently completed a book on Thomas Raddall.

ACKNOWLEDGEMENTS

Grateful Acknowledgement is made to the following:
Lee Briscoe Thompson for "In Search of Order: The Structure of Grove's *Settlers of the Marsh*". This is an altered version of an essay that originally appeared in the *Journal of Canadian Fiction*. Reprinted by Permission.
Henry Makow for "Grove's 'Garbled Extract': The Bibliographical Origins of *Settlers of the Marsh*".
Stanley S. Atherton for "Ostenso Revisited".
Wilfred Cude for "Morley Callaghan's Practical Monsters" Downhill from Where and When?"
John Moss for "Mrs. Bentley and the Bicameral Mind: A Hermeneutical Encounter with *As For Me and My House*".
David Arnason and the *Journal of Canadian Fiction* for "Canadian Nationalism in Search of a Form: Hugh MacLennan's *Barometer Rising*".
Elspeth Cameron for "Of Cabbages and Kings: The Concept of Hero in *The Watch That Ends the Night*".
Lorraine McMullen for "Elizabeth Smart's Lyrical Novel: *By Grand Central Station I Sat Down and Wept*".
John Goddard for "An Appetite for Life: The Life and Love of Elizabeth Smart". This article originally appeared in *Books in Canada*, JuneJuly 1982. Reprinted by Permission.
Donna E. Smyth for "Maggie's Lake: The Vision of Female Power in *Swamp Angel*".
George Woodcock for "Innocence and Solitude: The Fictions of Ethel Wilson".
Alan R. Young and the *Journal of Canadian Fiction* for "The Genesis of Ernest Buckler's *The Mountain and the Valley*". Reprinted by Permission.
George Bowering for "Sheila Watson, Trickster".
Ken Mitchell and the *Lakehead University Review* for "The Universality of W. O. Mitchell's *Who Has Seen the Wind*". Reprinted by Permission.
Catherine McLay for "*The Vanishing Point*: From Alienation to Faith". This essay was originally accepted for publication by the editor in 1976.

PHOTO CREDITS